D.A. Gunnersen.

A Colour Atlas & Textbook of Oral Anatomy

B K B Berkovitz
Lecturer in Anatomy
(Oral Biology)
University of Bristol

G R Holland
formerly Assistant Professor
Dows Institute
Department of Endodontics
University of Iowa*

B J Moxham
Lecturer in Anatomy
(Oral Biology)
University of Bristol

*Now Assistant Professor
Department of Anatomy
(Oral Biology)
University of Manitoba

Wolfe Medical Publications Ltd

Copyright © B K B Berkovitz, G R Holland, B J Moxham, 1978
Published by Wolfe Medical Publications Ltd, 1978
Printed by Smeets-Weert, Holland
ISBN 0 7234 0719 3
2nd impression 1981

This book is one of the titles in the series
of Wolfe Medical Atlases, a series which brings
together probably the world's largest systematic
published collection of diagnostic colour
photographs.
   For a full list of Atlases in the series,
plus forthcoming titles and details of our surgical, dental and veterinary atlases, please
write to Wolfe Medical Publications Ltd,
3 Conway Street, London W1P 6HE

All rights reserved. The contents of this book, both
photographic and textual, may not be reproduced in any form,
by print, photoprint, phototransparency, microfilm,
microfiche, or any other means, nor may it be included in any
computer retrieval system, without written permission from the
publisher.

Preface

The demands placed upon students of dentistry to assimilate information regarded as crucial to the satisfactory development of their careers increase as the tempo of scientific enquiry increases. It is unfortunate that this, together with the defects of compartmentalisation of the subject, has conspired against the dental student to make the learning of oral anatomy less easy than it should be. Our aim in writing this book has been to gather together the diverse elements of oral anatomy which, in the past, have been scattered through many different textbooks, and to arrive at an integrated perspective of the subject. We were further persuaded to our task by the feeling that the time was ripe for such an encyclopaedic approach to oral anatomy; it is not so much that the rapid advances in the subject seem to be abating but that the variety of experimental approaches used in dental research seem to be converging to produce fewer deficiencies in our interpretations.

We have subdivided our book into four sections – the macroscopic appearance of the oral cavity and related structures, the microscopic appearance of oro-dental tissues, the development of oro-dental tissues and comparative dental anatomy. Thus, the book covers all the basic material generally used to teach oral anatomy in most dental schools. Indeed, the material has formed the basis of our own course in oral anatomy at Bristol University.

Since in our view oral anatomy occupies a central position in the dental curriculum, looking forward to much which is basic in the clinical world, we have included such topics as radiographic anatomy of the jaws and teeth, cephalometry and occlusion which, although anatomical, are not always taught to preclinical students (although it is our contention that they should be).

We have also striven to adopt the best features of the textbook and the atlas, without, we hope, their deficiencies. It may seem at times that we have adopted a dogmatic approach to the subject, preferring consensus views where there is uncertainty. However, we have not avoided controversy, merely avoided courting it. We have tried to suppress our own personal views where these are in the formative or hypothetical stages, although we appreciate that such views may come out if only through nuance of style. We hope that the suggestions for further reading at the back of the book will correct any bias.

Finally, in a book of this scope it is difficult to avoid errors. We crave the indulgence of the reader should he not agree with what is written, and trust that he will not hesitate to inform us of our mistakes.

B K B Berkovitz
G R Holland
B J Moxham

Bristol 1977

Acknowledgements

Our labours have been much lightened by help from many of our colleagues and friends. In the list of acknowledgements which follows, except where otherwise indicated, the contributors are from the University of Bristol.

We express our warm appreciation to Professor A I Darling for his kindness in making available material from the Dental School and M.R.C. Dental Unit, at the University of Bristol.

Thanks are owing to P F Heap, E Katchburian (London Hospital Medical School), J H Musgrave, H N Newman (Institute of Dental Surgery, London), D F G Poole, P R Shellis, C Squier (University of Iowa), C D Stevens, and C Stringer (British Museum of Natural History) for allowing us to draw freely from their knowledge and experience. Their encouragement and criticism of our efforts is highly valued. However, responsibility for the views expressed in this book lies entirely with us.

We are indebted to the many who provided us with material and who gave their permission to publish their photographs in this book:

D Adams, University of Wales, Cardiff (256, 266, 280, 342, 347, 399, 439, 440, 445, 526).

E H Batten (364, 365, 371, 372, 375, 376). D C Berry (76, 77). A D Beynon, University of Newcastle-Upon-Tyne (286, 294). E W Bradford (218, 248, 491, 516). M Byers, University of Washington, Seattle (299B, C).

J S Cooper (468, 479, 480, 481, 501, 502, 503, 518, 520, 521, 522).

G C Downer (99).

P Glick, University of Iowa (223, 242, 428, 429, 431, 432). A J Gwinnett, State University of New York, Stonybrook (182).

J D Harrison and B M Eley, Kings College Hospital Dental School (299). P F Heap (366, 367, 368, 369, 373, 374). R M Hopps, London Hospital Dental School (323B).

N W Johnson, London Hospital Dental School (175, 219, 323B).

E Katchburian, London Hospital Medical School (414, 416, 417, 420).

B G H Levers (188, 192, 240, 246, 445). D A Lunt, University of Glasgow (154B).

I Mackenzie, University of Iowa (324, 325). A H Meckel, W J Griebstein and R J Neal, Procter & Gamble, Cincinnati (165), B R R N Mendis (214, 220, 221, 222, 228, 434).

H N Newman, Institute of Dental Surgery, London (183, 184, 190, 196, 197, 198, 199, 200, 203, 204, 205, 206, 207, 208, 209, 210, 211).

H J Orams*, P P Phakey† and W A Rachinger†, Universities of Melbourne* and Monash† (163, 164). P D A Owens, Queens University, Belfast (274, 278, 301).

D F G Poole (158, 159, 161, 167, 172, 176, 183, 184, 190, 196, 197, 198, 199, 200, 475, 476, 480, 481). W D L Ride, Western Australian Museum (411).

J Searles, University of Iowa (239). R P Shellis (421, 437, 467, 471, 473, 474, 477, 485, 486, 490, 492, 493, 495, 496, 507, 508). L M Silverstone, University of Iowa (168, 169, 170). P Sloan (173, 290, 291, 292, 309, 318). J V Soames, University of Manchester (339, 340, 341). C Squier, University of Iowa (323, 336, 338, 354). C D Stevens (3, 122).

D K Whittacker, University of Wales, Cardiff (186, 189, 193, 279B, 280, 419, 445).

Acknowledgement is also owing to:

American Dental Association (for permission to reprint 456). Mammal section of the Zoology Department, British Museum of Natural History (563, 565, 566, 568, 569, 570, 571). National Geographic Society (592). National Museum, Dar-es-Salaam (589, 590). National Museum, Nairobi (586). Transvaal Museum, Pretoria (587). Trustees of the British Museum of Natural History (584, 585, 588, 591, 593, 594, 595, 596, 597, 598). Wenner-Gren Foundation (586, 587, 589, 590).

We thank the Editors of the following publications for permission to reproduce illustrations:

Archives of Oral Biology (183, 209, 290, 292). Journal of Cell Science (416, 417). Journal of Periodontal Research (299). Journal of Zoology (472, 480, 481, 514). Structural and Chemical Organisation of Teeth. Vol. I. 1967. Academic Press, London (182). Tooth Enamel. I. 1965. Wrights, Bristol (165).

We have modified diagrams originally published by the following:

B C W Barker and P L Davies (113). A Boyde (422, 483). R B Carter and E N Keen (95). H S M Crabb and A I Darling (425). H R B Fenn, K P Liddelow and A P Gimson (326). D Grant and S Bernick (446).

J C B Grant (92). L B Halstead (527). W H Hollingshead (87, 96, 97, 381). H C Killey, G R Seward and L W Kay (114). B S Kraus, R E Jordan and L Abrams (52). R C Page, W F Ammons, L R Schectman and L A Dillingham (346C). G J Romanes (82, 90). A S Romer (469, 470). H Sicher and E L Dubrul (84). C H Tonge and D A Luke (379). R C Wheeler (22, 31, 36, 41).

We are grateful to T Ovendon for radiographic assistance, B Rittman (University of Iowa) for preparing some of the histological material, D Coles, M H Gillett, C Ingham, and C C Jeal for photographic assistance, and M Appleby, D Ellis, R A Moxham and C Wood for preparing the manuscript. Above all, we acknowledge with much gratitude A Featherstone who was responsible for photographing most of the material in this book presented as colour illustrations.

Contents

Preface	iii
Acknowledgements	v
Macroscopic appearance of the oral cavity and environs	9
The *in vivo* appearance of oral tissues	10–12
Dento-osseous structures	13–46
The jaws	13–16
Tooth morphology	17–34
The alignment and occlusion of teeth	35–41
Mandibular posture	42
The temporomandibular joint	43–46
Oro-facial soft tissues	46–56
The muscles of mastication	46–47
The circum-oral muscles of facial expression	48
Muscles of the tongue	49
Muscles of the soft palate	50
Muscles at the oro-pharyngeal isthmus	51
Innervation of oro-dental tissues	51–54
Blood supply to oro-dental tissues	54–55
Venous drainage of oro-dental tissues	55
Lymphatic drainage of oro-dental tissues	56
Regional topography of the oral cavity and related areas	57–61
Tissue spaces around the jaws	62–63
The radiographic appearance of jaws and teeth	64–76
Extra-oral radiographic projections of jaws and related structures	65–71
inc. cephalometric analysis of lateral skull radiographs	68–70
Intra-oral radiographic projections of jaws and teeth	72–76
Microscopic appearance of oro-dental tissues	
Enamel	79–88
Investing organic layers on enamel surfaces	89–91
Dentine	91–101
Pulp	102–106
Cementum	107–111
Periodontal ligament	111–119
Alveolar bone	120–123
Oral mucosa	124–136
Temporomandibular joint	137
Salivary glands	138–142
Development of oro-dental tissues	
Development of face	144–145
Development of palate	146–147
Development of jaws	148–152
Development of tongue	152
Early tooth development	153–157
Amelogenesis	158–163
Dentinogenesis	164–167
Development of the pulp	168
Development of the root and periodontal ligament	169–172
Development of the dentitions	173–179
Development of occlusion	180

Comparative dental anatomy	182–185
Evolution of the jaws and teeth	185–190
Comparative histology of the dental tissues	185–187
Enameloid	187–188
Aprismatic enamel	188–189
Prismatic enamel (inc. tubular enamel)	189–190
Dentine	191–193
Types of tooth attachments	193–195
Tooth replacement	195–223
Features of vertebrate dentitions	195–198
Dentitions of fishes	195
Agnatha	196–197
Chondrichthyes	197–198
Osteichthyes	198
Dentitions of amphibia	199–201
Dentitions of reptiles	201–223
Dentitions of mammals	203
Prototheria	203–204
Metatheria	205–223
Eutheria	205
Insectivora	205–206
Chiroptera	206–207
Rodentia	207
Lagomorpha	208–209
Carnivora	209–210
Arteriodactyla	210
Perissodactyla	211
Proboscidea	211
Cetacea	212
Edentata	212
Sirenia	212
Hyracoidea	212
Tubulidentata	212
Pholidota	212–223
Primates	213–215
Prosimii	215–223
Anthropoidea	219–223
(inc. Hominidae)	225–229
Suggestions for further reading	231–248
Index	

Macroscopic appearance of the oral cavity and environs

1 The oral cavity extends from the lips and cheeks externally to the pillars of the fauces internally, where it is continuous with the oropharynx. It may be subdivided into the vestibule external to the teeth and the oral cavity proper internal to the teeth. The palate forms the roof of the mouth, separating it from the nasal cavity. The floor of the oral cavity is formed by the mylohyoid muscle and is occupied primarily by the tongue. The lateral walls of the oral cavity are defined by the cheeks and retromolar regions.

The functions of the mouth are primarily those concerned with ingestion, mastication and phonation and secondarily with ventilation.

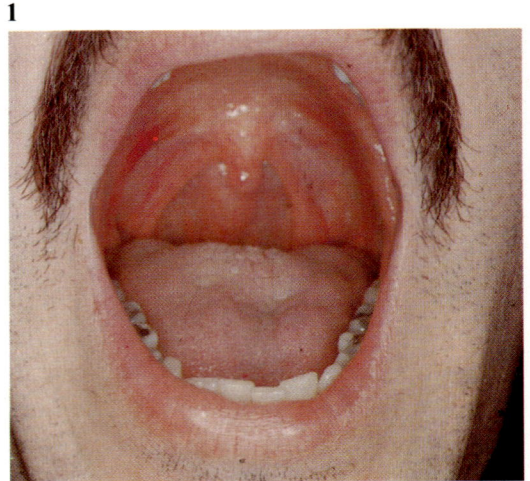

2 The lips are composed of a muscular skeleton – the orbicularis oris muscle – and connective tissue and are covered externally by skin and internally by mucous membrane. The red zone of the lip is a feature characteristic of man. The sharp junction of the red zone and the skin is termed the vermilion border. In the upper lip, the red zone protrudes in the midline to form the tubercle. The lower lip shows a slight depression in the midline corresponding to the tubercle. From the midline to the corners of the mouth the lips widen and then narrow. Laterally, the upper lip is separated from the cheeks by nasolabial grooves. With age, similar grooves appear at the corners of the mouth delineating the lower lip from the cheeks (labiomarginal sulcus). A labiomental groove separates the lower lip from the chin. In the midline of the upper lip runs the philtrum. The corners of the lips, the labial commissures, are usually adjacent to the maxillary canine and mandibular first premolar. The lips exhibit sexual dimorphism; as a general rule the skin of the male is thicker, firmer, less mobile and hirsute. The lips shown are said to be 'competent' in that at rest they are lightly closed.

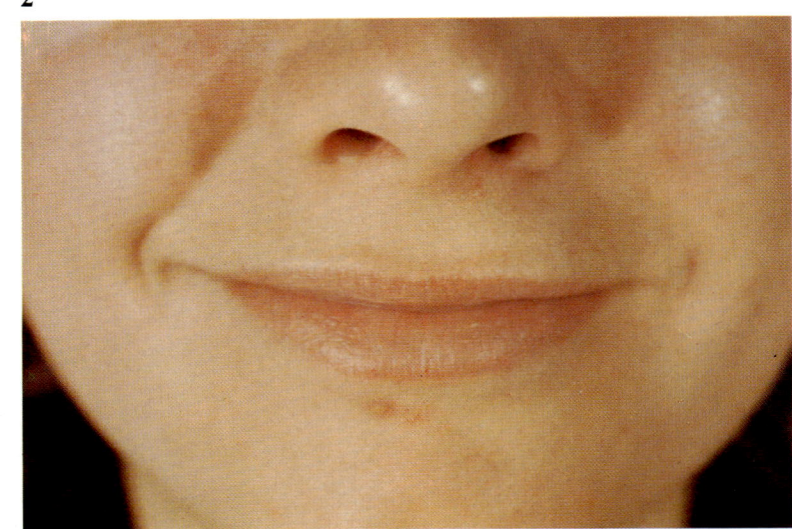

3 Incompetent lips describes a lip posture which at rest, with the facial muscles relaxed, does not produce an anterior seal. The position and activity of the lips are important in controlling the degree of protrusion of the incisors. With competent lips, the tips of the maxillary incisors lie below the upper border of the lower lip, this arrangement controlling the inclination of the incisors. With incompetent lips, the tips of the maxillary incisors may not be so controlled and the lower lip may even lie behind them, thus producing an exaggerated proclination of the maxillary incisors. During swallowing, it may not be possible to produce an anterior oral seal without the aid of the tongue. This behaviour termed 'tongue thrusting' may produce further forces tending to protrude the incisors. A tight or over-active lip musculature may produce sufficient forces to retrocline the incisors.

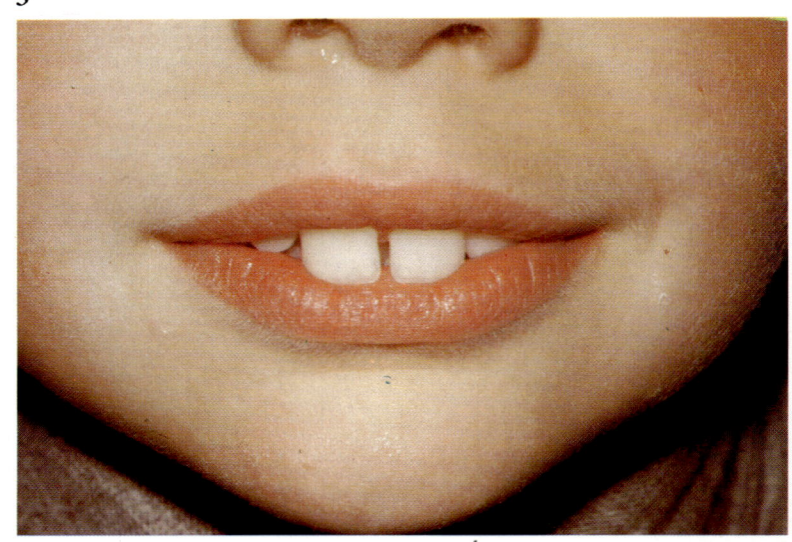

4 The oral vestibule is a slit-like space between the lips and cheeks and the teeth and alveolus. At rest, or with the mouth open, the vestibule and oral cavity proper directly communicate between the teeth. When the teeth occlude (as illustrated) the vestibule is a closed space which only communicates with the oral cavity proper in the retromolar regions. Where the mucosa covering the alveolus is reflected on to the lips and cheeks, a trough or sulcus is formed, the fornix vestibuli. In some regions of the sulcus the mucosa may show distinct sickle-shaped folds running from the cheeks and lips to the alveolus. The upper and lower labial frena or frenula are such folds in the midline. Other folds of variable dimensions may traverse the sulcus in the regions of the canines or premolars. Such frena are said to be more pronounced in the lower sulcus. All folds contain loose connective tissue and are neither muscle attachments nor sites of large blood vessels.

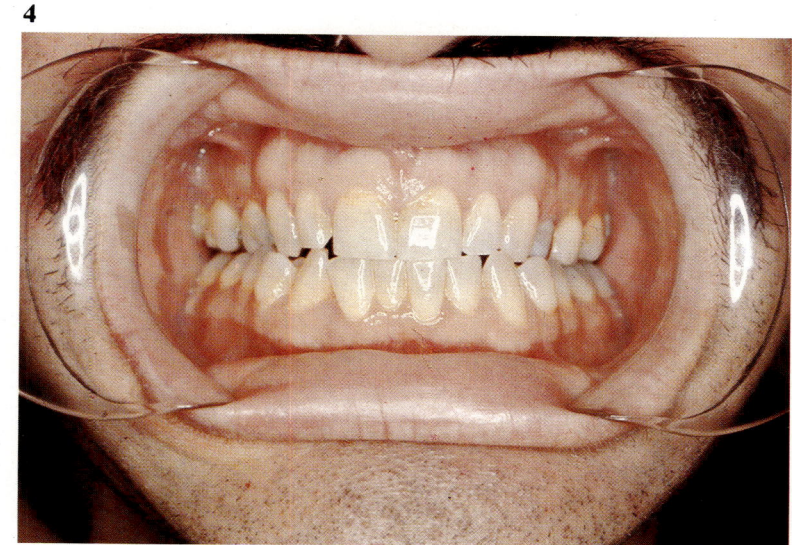

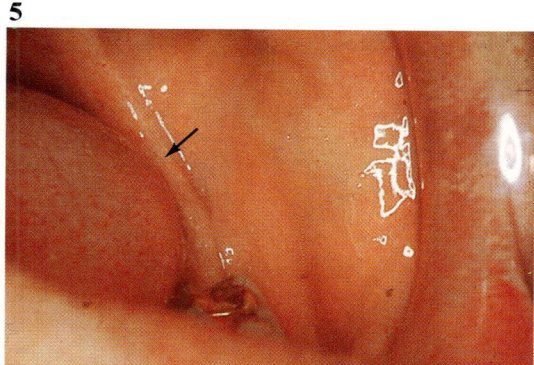

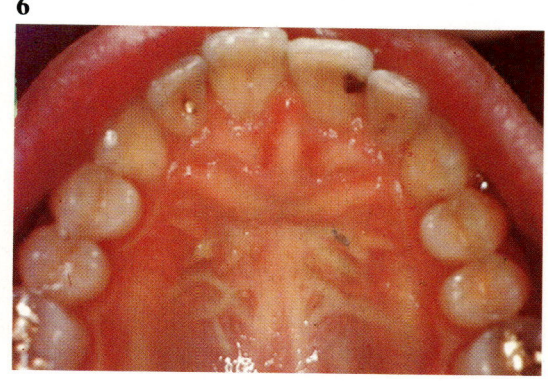

5 The cheek and mandibular retromolar region. Viewed from the oral cavity, the cheeks extend from the labial commissures anteriorly to the ridge of mucosa overlying the ascending ramus of the mandible posteriorly, and are bounded superiorly and inferiorly by the upper and lower vestibular sulci. The mucosa, being tightly adherent to the buccinator muscle, is stretched when the mouth is opened and wrinkled when closed. Ectopic sebaceous glands may be evident as yellowish patches, Fordyce's spots. Few structural landmarks are visible: the parotid duct drains into the cheek opposite the maxillary second molar tooth and a hyperkeratinised line, the linea alba, may be seen at a position related to the occlusal plane. In the retromolar region, in front of the pillars of the fauces, a fold of mucosa (*arrow*), containing the pterygomandibular raphe, extends from the upper to the lower alveolus. The pterygomandibular space, in which the lingual and inferior dental nerves run, lies lateral to this fold and medial to the ridge produced by the mandibular ramus.

6 The palate is divided into the immovable hard palate anteriorly and the movable soft palate posteriorly. As their names suggest, the skeleton of the hard palate is bony while that of the soft palate is fibrous. The hard palate (here illustrated) shows a distinct prominence immediately behind the maxillary central incisors, the incisive papilla, which covers the nasopalatine nerves as they emerge from the incisive foramen. From the papilla, extending posteriorly in the midline, runs a ridge, the palatine raphe. The palatine rugae are irregular folds which radiate transversely from the incisive papilla and the anterior part of the palatine raphe. At the junction of the palate and the alveolus lies a mass of soft tissue in which run the anterior palatine nerves and vessels. The shape and size of the dome of the palate varies considerably, being relatively shallow in some cases, and having considerable depth in others.

The soft palate is illustrated in figure 1. The boundary between the hard and soft palate is readily palpable and may be distinguished by a contrast in colour, the soft palate being a darker red with a yellowish tint. Extending laterally from the free border of the soft palate are the palatoglossal and palatopharyngeal folds, the palatoglossal folds being more anterior. These folds cover the palatoglossus and palatopharyngeus muscles and between them lie the tonsillar crypts housing the palatal tonsils. Extending backwards from the free edge of the soft palate in the midline lies the palatal uvula.

7 The floor of the mouth is a small horseshoe-shaped region above the mylohyoid muscle and beneath the movable part of the tongue. In the midline near the base of the tongue a fold of tissue, the lingual frenum (A), extends on to the inferior surface of the tongue. Rarely, the lingual frenum extends across the floor of the mouth to be attached to the mandibular alveolus. The sublingual papilla (B), on to which the submandibular salivary ducts open into the mouth, is a large centrally positioned protuberance at the base of the tongue. On either side of this papilla are the sublingual folds (C) beneath which lie the submandibular ducts and sublingual salivary glands.

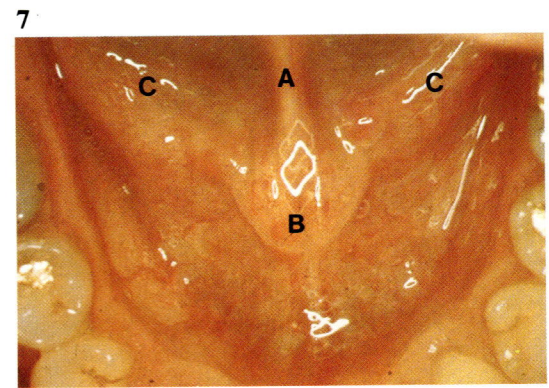

The tongue is a muscular organ with its base attached to the floor of the mouth.

8 The inferior surface of the tongue, related to the floor of the mouth, is covered by a thin lining of non-keratinised mucous membrane which is tightly bound to the underlying muscles. In the midline, extending on to the floor of the mouth, lies the lingual frenum (A). Lateral to the frenum lie irregular, fringed folds of mucous membrane, the fimbriated folds (B). Also visible through the mucosa are the large sublingual veins (C).

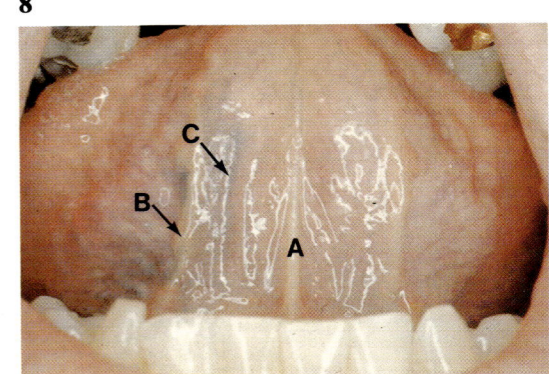

9 The dorsum of the tongue may be subdivided into the anterior two-thirds or palatal part of the tongue and the posterior third or pharyngeal part. The junction of the palatal and pharyngeal parts is marked by a shallow V-shaped groove, the sulcus terminalis. The angle (or V) of the sulcus terminalis is directed posteriorly. In the midline, near the angle, may be seen a small pit, the foramen caecum. The foramen caecum is the primordial site of development of the thyroid gland. The mucosa of the palatal part of the tongue is partly keratinised and is characterised by the abundance of papillae (for histology see pages 134–135). The most conspicuous papillae on the palatal surface of the tongue are the circumvallate papillae which lie immediately in front of the sulcus terminalis. The pharyngeal surface of the tongue is covered with large rounded nodules, the lingual follicles. These follicles are composed of lymphatic tissue (the lingual tonsil). The posterior part of the tongue slopes towards the epiglottis where a midline fold of mucous membrane, the glossoepiglottic fold, joins the two. The anterior pillars of the fauces (the palatoglossal arches) extend from the soft palate to the sides of the tongue near the circumvallate papillae. In order to show the above features a dissected specimen is illustrated; *in vivo* the posterior part of the tongue not being readily demonstrated.

The appearance of the teeth is described on pages 17–33, and the gums or gingivae on page 129.

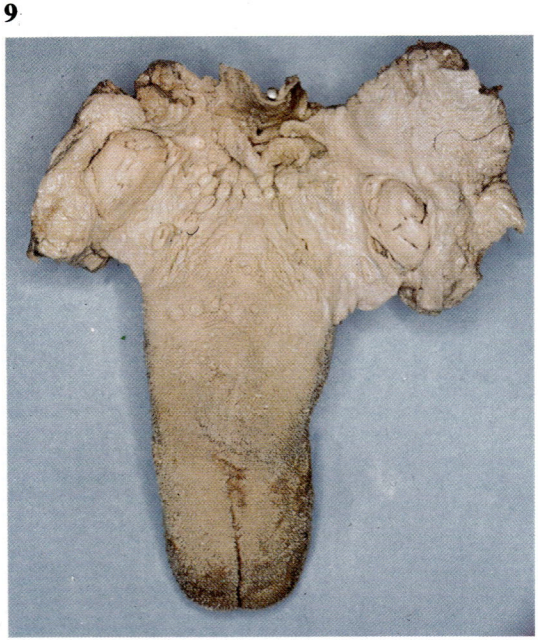
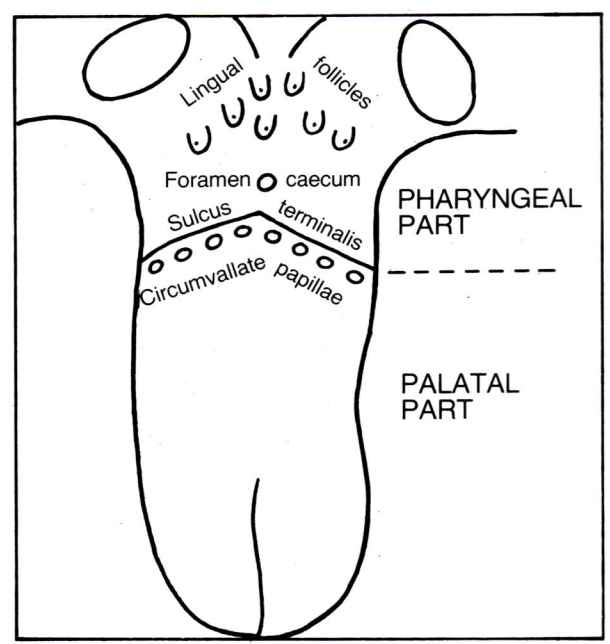

Dento-osseous structures

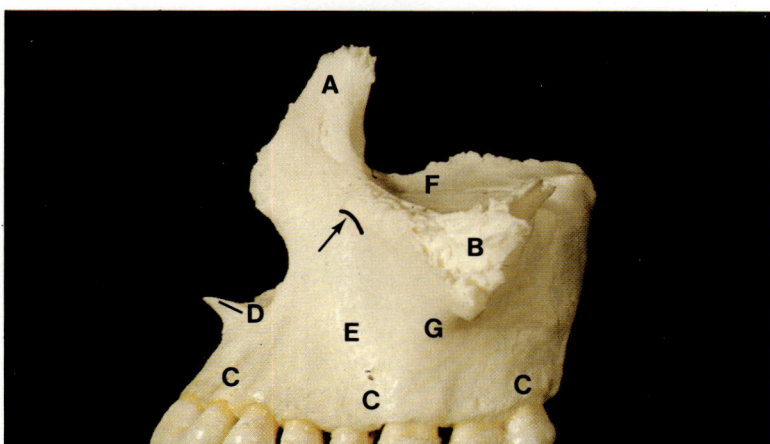

10 The maxilla (upper jaw) – lateral view. The maxilla consists of a body and four processes, the frontal (A), zygomatic (B), alveolar (C) and palatine processes, only the latter not being shown in this view. The anterolateral surface, the malar surface, forms the skeleton of the anterior part of the cheek. In the midline, the alveolar processes of the two maxillae meet at the intermaxillary suture whence they diverge laterally to form the opening of the nasal fossa, the piriform aperture. At the lower border of the aperture, in the midline, lies the sharp bony projection termed the anterior nasal spine (D). The malar surface of the body of the maxilla is concave – the canine fossa (E). Superiorly, the malar surface becomes continuous with the orbital plate of the maxilla (F) which forms the floor of the orbit. Anterior to the orbital plate, the frontal process extends above the piriform aperture to meet the nasal and frontal bones. Below the infraorbital rim lies the infraorbital foramen (*arrow*) through which the infraorbital branch of the maxillary nerve and the infraorbital artery from the maxillary artery emerge on to the face. The posterolateral surface of the maxilla, the infratemporal surface, forms the anterior wall of the infratemporal fossa. The malar and infratemporal surfaces meet at a bony ridge extending from the zygomatic process to the alveolus adjacent to the first molar tooth, the zygomaticoalveolar or jugal crest (G). The posterior convexity of the infratemporal surface, called the maxillary tuberosity, presents several small foramina associated with the posterior superior dental nerves (supplying the posterior maxillary teeth). The zygomatic process extends both from the malar and infratemporal surfaces of the maxilla. From the entire lower surface of the body arises the alveolar process which supports the maxillary teeth.

11 The medial aspect of the maxilla forms the lateral wall of the nose. In this specimen, the central hollow of the body of the maxilla, the maxillary air sinus or antrum, is divided longitudinally by a bony septum. In front of the antrum lies a smooth, deep, vertical groove, the lacrimal sulcus (A) which, with the lower edge of the lacrimal bone, forms the nasolacrimal canal. Behind the antrum lies the palatine groove (B) which is converted into a canal carrying the anterior palatine nerve and artery by the perpendicular plate of the palatine bone. The maxillary palatine process (C) extends horizontally from the medial surface of the maxilla where the body meets the alveolar process.

12 Inferior view of the maxillae and elements comprising the skeleton of the hard palate. The bones contributing to the hard palate are the palatine processes of the maxillae (A) and the horizontal plates of the palatine bones (B). As mentioned above, the maxillary palatine processes arise as horizontal plates at the junction of the bodies and alveolar processes of the maxillae. Only posteriorly is the boundary between the palatine and alveolar processes sharp. Anteriorly, the angle between the two is less well defined. The junction between the palatine processes in the midline is termed the median palatine suture. Anteriorly behind the central incisors this junction is incomplete, thus forming the incisive foramen through which pass the nasopalatine nerves. Unlike the nasal surface, the oral surface of the palatine process is rough and irregular. The posterior edges of the palatine processes articulate with the horizontal plates of the two palatine bones to form the transverse palatine suture. Laterally, this junction is incomplete, forming the greater palatine foramina. Through these foramina pass the anterior palatine nerves and vessels. Behind the greater palatine foramina lie the lesser palatine foramina, through which pass the posterior palatine nerves and vessels. The junction of the two palatine bones in the midline completes the median palatine suture. The posterior borders of the horizontal palatine plates are concave and in the midline form a sharp ridge of bone, the posterior nasal spine. To the posterior edge of the hard palate is attached the fibrous palatine aponeurosis of the soft palate which is formed by the tendons of the tensor palati muscles.

13 The maxillary alveolus and the arrangement of the tooth sockets. The maxillary alveolar processes extend inferiorly from the bodies of the maxillae and support the teeth within bony sockets. Each maxilla can contain a full quadrant of 8 permanent teeth or 5 deciduous teeth. The form of the alveolus is related to the functional demands put upon the teeth. When the teeth are removed the alveolus resorbs. Essentially, the alveolar process consists of two parallel plates of cortical bone, the buccal and palatal alveolar plates, between which lie the sockets of individual teeth. Between each socket lie interalveolar or interdental septa. The floor of the socket has been termed the fundus, its rim the alveolar crest. The form and depth of each socket is defined by the form and length of the root it supports and thus shows considerable variation. In multirooted teeth, the sockets are divided by interradicular septa. The apical regions of the sockets of anterior teeth are closely related to the nasal fossae, while those of posterior teeth are closely related to the maxillary antra. The position of the sockets in relation to the buccal and palatal alveolar plates is shown in figure **19**.

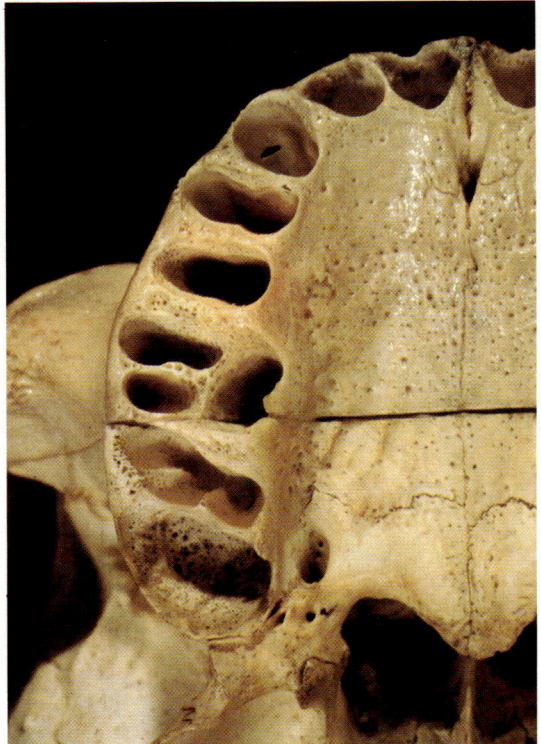

14 Lateral view of the maxillary teeth *in situ* within the alveolus, demonstrated by the removal of buccal bone around the roots of the teeth above the alveolar crests. Note the close relationship of the root apices of the premolars and molars to the floor of the maxillary antrum and those of the incisors and canine to the floor of the nasal fossa.

15 The mandible (lower jaw) – lateral view. The mandible consists of a horizontal horseshoe-shaped component, the body of the mandible (A), and two vertical components, the rami (B). The rami join the body posteriorly at obtuse angles. The body of the mandible carries the mandibular teeth and their associated alveolar processes. Before birth, the body consists of two lateral halves which subsequently fuse in the midline to form the symphysis. On either side of the symphysis close to the inferior margin of the body lies a distinct prominence, the mental tubercle, which together with the lower part of the symphysis comprises the mental protuberance or chin. Above the mental protuberance lies a shallow depression called the incisive fossa (C). Behind this fossa, the canine eminence overlies the root of the mandibular canine. Midway in the height of the body of the mandible, related to the premolar teeth, is the mental foramen (D). The mental branches of the inferior dental nerve and artery pass on to the face through this foramen. According to most standard textbooks, the mental foramen lies between the root apices of the mandibular premolars. However, a recent study indicates that the most common position for the foramen is on a vertical line passing through the mandibular second premolar. During the first and second years of life as the prominence of the chin develops, the opening of the mental foramen alters in direction from

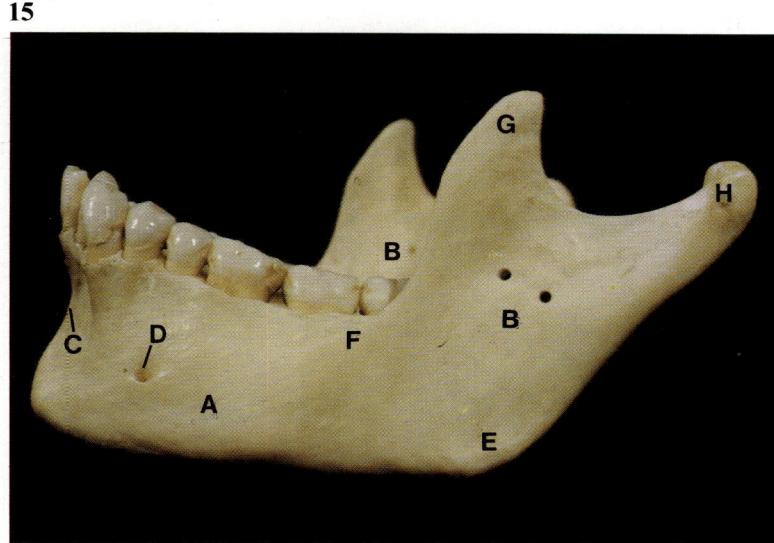

facing forwards to facing upwards and backwards. Rarely, there may be multiple mental foramina. The inferior margin of the body meets the posterior margin of the ramus at the angle of the mandible (E). This area is irregular, being the site of insertion of the masseter muscle and stylomandibular ligament. The alveolus forms the superior margin of the mandibular body. The junction of the alveolus and ramus is demarcated by a ridge of bone, the external oblique line (F), which continues downwards and forwards across the body of the mandible terminating below the mental

foramen. As this line progresses upwards, it becomes the anterior margin of the ramus and ends as the tip of the coronoid process. The coronoid (G) and the condylar (H) processes form the two processes of the superior border of the ramus. The coronoid process provides attachment for the temporalis muscle. The condylar process has a neck supporting an articular surface which fits into the glenoid fossa of the temporal bone to form a movable synovial joint, the temporomandibular joint. The concavity between the coronoid and condylar processes is the mandibular notch.

16 Posterolateral view of the medial surface of the mandible. Close to the midline on the inferior surface of the mandibular body lie two shallow depressions, the digastric fossae, to which are inserted the anterior bellies of the digastric muscles. Above these fossae in the midline are the genial spines or tubercles (A) – there are generally two inferior and two superior tubercles. The inferior tubercles serve as attachments for the geniohyoid muscles and the superior tubercles for the genioglossus muscles. Passing upwards and backwards across the medial surface of the body of the mandible is a prominent ridge, the mylohyoid or internal oblique ridge (B) from which the mylohyoid muscle takes origin. This ridge arises between the genial tubercles and digastric fossa and increases in prominence as it passes backwards to end on the anterior surface of the ramus. Since the mylohyoid muscle forms the floor of the mouth, the bone above the mylohyoid ridge forms the anterior wall of the oral cavity proper, while that below the ridge forms the lateral wall of the submandibular space.

The following features may be seen on the medial surface of the ramus: Around the angle of the mandible the bone is roughened (C) for the attachment of the medial pterygoid muscle.

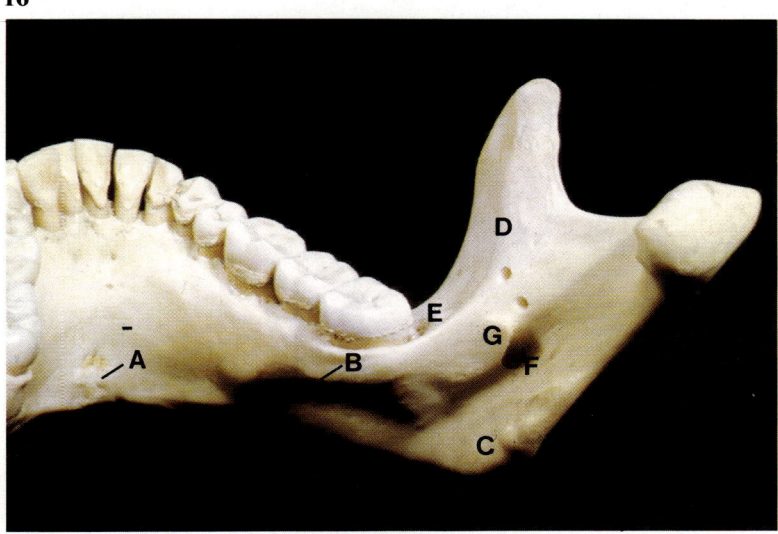

Commencing at the tip of the coronoid process, a ridge of bone, the temporal crest (D), runs down the anterior surface of the ramus to end behind the mandibular molars at the retromolar triangle (E). In the centre of the medial surface of the ramus lies the mandibular foramen (F) through which the inferior dental

nerve and artery pass into the mandibular canal. A bony process, the lingula (G), extends from the anterosuperior surface of the foramen. A groove, the mylohyoid groove, may be seen running down from the posteroinferior surface of the foramen.

17 The mandibular alveolus and the arrangement of the tooth sockets. Like the maxilla, the mandibular alveolus consists of buccal and lingual alveolar plates joined by interdental and interradicular septa. In the region of the second and third molars, the external oblique line is superimposed upon the buccal alveolar plate. As in the upper jaw, the form and depth of the tooth sockets is related to the morphology of the roots of the mandibular teeth and the functional demands placed upon them.

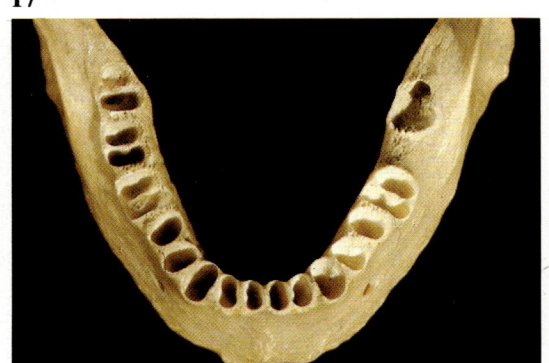

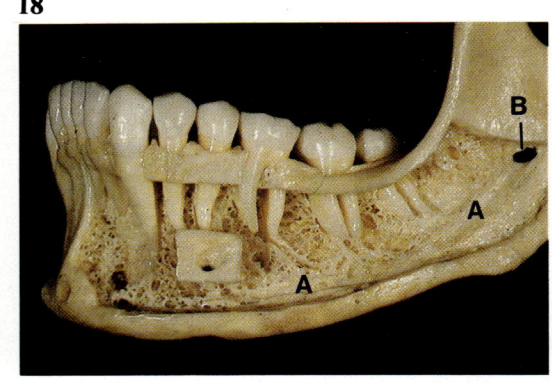

18 Lateral view of the mandibular teeth *in situ* within the alveolus and their relationship with the mandibular canal (A). The mandibular canal, which transmits the inferior dental nerve, artery and veins, begins at the mandibular foramen (B) and extends to the region of the premolar teeth where it bifurcates into the mental and incisive canals. The course of the mandibular canal and its relationship with the teeth is variable and this variation is illustrated in connection with the course of the inferior dental nerve in figure **95**.

19 Buccolingual sections through the teeth. These demonstrate the directional axes and bony relationships of the teeth and their alveoli and the relative thickness of the buccal and lingual alveolar plates.
A The central incisor region.
B The premolar region.
C The first molar region.
D The third molar region.
Stippled shading = cancellous bone.
Solid shading = compact bone.
Note the relationships of the mandibular teeth to the mandibular canal, and the maxillary teeth to the antrum (a). The deep groove on the palatal side of the maxillary third molar is related to the anterior palatine nerve and vessels.

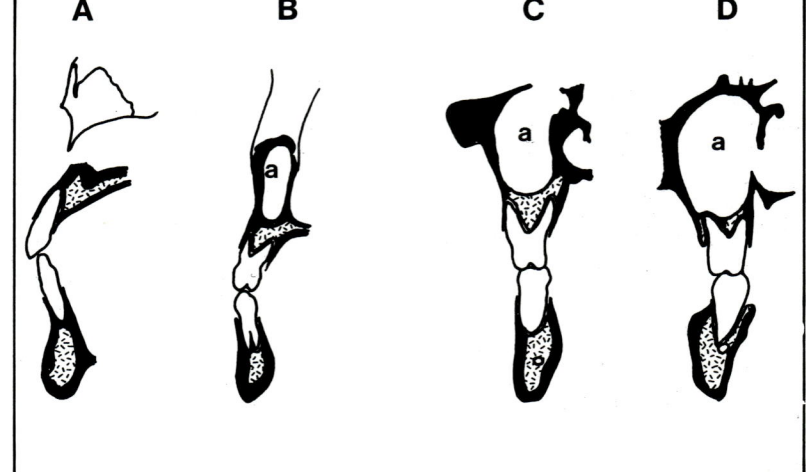

20 Relationship between the jaws and the remainder of the skull.
A Lateral view. B Anterior view.
The black outline describes the boundaries of a maxillary bone.

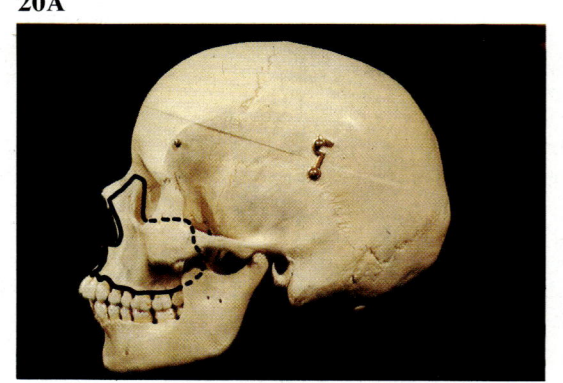

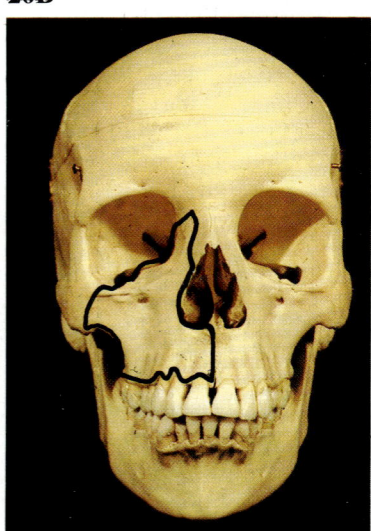

Tooth morphology

Man has two generations of teeth, the deciduous or primary dentition and the permanent or secondary dentition. There are no teeth in the mouth at birth but by the age of 3 years the deciduous dentition is complete. By 6 years, the first permanent teeth appear and thence the deciduous teeth are exfoliated one by one to be replaced by their permanent successors. A complete permanent dentition is present at or about the age of 18 years. Thus, given the average life of 70 years, the functional life span of the deciduous dentition is only 6 per cent of this total, while with care and luck it can be over 90 per cent for the permanent dentition. In the complete deciduous dentition there are 20 teeth – 10 in each jaw. In the complete permanent dentition there are 32 teeth – 16 in each jaw. In both dentitions, there are three basic tooth forms, incisiform, caniniform and molariform. Incisiform teeth (incisors) are cutting teeth having thin, blade-like crowns. Caniniform teeth (canines) are piercing or tearing teeth, having a single, stout, pointed, cone-shaped crown. Molariform teeth (molars and premolars) are grinding teeth possessing a number of cusps on an otherwise flattened biting surface. Premolars are bicuspid teeth which are peculiar to the permanent dentition and which replace the deciduous molars.

Some terms used for the description of tooth form:

Crown — Clinical crown – that portion of a tooth visible in the oral cavity.
Anatomical crown – that portion of a tooth covered with enamel.

Root — A clinical and anatomical root may be defined, the clinical root being that portion of a tooth which lies within the alveolus, the anatomical root being that portion of a tooth covered by cementum.

Cervical margin — The junction of the anatomical crown and root.

Occlusal surface — The biting surface of a molar or premolar.

Incisal margin — The cutting edge of anterior teeth, analogous to the occlusal surface of the cheek teeth.

Cusp — A pronounced elevation on the occlusal surface of a posterior tooth.

Tubercle — A small elevation on the crown which may or may not be typical.

Cingulum — A bulbous convexity near the cervical region of a tooth.

Ridge — A linear elevation on the surface of a tooth.

Marginal ridge — A ridge at the mesial or distal edge of the occlusal surface of posterior teeth. Some anterior teeth have equivalent ridges.

Fissure — A long cleft between cusps or ridges.

Fossa — A rounded depression in a surface of a tooth.

Buccal — Towards or adjacent to the cheek. The term buccal surface is reserved for that surface of a premolar or molar which is positioned immediately adjacent to the cheek.

Labial — Towards or adjacent to the lips. The term labial surface is reserved for that surface of an incisor or canine which is positioned immediately adjacent to the lips.

Palatal — Towards or adjacent to the palate. The term palatal surface is reserved for that surface of a maxillary tooth which is positioned immediately adjacent to the palate.

Lingual — Towards or adjacent to the tongue. The term lingual surface is reserved for that surface of mandibular tooth which lies immediately adjacent to the tongue.

Mesial — Towards the median. The mesial surface is that surface which faces towards the median line following the curve of the dental arch.

Distal — Away from the median. The distal surface is that surface which faces away from the median line following the curve of the dental arch.

The types and numbers of teeth in any mammalian dentition can be expressed using dental formulae which, whatever the species, conform to a standard format. The type of tooth is represented by its initial letter, i.e. I for incisors, C for canines, P for premolars and M for molars. The deciduous dentition is indicated by the letter D. The formula for the deciduous dentition of man is $DI\frac{2}{2}DC\frac{1}{1}DM\frac{2}{2} = 10$, and for the permanent dentition $I\frac{2}{2}C\frac{1}{1}P\frac{2}{2}M\frac{3}{3} = 16$, where the numbers following each letter refer to the number of teeth of each type in the upper and lower jaws on one side only.

Identification of teeth is made not only according to the dentition to which they belong and to basic tooth form, but also according to their anatomical location within the jaws. The tooth-bearing region of the jaws can be divided into four quadrants, the right and left maxillary and mandibular quadrants. A tooth may thus be identified according to the quadrant in which it is located, e.g. a right maxillary deciduous incisor or a left mandibular permanent molar. In both the permanent and deciduous dentitions, the incisors may be distinguished according to their relationship to the midline. Thus, the incisor nearest the midline is the central or first incisor, the incisor which is more laterally positioned being termed the lateral or second incisor. The permanent premolars and the permanent and deciduous molars can also be distinguished according to their mesiodistal relationships. The molar most mesially positioned is designated the first molar, the one behind it being the second molar. In the permanent dentition, the tooth most distally positioned is the third molar. The mesial premolar is the first premolar, the premolar behind it being the second premolar.

A dental shorthand may be used in the clinic to simplify tooth identification. The permanent teeth in each quadrant are numbered 1 to 8 and the deciduous teeth in each quadrant are lettered A to E.

The symbols for the quadrants are derived from an imaginary cross with the horizontal bar placed between the upper and lower jaws and the vertical bar running between the upper and lower central incisors.

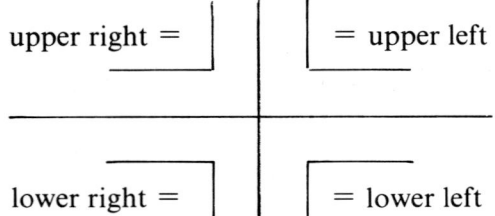

Thus, the maxillary right first permanent molar is allocated the symbol, 6⌋ and the mandibular left deciduous canine, ⌈C. This system of dental shorthand is termed the Zsigmond System. An alternative scheme has been devised by the Federation Dentaire Internationale in which the quadrant is represented by a number

1 = maxillary right quadrant
2 = maxillary left quadrant
3 = mandibular left quadrant
4 = mandibular right quadrant } Permanent
5 = maxillary right quadrant
6 = maxillary left quadrant
7 = mandibular left quadrant
8 = mandibular right quadrant } Deciduous

which prefixes a tooth number. According to this system, the maxillary right first permanent molar is symbolised as 1,6 and the mandibular left deciduous canine as 7,3.

The diagram below illustrates some of the descriptive terms used in tooth morphology and summarises the systems employed for the identification of teeth according to their location in the jaws.

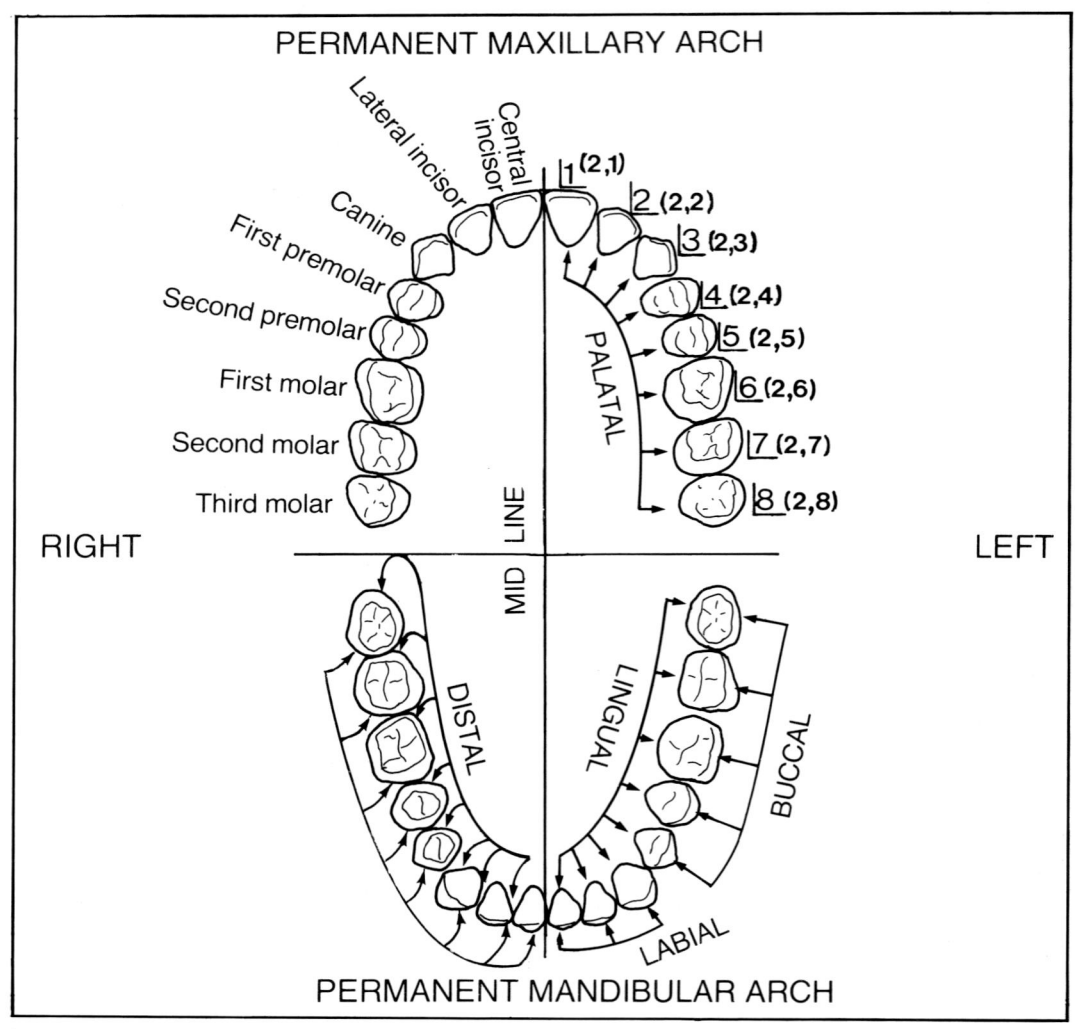

24 Maxillary second (lateral) permanent incisor. The lateral incisor is one of the most variable teeth in the dentition though generally it is morphologically a diminutive form of the maxillary central incisor with slight modifications. The lateral incisor crown is much narrower and shorter than the central incisor, though the crown root length ratio is considerably decreased. From the *incisal* aspect (A), the crown has a more rounded outline than the adjacent central incisor. Viewed *labially* (B), the mesioincisal and distoincisal angles and the mesial and distal crown margins are more rounded than those of the central incisor. The *palatal* aspect (C) of the crown is similar to that of the central incisor though the marginal ridges and cingulum are often more pronounced. Consequently, the palatal concavity appears deeper. Lying in front of the cingulum is a pit, the foramen cacumen, which may extend some way into the root. The *mesial* (D) and *distal* (E) aspects of the lateral incisor differ little from those of the central incisor. A common morphological variation is the so-called peg-shaped lateral incisor which has a thin root surmounted by a small conical crown. The course of the cervical margin and the shape of the root is similar to the central incisor. However, the root is often slightly compressed and grooved on the mesial and distal surfaces.

The mandibular incisors have the smallest mesiodistal dimensions of any teeth in the permanent dentition. They can be distinguished from the maxillary incisors not only by their size but also by the marked lingual inclination of the crowns over the roots, the mesiodistal compression of their roots and the poor development of the marginal ridges and cingula.

25 Mandibular first (central) permanent incisor. Viewed *incisally* (A), the tooth has a bilaterally symmetrical triangular shape. The incisal margin in this specimen has been worn and appears flat, though in the newly-erupted tooth, three mamelons are usually present. The incisal margin is at right angles to a line bisecting the tooth labiolingually. Viewed *labially* (B), the crown of the incisor is almost twice as long as it is broad. The unworn incisal margin is straight and approximately at right angles to the long axis of the tooth. The mesioincisal and distoincisal angles are sharp and the mesial and distal surfaces are approximately at right angles to the incisal margin. The profiles of the mesial and distal surfaces appear very similar, being convex in their incisal thirds and relatively flattened in the middle and cervical thirds. The *lingual* surface (C) is smooth and slightly concave, the lingual cingulum and mesial and distal marginal ridges appearing less distinct than those of the maxillary incisors. The *mesial* (D) and *distal* (E) views show the characteristic wedge-shape of the incisor and the inclination of the crown lingually over the root.

The cervical margins on the labial and lingual surfaces show their maximum convexities midway between the mesial and distal borders of the root. The cervical margin on the distal surface is said to be less curved than that on the mesial surface. The root is narrow and conical though flattened mesiodistally. It is frequently grooved on the mesial and distal surfaces, the distal groove generally being more marked and deeper.

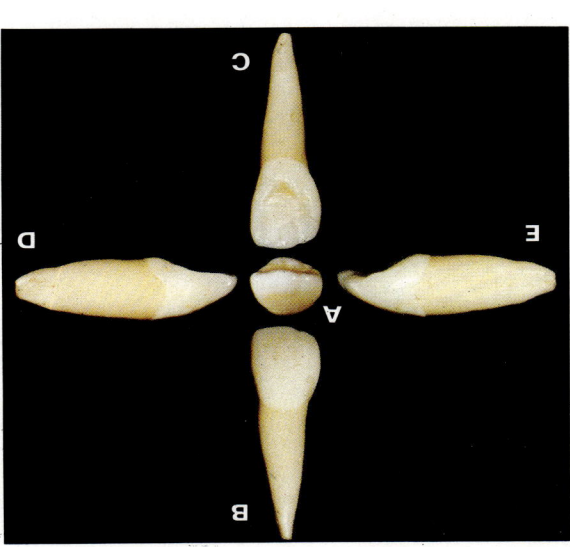

26 The mandibular second (lateral) permanent incisor closely resembles the mandibular central incisor. However, it is slightly wider mesiodistally and is more asymmetrical in shape. The distal surface diverges at a greater angle from the long axis of the tooth giving it a fan-shaped appearance and the distoincisal angle is more acute and rounded. Another distinguishing characteristic is the angulation of the incisal margin relative to the labiolingual axis of the root. In the central incisor, the incisal margin forms a right angle with the labiolingual axis, whereas that of the lateral incisor is 'twisted' distally in a lingual direction.

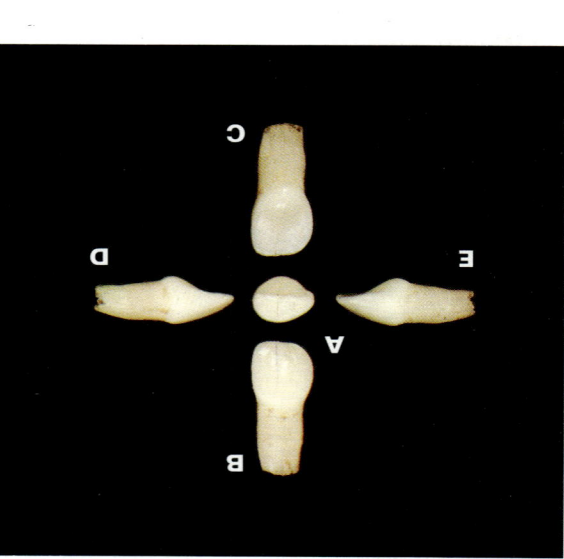

27 Maxillary first (central) deciduous incisor. This tooth is similar morphologically to the corresponding permanent tooth. However, since the transverse diameter of the crown of the deciduous incisor nearly equals the vertical diameter, it appears plumper than its permanent successor. From the *incisal* view (A) the straight incisal margin appears to be centred over the bulk of the crown. Unlike the permanent teeth, no mamelons are seen on the incisal margin of the newly erupted deciduous incisor. The *labial* surface (B) is slightly convex in all planes and unmarked by grooves, lobes or depressions. The mesioincisal angle is sharp and acute, while the distoincisal angle is more rounded and obtuse. On the *palatal* surface (C), the cingulum is a very prominent bulge which extends some way up the crown, sometimes to the incisal margin to form a ridge. Unlike its permanent successor, the marginal ridges are ill-defined and the concavity of the palatal surface shallow. *Mesial* (D) and *distal* (E) views show the typical incisal form of the crown. Note the low, rounded cingulum at the margin of the labial surface.

As with all deciduous teeth, the cervical margins are more pronounced but less sinuous than their permanent successors. The fully-formed root is conical in shape, tapering apically to a rather blunt apex. Compared with the corresponding permanent tooth, the root is longer in proportion to the crown. In the specimen shown, however, the root has not fully formed.

28 The maxillary second (lateral) deciduous incisor is similar in shape though smaller than the maxillary first deciduous incisor. One obvious difference is the more acute mesioincisal angle and the more rounded distoincisal angle. The palatal surface is more concave and the marginal ridges are more pronounced. Viewed *incisally* (A), the crown appears almost circular in contrast to the central incisor which appears diamond-shaped. As the first deciduous incisor, there is a rounded, labial cingulum cervically. The palatal cingulum is generally lower than that of the central incisor.

The course of the cervical margin and the shape of the root is similar to the first deciduous incisor.

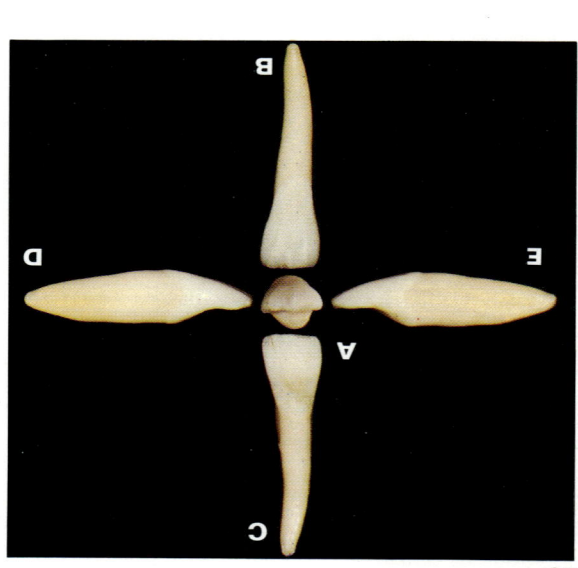

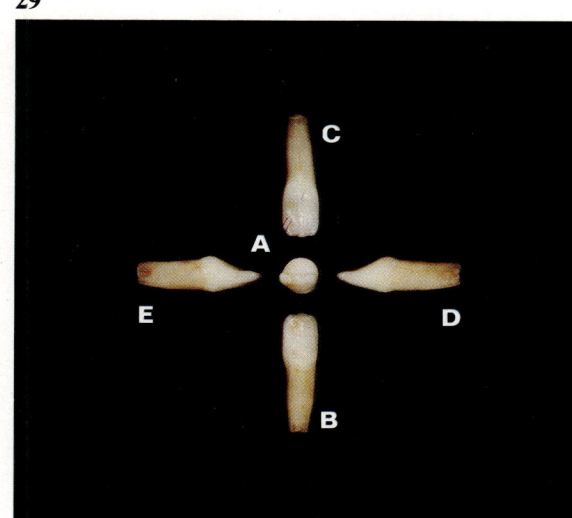

29 The mandibular first (central) deciduous incisor is morphologically similar to its permanent successor. However, it is much shorter and has a low labial cingulum. The mesioincisal and distoincisal angles are sharp right angles and the incisal margin is straight in the horizontal plane. While there are generally no mammelons or grooves on the incisal margin, in this specimen three mammelons may be discerned. The palatal cingulum and the marginal ridges are poorly defined.

The single root is more rounded than the corresponding permanent tooth and when complete tapers and tends to incline distally.

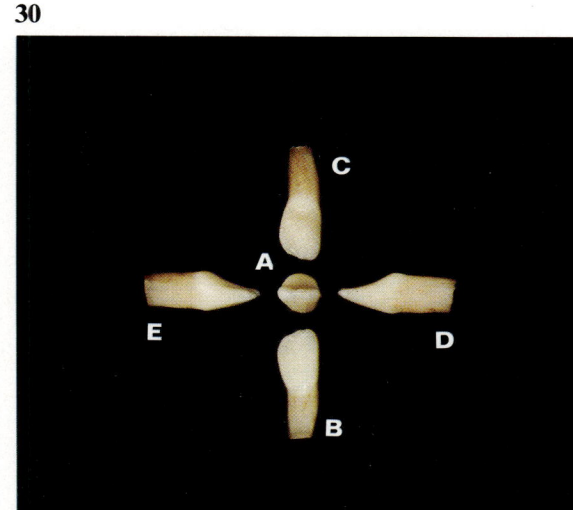

30 The mandibular second (lateral) deciduous incisor is a bulbous tooth which resembles its permanent successor. It is wider than the mandibular first deciduous incisor and is asymmetrical. The mesioincisal angle is more obtuse and rounded than that of the mandibular first deciduous incisor and the incisal margin slopes downward distally. Should the distoincisal angle be markedly rounded then the tooth may be difficult to distinguish from a maxillary second deciduous incisor.

Unlike the permanent successor, the root is rounded. When complete it is longer than the root of the mandibular first deciduous incisor.

The canines

Canines are the only teeth in the dentition with a single cusp. Morphologically, they can be considered transitional between incisors and premolars.

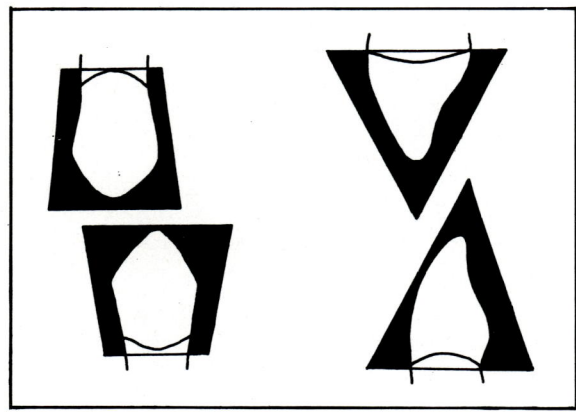

31 Schematic drawings of canine crown form illustrating the relationship between anatomic and geometric form. Like the incisors, the crowns of canines are roughly triangular in shape when viewed mesially or distally and trapezoidal buccally and lingually.

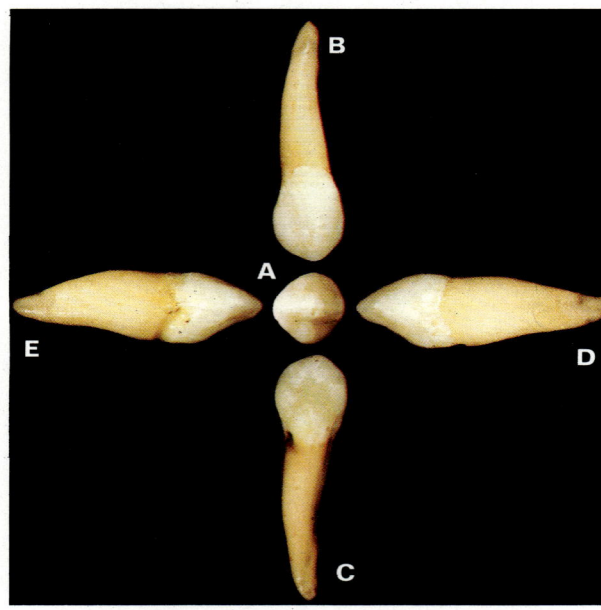

32 Maxillary permanent canine. This is a stout tooth with a well-developed cingulum and the longest root of any tooth. Viewed from its *'incisal'* aspect (A), it appears asymmetrical. If a plane is envisaged passing through the apex of the cusp to the cingulum on the palatal surface, then the distal portion of the crown is much wider than the mesial portion. It is thought that the pointed shape of the canine tooth is related to an increase in size of a central mammelon at the expense of mesial and distal mammelons. Prominent longitudinal ridges pass from the cusp tip down both the labial and palatal surfaces. A relatively frequent variation in the morphology of the incisal ridge is the development of an accessory cusp on its distal arm. The *labial* surface (B) of the canine is marked by the longitudinal ridge which extends from the cusp towards the cervical margin. The incisal part of the crown occupies at least one-third of the crown height. Note that from this view, the mesial arm of the incisal margin is shorter than the distal arm and the distoincisal angle is more rounded than the mesioincisal angle. The profiles of the mesial and distal surfaces converge markedly towards the cervix of the tooth. The mesial profile is slightly convex, the distal profile markedly convex. The mesial surface of the crown forms a straight line with the root. The distal surface meets the root at an obtuse angle. The *palatal* surface (C) shows distinct mesial and distal marginal ridges and a well-defined cingulum. The longitudinal ridge from the tip of the cusp meets the cingulum and is separated from the marginal ridges on either side by distinct grooves or fossae. Viewed *mesially* (D) or *distally* (E), the distinctive feature is the stout character of the crown and the great width of the cervical third of both the crown and root.

The cervical margin of this tooth follows a similar course to the incisors, though the curves are less pronounced. The curvature of the cervical margin on the distal surface is less marked than that on the mesial surface. The root is the largest and stoutest in the dentition, being in cross-section triangular in shape, its labial surface being wider than its palatal surface. The mesial and distal surfaces of the root are often grooved longitudinally.

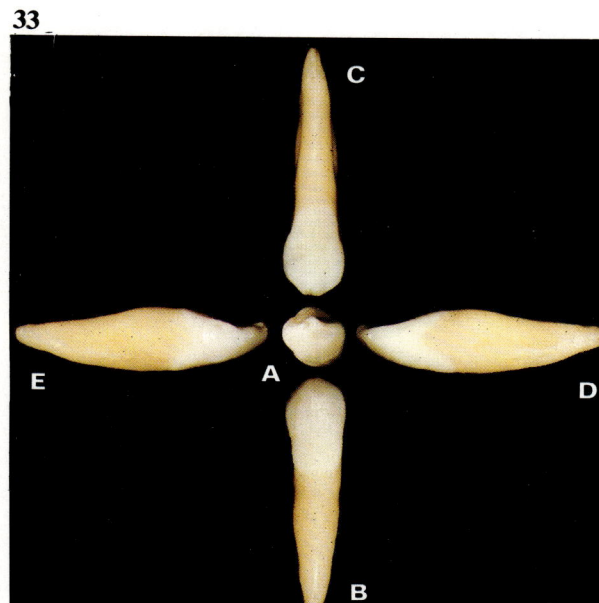

33 **The mandibular permanent canine** is similar to the maxillary canine, but is a smaller, slender, more symmetrical tooth. The cusp is generally less well-developed. Indeed, with attrition, the low cusp may be lost and the tooth may resemble a maxillary second permanent incisor. From the *incisal* aspect (A), no distinct longitudinal ridges can be seen running from the tip of the cusp on to the labial and lingual surfaces. Viewed *labially* (B), the incisal margin occupies only one-fifth of the crown height and the cusp is less pointed. The crown is narrower mesiodistally than the maxillary canine so that it appears longer, narrower and more slender. The mesial and distal profiles tend to be parallel or only slightly convergent towards the cervix. The labial and mesial surfaces are clearly defined, being inclined acutely to each other, whereas the labial surface merges gradually into the distal surface. On the *lingual* surface (C), the cingulum, marginal ridges and fossae are indistinct. The lingual surface is flatter than the corresponding palatal surface of the maxillary permanent canine and simulates the lingual surface of the mandibular incisors. Viewed *mesially* (D) and *distally* (E), the wedge-shaped appearance of the canine can be clearly seen. These proximal surfaces are longer than those of the maxillary canine. The labiolingual diameter of the crown near the cervix is less than the corresponding labio-palatal diameter of the maxillary canine.

The cervical margin of this tooth follows a similar course to the incisors. The crownward convexity on the mesial surface is generally more marked than that on the distal surface. The root is normally single, though occasionally it may bifurcate. In cross-section, the root is oval, being flattened mesially and distally. The root is grooved longitudinally on both its mesial and distal surfaces.

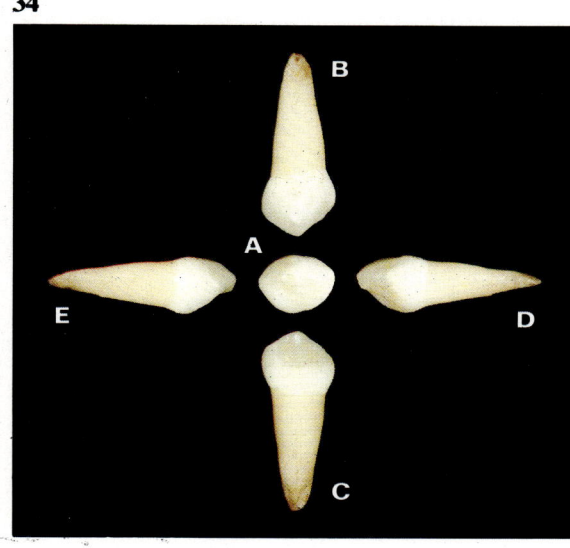

34 **The maxillary deciduous canine** has a fang-like appearance, being similar morphologically to its permanent successor (though more bulbous). It is generally symmetrical, but where there is asymmetry, it is usual for the mesial slope of the cusp to be longer than the distal slope. Bulging of the tooth gives the crown a diamond-shaped appearance when viewed *labially* (B) or *palatally* (C), with the crown margins overhanging the root profiles. The mesiodistal dimension of the crown is greater than its height. On the labial surface, there is a low cingulum cervically from which runs a longitudinal ridge up to the tip of the cusp. A similar longitudinal ridge also runs on the palatal surface. This ridge extends from the cusp apex to the palatal cingulum and divides the palatal surface into two shallow pits. The marginal ridges on the palatal surface are low and indistinct.

The root is long compared with the crown height and is triangular in cross-section.

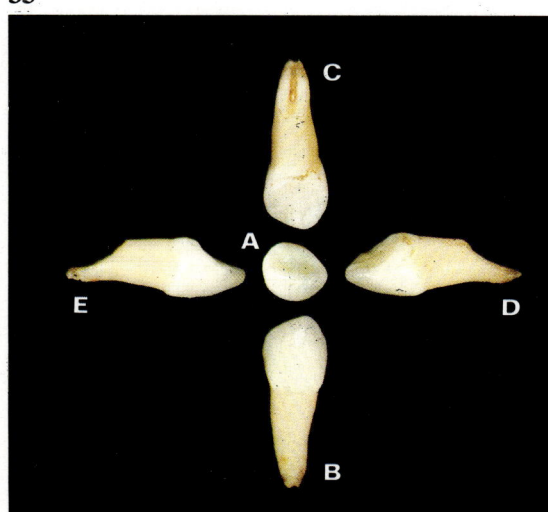

35 **The mandibular deciduous canine** is more slender than the maxillary deciduous canine. The crown is asymmetrical with the cusp tip displaced mesially. Consequently, the mesial arm is shorter and more vertical than the distal arm. On the *labial* surface (B), there is a low, labial cingulum. On the *lingual* surface (C), the cingulum and marginal ridges are less pronounced than the corresponding structures on the palatal surface of the maxillary deciduous canine. The longitudinal ridges on both the labial and lingual surfaces are poorly developed. The mesiodistal dimension is less than the height.

The root is single and tends to be triangular in cross-section.

The premolars

Premolars are unique to the permanent dentition. They are sometimes referred to as 'bicuspids', having two main cusps, a buccal and a palatal or lingual cusp, which are separated by a mesiodistal occlusal fissure. The buccal surface of the buccal cusp is similar in shape, and may be considered analogous to the cusp of a canine, while the palatal or lingual cusp corresponds developmentally to the cingulum of the anterior teeth. Thus, premolars are considered to be transitional between canines and molars.

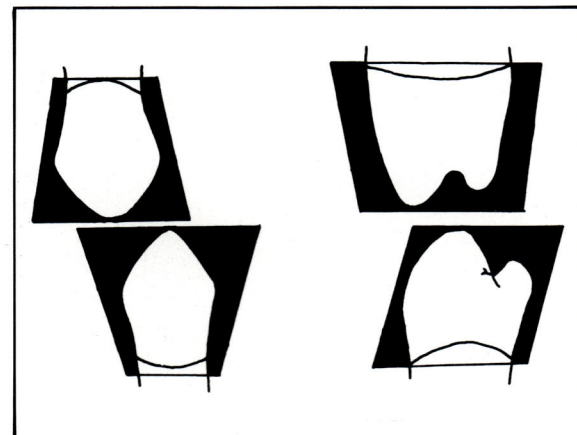

36 Schematic drawings of premolar crown form illustrating the relationship between anatomic and geometric form. Viewed mesially or distally, the maxillary premolars are trapezoidal in shape, the longest side of the trapezoid being the base of the crown at the cervical margin. Functionally, it is thought that because the occlusal surface is not as wide as the base of the crown, the tooth can penetrate the food more easily, while minimising the occlusal forces. The mandibular premolars, however, are roughly rhomboidal in shape. The rhomboidal outline is inclined lingually, thus allowing correct intercuspal contact with their maxillary antagonists. Viewed buccally or lingually, all the premolars are trapezoidal, the shortest of the uneven sides being the bases of the crowns cervically.

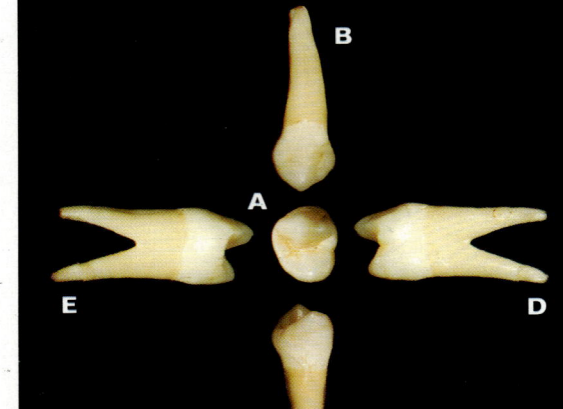

37 Maxillary first premolar. From the *occlusal* aspect (A), the crown appears ovoid, being broader buccally than palatally. Thus, the profiles of the mesial and distal surfaces converge palatally. The mesiobuccal and distobuccal corners are less rounded than the mesiopalatal and distopalatal corners. The mesial and distal borders of the occlusal surface are marked by distinct ridges, the mesial and distal marginal ridges. The buccal and palatal cusps are separated by a central occlusal fissure which runs in a mesiodistal direction. The occlusal fissure crosses the mesial marginal ridge on to the mesial surface. On the distal side, the fissure terminates in a fossa before the distal marginal ridge. Supplementary grooves from the central fissure are rare. Viewed *buccally* (B), the first premolar bears a distinct resemblance to the adjoining canine. A longitudinal ridge may be seen passing down the buccal cusp. The mesial and distal ridges of the buccal cusp each form a 30 degree slope and the mesio- and disto-occlusal angles are prominent, giving the crown a 'bulging-shouldered' ovoid appearance. The mesial slope is generally longer than the distal slope. Viewed *palatally* (C), the buccal part of the crown appears larger in all dimensions than the palatal part so that the entire buccal profile of the crown is visible from the palatal aspect. The palatal cusp is lower, and its tip lies more mesially than the tip of the buccal cusp. From the *mesial* aspect (D), the unequal height of the cusps is clearly seen. Note the canine groove extending across the marginal ridge from the occlusal surface. The cervical third of the mesial surface is marked by a distinct concavity, the canine fossa. The *distal* aspect (E) of the crown differs from the mesial aspect in that it lacks a canine groove and canine fossa.

The cervical margin follows a fairly level course around the crown, deviating slightly towards the root on the buccal and palatal surfaces and away from the root on the mesial and distal surfaces. There are usually two roots, a buccal and palatal root, though sometimes there may be a single root. However, even when it is single, it is deeply grooved on its mesial and distal surfaces.

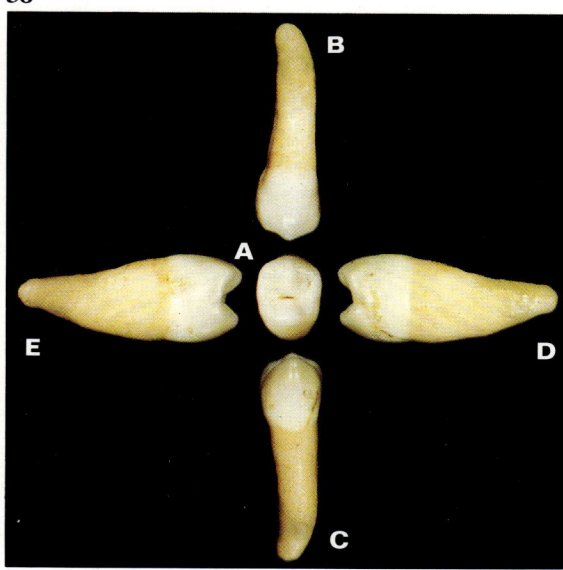

38 The **maxillary second premolar** is similar in shape to the maxillary first premolar except for the following features. Viewed *occlusally* (A), the mesiobuccal and distobuccal corners are more rounded and the mesial and distal profiles do not converge lingually, being nearly parallel. The occlusal surface appears more compressed, the mesiodistal dimension of the crown being smaller. The central fissure appears shorter and does not cross the mesial marginal ridge. From the *buccal* aspect (B), the mesio- and disto-occlusal angles are less prominent. These features give the crown a 'narrow-shouldered' appearance. The two cusps are smaller and more equal in size than those of the first premolar. The height of the buccal cusp is 1/4 of the height of the crown measured from the base of the occlusal fissure, while the height of the buccal cusp of the first premolar is up to 1/2 the height of the crown. Viewed *palatally* (C), less of the buccal profile is visible. *Mesially* (D) and *distally* (E), the tooth appears similar to the first premolar but there is no canine fossa or canine groove on the mesial surface. Note also the more equal size of the cusps.

The cervical margin appears similar to that of the maxillary first premolar but is slightly less undulating. The root is single.

The mandibular premolars differ from the maxillary premolars in that, occlusally, the crowns appear rounder and the cusps are of unequal size, the buccal cusp being the most prominent. Furthermore, unlike the maxillary premolars, the first and second premolars differ more markedly.

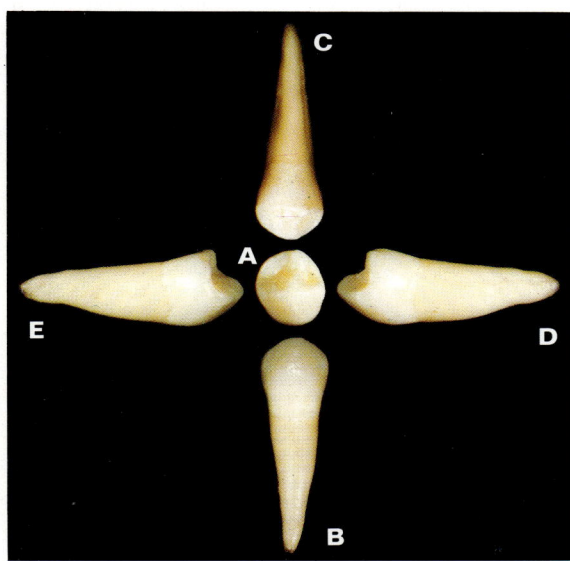

39 The **mandibular first premolar** is the smallest premolar. Since it is comprised of a dominant buccal cusp and a very small lingual cusp which appears not unlike a cingulum, some consider it to be a modified canine. From the *occlusal* aspect (A), more than two-thirds of the buccal surface is visible though only a small portion of the lingual surface can be seen. The occlusal outline is diamond-shaped and the occlusal table, outlined by the cusps and marginal ridges, is triangular. The buccal cusp is a broad cusp with its apex approximately overlying the midpoint of the crown. The lingual cusp is less than half the size of the buccal cusp. The buccal and lingual cusps are connected by a blunt, transverse ridge which divides the poorly developed mesiodistal occlusal fissure into mesial and distal fossae. The mesial fossa is generally smaller than the distal fossa. A canine groove often extends from the mesial fossa over the mesial marginal ridge on to the mesiolingual surface of the crown. Viewed *buccally* (B), the crown is seen to be nearly symmetrical though the mesial profile is more curved than the distal. The buccal surface is markedly convex in all planes. From the *lingual* aspect (C), the entire buccal profile and the occlusal surface are visible. Thus, the mandibular first premolar differs from other premolars in that the occlusal plane does not lie perpendicular to the long axis of the tooth. The tilt of the occlusal plane can also be appreciated from the *mesial* (D) and *distal* (E) aspects. Note also the pronounced convexity of the buccal surface and the position of the apex of the buccal cusp over the crown.

The cervical line follows an almost level course around the tooth. The root is single, conical and oval to nearly round in cross section. The root is grooved longitudinally both mesially and distally, the mesial groove being the more prominent.

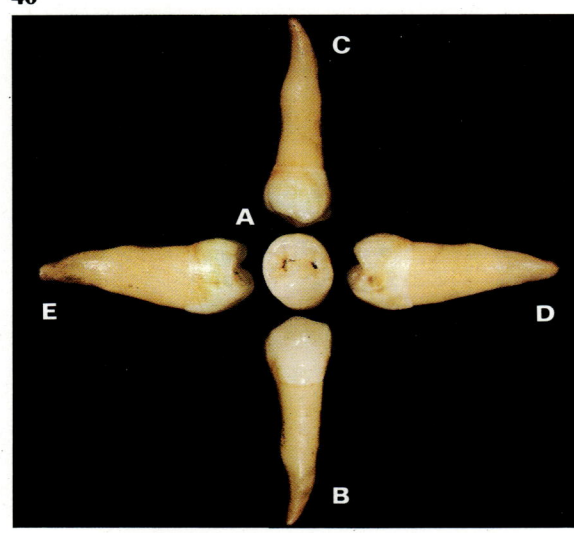

40 The mandibular second premolar differs from the mandibular first premolar in the following respects. Its crown is generally larger. The lingual cusp is better developed although it is not quite as large as its buccal cusp which appears correspondingly reduced in size. From the *occlusal* aspect (A), its outline appears round or square, the mesial and distal profiles being straight and parallel. The mesiodistal occlusal fissure between the cusps is well-defined. However, like the first premolar, the fissure ends in mesial and distal fossae, the distal fossa being generally larger than the mesial fossa. Unlike the first premolar, the apices of the cusps are not usually joined by a transverse ridge. Accessory cusplets are frequent on both buccal and lingual cusps. Usually, the lingual cusp is subdivided into mesiolingual and distolingual cusps, the mesiolingual cusp being wider and higher than the distolingual cusp. The groove separating the mesiolingual and distolingual cusps lies opposite the tip of the buccal cusp. From the *buccal* aspect (B), the crown of the second premolar is symmetrical. From this view, the buccal cusp generally appears shorter and more rounded than that of the mandibular first premolar. *Lingually* (C), little if any of the occlusal surface and the buccal profile is visible. From the *mesial* (D) and *distal* (E) aspects, note that the occlusal surface is horizontal to the long axis of the tooth. The crown appears wider buccolingually than that of the first premolar and the buccal cusp does not incline so far over the root. Note the relative size of the lingual cusp(s) from this view.

The cervical margin follows an almost level course around the tooth. The root is single, conical and nearly round in cross-section.

The molars

Molars present the largest occlusal surfaces of all teeth. They have three to five major cusps (though the maxillary first deciduous molar has only two). Molars are the only teeth which have more than one buccal cusp. Generally, the lower molars have two roots, the upper, three. The permanent molars do not have deciduous predecessors.

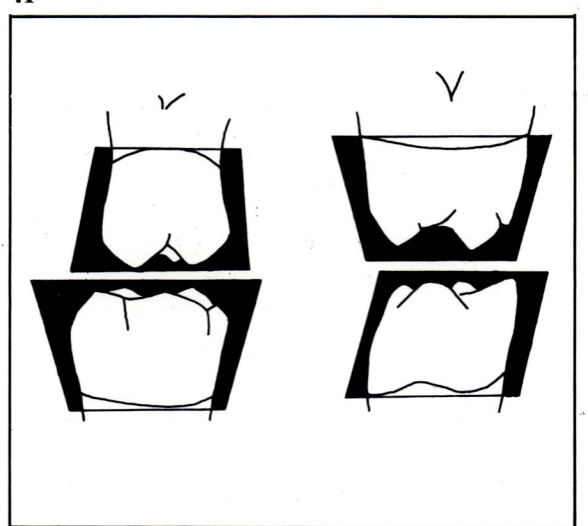

41 Schematic drawings of molar crown form illustrating the relationship between anatomic and geometric form. Like the premolars, the maxillary molars are roughly trapezoidal when viewed mesially and distally, the mandibular molars rhomboidal. Viewed buccally or lingually, the molars are trapezoidal.

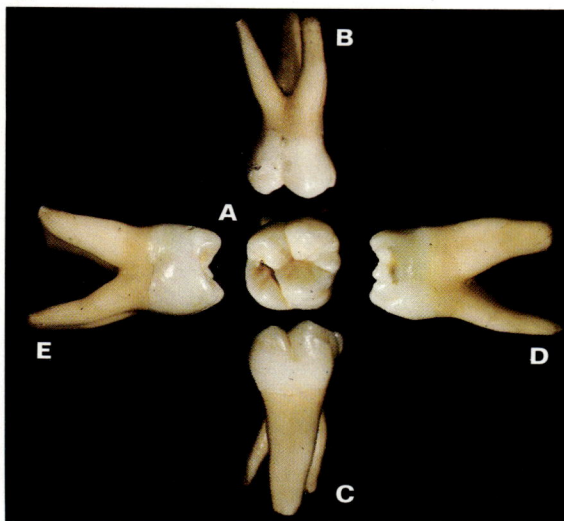

42 Maxillary first permanent molar. The first permanent molar is usually the largest molar in each quadrant. Viewed *occlusally* (A), the crown is rhombic in outline. The mesiopalatal and distobuccal angles are obtuse. The longest diameter of the crown runs from the mesiobuccal to the distopalatal corners. It has four major cusps separated by an irregular H-shaped occlusal fissure. The occlusal table may be divided into two distinct components, the trigon and talon, by an oblique ridge which passes diagonally across the occlusal table from the mesiopalatal cusp to the distobuccal cusp. The trigon bears the mesiobuccal, mesiopalatal and distobuccal cusps, and the talon bears the distopalatal cusp. The trigon is characteristically triangular in shape, the apex of the triangle being directed palatally. The mesiopalatal cusp is the largest, the buccal cusps being smaller and of approximately equal size. The buccal cusps form the base of the trigon. The mesial marginal ridge forms the mesial side of the trigon and its distal side is formed by the oblique ridge. An accessory cusplet of variable size may be seen on the palatal surface of the mesiopalatal cusp. This cusplet is termed the tubercle of Carabelli and is found on about 60 per cent of maxillary first permanent molars. The trigon has a central fossa from which a fissure extends mesially to terminate in a mesial pit before the mesial marginal ridge. Another fissure extends buccally from the central fossa to pass on to the buccal surface of the crown between the two buccal cusps. The distopalatal cusp of the talon is generally the smallest cusp of the tooth and is separated from the mesiopalatal cusp by a distopalatal fissure which curves distally to end in a distal pit before the distal marginal ridge. The oblique ridge may be crossed by a shallow fissure which thus connects the central fossa of the trigon with the distopalatal fissure and distal pit of the talon, completing the H-shaped fissure pattern. That the tips of the palatal cusps are situated nearer the mid-mesiodistal diameter of the crown than those of the buccal cusps is characteristic of maxillary molars. From the *buccal* aspect (B), the buccal cusps are seen to be approximately equal in height, though the mesiobuccal cusp is wider than the distobuccal cusp. The buccal surface is convex in its cervical third but relatively flat in its middle and occlusal thirds. Note the buccal groove extending from the occlusal table passing between the cusps to end about halfway up the buccal surface. The mesial profile is convex in its occlusal and middle thirds but flat, or even concave, in the cervical third. The distal profile on the other hand is convex in all regions. Viewed *palatally* (C), the disproportion in size between the mesiopalatal and distopalatal cusps is most evident. The mesiopalatal cusp is blunt and occupies approximately three-fifths of the mesiodistal width of the palatal surface. The palatal surface is more or less uniformly convex in all regions. A palatal groove extends from the distal pit on the occlusal surface between the palatal cusps to terminate approximately halfway up the palatal surface. From the *mesial* (D) and *distal* (E) aspects, the maximum buccopalatal dimension is at the cervical margin from which the buccal and palatal profiles converge occlusally. The mesial marginal ridge is more prominent than the distal ridge. The mesial marginal ridge may have a number of distinct tubercles. Such tubercles are rare on the distal marginal ridge.

The cervical line follows a fairly even contour around the tooth. There are three roots, two buccal and one palatal, which arise from a common root stalk. The palatal root is the longest and strongest and is circular in cross-section. The buccal roots are more slender and are flattened mesiodistally; the mesiobuccal root is usually the larger and wider of the two. At the root stalk, the palatal root is more commonly related to the distobuccal root than to the mesiobuccal root.

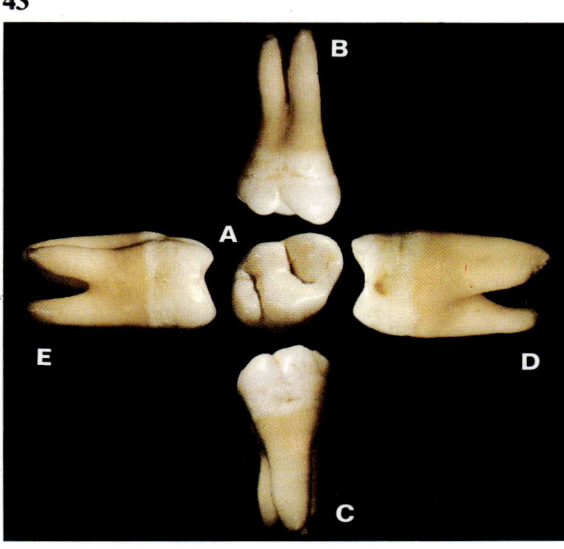

43 The maxillary second permanent molar closely resembles the maxillary first permanent molar but shows some reduction in size and slightly different cusp relationships. *Occlusally* (A), the rhomboid form is more pronounced than the first molar and the oblique ridge is smaller. The talon (distopalatal fissure cusp) is considerably reduced. The occlusal fissure pattern is similar to the first molar but is more variable and supplemental grooves are more numerous. Two features of the *buccal* surface (B) differentiate the second molar, namely the smaller size of both the crown and the distobuccal cusp. *Palatally* (C), note the reduction in size of the distopalatal cusp. A tubercle of Carabelli is not usually found on the mesiopalatal cusp. The *mesial* (D) and *distal* (E) surfaces differ little from those of the first molar save that the tubercles on the mesial marginal ridge are less numerous and less pronounced.

Like the first molar, the second molar has three roots, two buccal and one palatal. However, they are shorter and less divergent than those of the first molar and may be partly fused. The apex of the mesiobuccal root is generally in line with the centre of the crown, unlike that of the first molar which generally lies in line with the tip of the mesiobuccal cusp.

Variations in morphology of the maxillary second permanent molar are quite common. Total reduction of the distopalatal cusp is frequent so that only the trigon remains. Less frequently, the crown may appear compressed because of fusion of the mesiopalatal and distobuccal cusps resulting in an oval crown possessing three cusps in a straight line.

Maxillary third permanent molar. This tooth being the most variable in the dentition, is not illustrated. Its morphology may range from that characteristic of the adjacent maxillary permanent molars to a rounded triangular crown shape with a deep central fossa from which numerous, irregular fissures radiate outwards. Most commonly, the crown is triangular in shape having the three cusps of the trigon but no talon. The roots are often fused and irregular in form.

The mandibular molars differ from the maxillary molars in the following respects:
1 the mandibular molars have two roots, one mesial and one distal;
2 they are considered to be derived from a five-cusped form;
3 the crowns of the lower molars are oblong, being broader mesiodistally than buccolingually;
4 the fissure pattern is cross-shaped;
5 the lingual cusps are of more equal size;
6 the tips of the buccal cusps are shifted lingually so that from the occlusal view the whole of the buccal surface is visible.

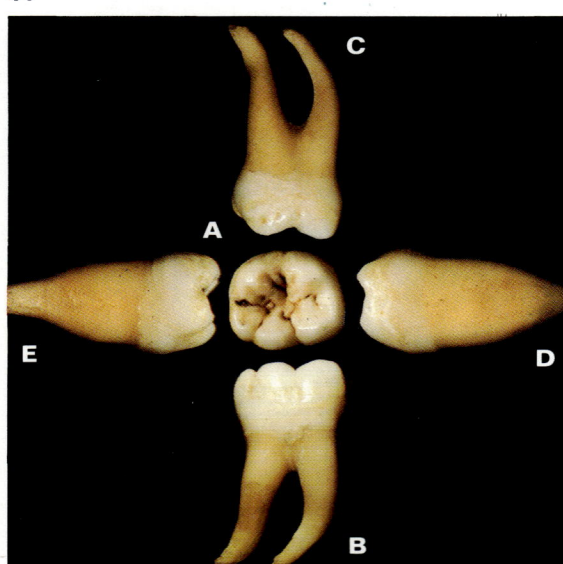

44

44 Mandibular first permanent molar. Viewed *occlusally* (A), the crown of this tooth is somewhat pentagonal in outline. It is broader mesiodistally than buccolingually. The occlusal surface is divided into buccal and lingual parts by a mesiodistal occlusal fissure which arises from a deep central fossa. The buccal side of the occlusal table has three distinct cusps, mesiobuccal, distobuccal and distal. Each cusp is separated by a groove which joins the mesiodistal fissure. On the lingual side are two cusps, mesiolingual and distolingual. The fissure separating the lingual cusps joins the mesiodistal fissure in the region of the central fossa. The lingual cusps tend to be the largest and are more pointed, though they are not disproportionately larger than the mesiobuccal and distobuccal cusps. The tips of the buccal cusps are displaced lingually, are rounded and are lower than the lingual cusps. The smallest cusp is the distal cusp which is displaced slightly towards the buccal surface. In 90 per cent of cases, the mesiolingual cusp is joined to the distobuccal cusp across the floor of the central fossa. This feature and the five cusped pattern is termed the *Dryopithecus* pattern. This 'primitive' pattern is characteristic of all the lower molars of the anthropoid apes and their early ancestors, the Dryopithecines. From the *buccal* aspect (B), note the three cusps, the distal cusp being the smallest. The fissure separating the mesiobuccal and distobuccal cusps arises from the central fossa on the occlusal surface and terminates halfway up the buccal surface in a buccal pit. The buccal surface appears markedly convex especially at the cervical third of the crown. This convexity is associated with the characteristic lingual inclination of the buccal cusps. From the *lingual* aspect (C), note that although the two lingual cusps are nearly equal in size, the mesiolingual cusp is slightly larger. The fissure between the lingual cusps arises from the central fossa on the occlusal surface but does not extend a significant way down the lingual surface. The lingual surface is convex in its occlusal and middle thirds but is flat or concave cervically. From the lingual aspect, part of the buccal profiles and proximal surfaces may be seen. Viewed *mesially* (D), the mesial marginal ridge joining the mesiobuccal and mesiolingual cusps is V-shaped, being notched at its midpoint. The mesial surface is flat or concave cervically and convex in its middle and occlusal thirds. From the *distal* aspect (E), the distal marginal ridge joining the distal and distolingual cusps also appears V-shaped. The cervical third of the distal surface is relatively flat, the middle and occlusal thirds being highly convex. Thus, the distal surface is more convex than the mesial surface due to the distal cusp. From the proximal views, note the highly convex slope of the buccal surface compared to the lingual surface.

The cervical margin follows a uniform contour around the tooth. The two roots, one mesial and one distal, arise from a common root stalk. They are both markedly flattened mesiodistally and the mesial root is usually deeply grooved. Both roots curve distally.

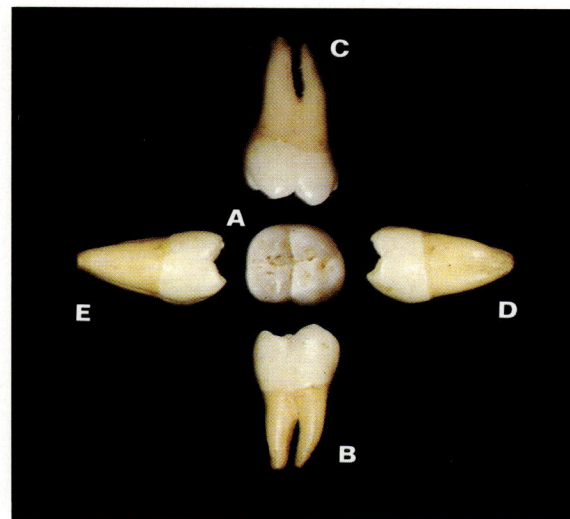

45 Mandibular second permanent molar. Viewed *occlusally* (A), the crown has a regular, rectangular shape. Thus, unlike the mandibular first permanent molar, the buccal profile is nearly equal in length to the lingual profile. There are four cusps, the mesiobuccal and mesiolingual cusps being slightly larger than the distobuccal and distolingual cusps. The cusps are separated by a cross-shaped occlusal fissure pattern, though it may be complicated by numerous supplemental grooves. From the *buccal* aspect (B), the crown appears smaller than that of the first molar. A fissure extends between the buccal cusps from the occlusal surface and terminates approximately halfway up the buccal surface. Like the mandibular first molar, the buccal surface is highly convex. *Lingually* (C), the buccal profiles and proximal surfaces are not visible and the crown is noticeably shorter occlusocervically than the first molar. The *mesial* (D) and *distal* (E) aspects of the second molar resemble those of the first molar though, because there is no distal cusp, the proximal surfaces are more equal in terms of their convexity. Note that the mesial and distal marginal ridges do not converge and are not so markedly notched at their midpoint.

The mesial and distal roots are flattened mesiodistally and are smaller and less divergent than those of the first molar. Indeed, they may be partly fused. The mesial root is not as broad as that of the first molar, and the distal inclination of the roots is usually more marked.

Mandibular third permanent molar. The morphology of this tooth is variable, though not as variable as that of the maxillary third permanent molar. The crown is usually the smallest of the mandibular molars, but occasionally it may be as large as the mandibular first molar. The crown usually has four or five cusps. In shape, it is normally a rounded rectangle or is circular. Its occlusal fissure pattern is generally very irregular. As a rule, the roots are greatly reduced in size and are fused. They show a marked distal inclination.

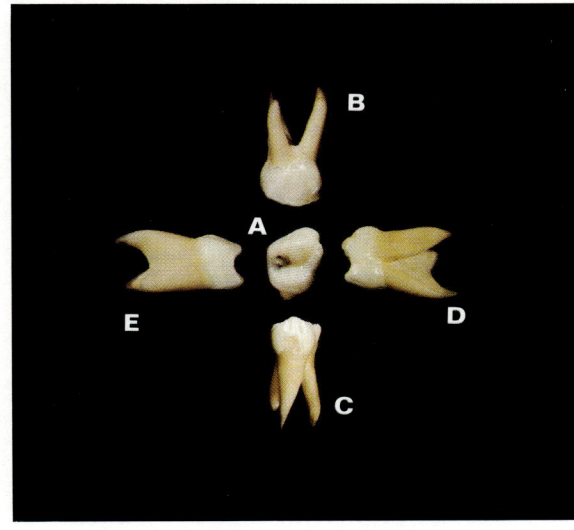

46 Maxillary first deciduous molar. This tooth is the most atypical of all molars, deciduous or permanent. In form, it appears to be intermediate between a premolar and a molar. It is the smallest molar. Viewed *occlusally* (A), the crown is an irregular quadrilateral with the buccal and palatal surfaces lying parallel to one another. However, the mesiobuccal corner is extended to produce a prominent bulge, the molar tubercle. The mesial surface thus slopes distally as it passes towards the palatal surface and the mesiopalatal angle is markedly obtuse. The tooth is generally bicuspid. The buccal and palatal cusps are separated by a mesiodistally-running occlusal fissure. The buccal cusp is the most pronounced cusp. A shallow buccal fissure may extend from the central mesiodistal fissure to divide the buccal cusp into two, the mesial part being the larger. The lingual cusp also may be subdivided into two. The tips of the cusps converge towards the midline so reducing the occlusal surface of the tooth. From the *buccal* aspect (B), the crown appears squat, its height being less than its width. On the mesial side lies the buccal cingulum which extends to the molar tubercle. From the *palatal* aspect (C), note that the palatal surface is shorter mesiodistally than the buccal surface whose profile can be seen from this view. The views from the *mesial* (D) and *distal* (E) aspects show the cervical bulbosity of the buccal and palatal surfaces. Note the prominent molar tubercle mesially. Marginal ridges link the buccal and palatal cusps. No fissure crosses the marginal ridges.

The tooth has three roots, two buccal and one palatal, which arise from a common root stalk. The mesiobuccal root is flattened mesiodistally. The distobuccal root is smaller and more circular. The palatal root is the largest and is round in cross-section. The distobuccal and palatal roots may be partly fused.

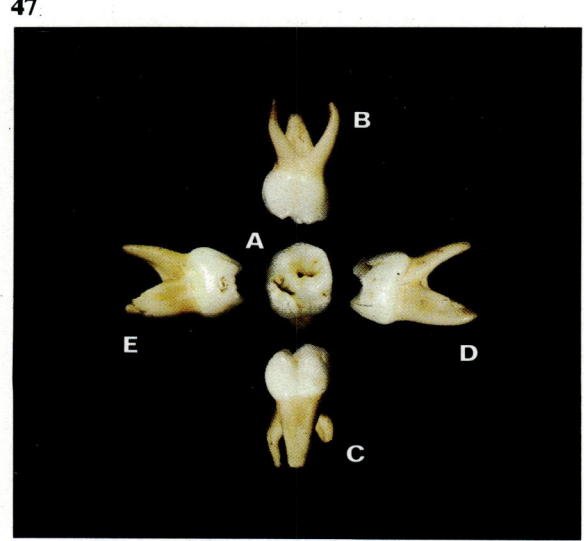

47 Maxillary second deciduous molar. This tooth closely resembles the maxillary first permanent molar (see figure 42), though its size, whiteness, widely diverging roots and low buccal cingulum ought to distinguish it. A tubercle of Carabelli on the mesiopalatal cusp is often well developed.

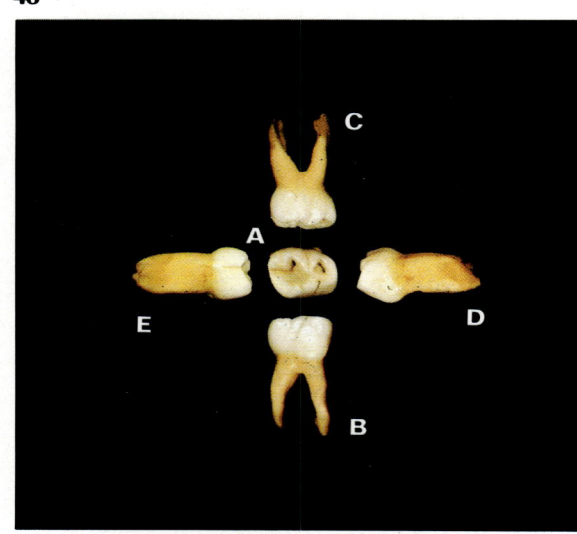

48 Mandibular first deciduous molar. Unlike the maxillary first deciduous molar, this tooth is molariform but has a number of unique features. From the *occlusal* aspect (A), the crown appears elongated mesiodistally and is an irregular quadrilateral, the buccal and lingual surfaces being parallel. Note that the mesiobuccal corner is extended, forming a molar tubercle, and that the mesial surface slopes distally as it passes lingually. The mesiolingual angle is markedly obtuse. The occlusal table can be divided into buccal and lingual parts by a mesiodistal fissure. The buccal part consists of two cusps, the mesiobuccal cusp being larger than the distobuccal cusp. The lingual part of the tooth is narrower than the buccal part and has two cusps separated by a lingual fissure, the mesiolingual cusp being larger than the distolingual cusp. The buccal cusps are larger than the lingual cusps. A transverse ridge may connect the mesial cusps, dividing the mesiodistal fissure into a distal fissure and a mesial pit. Often a distal pit may be found just mesial to the distal marginal ridge. A supplemental groove from the mesial pit may extend over the mesial marginal ridge. From the *buccal* aspect (B), the mesiobuccal cusp occupies at least two-thirds of the crown area and projects higher occlusally than the distobuccal cusp. The distal slopes of the buccal cusps are longer than the mesial. The profile of the mesial surface appears flat, that of the distal surface convex. Note the molar tubercle on the mesial corner of the buccal surface. From the *lingual* aspect (C), note the conical shape of the cusps. The distolingual cusp appears only as a bulging protuberance on the distal margin. *Mesially* (D) and *distally* (E), the buccal and lingual aspects are seen to converge towards the midline of the crown. The mesial marginal ridge is more prominent than the distal marginal ridge. Note the bulge associated with the buccal cingulum near the cervical margin of the mesiobuccal cusp.

The mandibular first deciduous molar has two divergent roots, mesial and distal, which are flattened mesiodistally. The mesial root is often grooved.

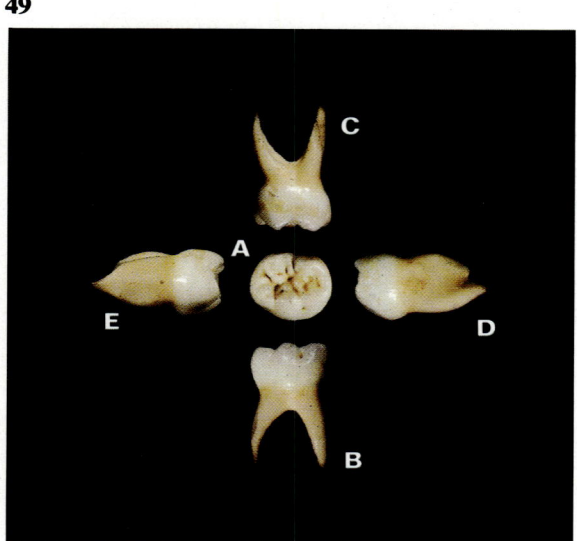

49 Mandibular second deciduous molar. This tooth is almost a model of the mandibular first permanent molar (see figure 44) though it is smaller, narrower, whiter and has widely diverging roots. Other distinguishing features are: the cingulum on the mesiobuccal corner of the crown, the greater convexity of the mesial and distal surfaces, the more extensive central fossa on the occlusal surface. The mesiolingual and distobuccal cusps are not usually joined to give the *Dryopithecus* pattern.

Average dimensions of permanent teeth

Tooth	Crown height	Length of root	Mesiodistal crown diameter	Labiolingual crown diameter
Maxillary	*mm*	*mm*	*mm*	*mm*
1	10.5	13.0	8.5	7.0
2	9.0	13.0	6.5	6.0
3	10.0	17.0	7.5	8.0
4	8.5	14.5	7.0	9.0
5	8.5	14.0	7.0	9.0
6	7.5	12.5	10.5	11.0
7	7.0	11.5	9.5	11.0
8	6.5	11.0	8.5	10.0
Mandibular				
1	9.0	12.5	5.0	6.0
2	9.5	14.0	5.5	6.5
3	11.0	15.5	7.0	7.5
4	8.5	14.0	7.0	7.5
5	8.0	14.5	7.0	8.0
6	7.5	14.0	11.0	10.0
7	7.0	12.0	10.5	10.0
8	7.0	11.0	10.0	9.5

Average dimensions of deciduous teeth

Tooth	Crown height	Length of root	Mediodistal crown diameter	Labiolingual crown diameter
Maxillary	*mm*	*mm*	*mm*	*mm*
A	6.0	10.0	6.5	5.0
B	5.6	10.2	5.2	4.0
C	6.5	13.0	6.8	7.0
D	5.1	10.0	7.1	8.5
E	5.7	11.7	8.4	10.0
Mandibular				
A	5.0	9.0	4.0	4.0
B	5.2	9.8	4.5	4.0
C	6.0	11.2	5.5	4.9
D	6.0	9.8	7.7	7.0
E	5.5	12.5	9.7	8.7

Pulp morphology

The pulp cavity consists of a pulp chamber in the crown from which canal(s) pass down into the root(s). As a general rule, the pulp cavities follow the contours of the teeth. Each root canal opens by a foramen or foramina at the apex of the root.

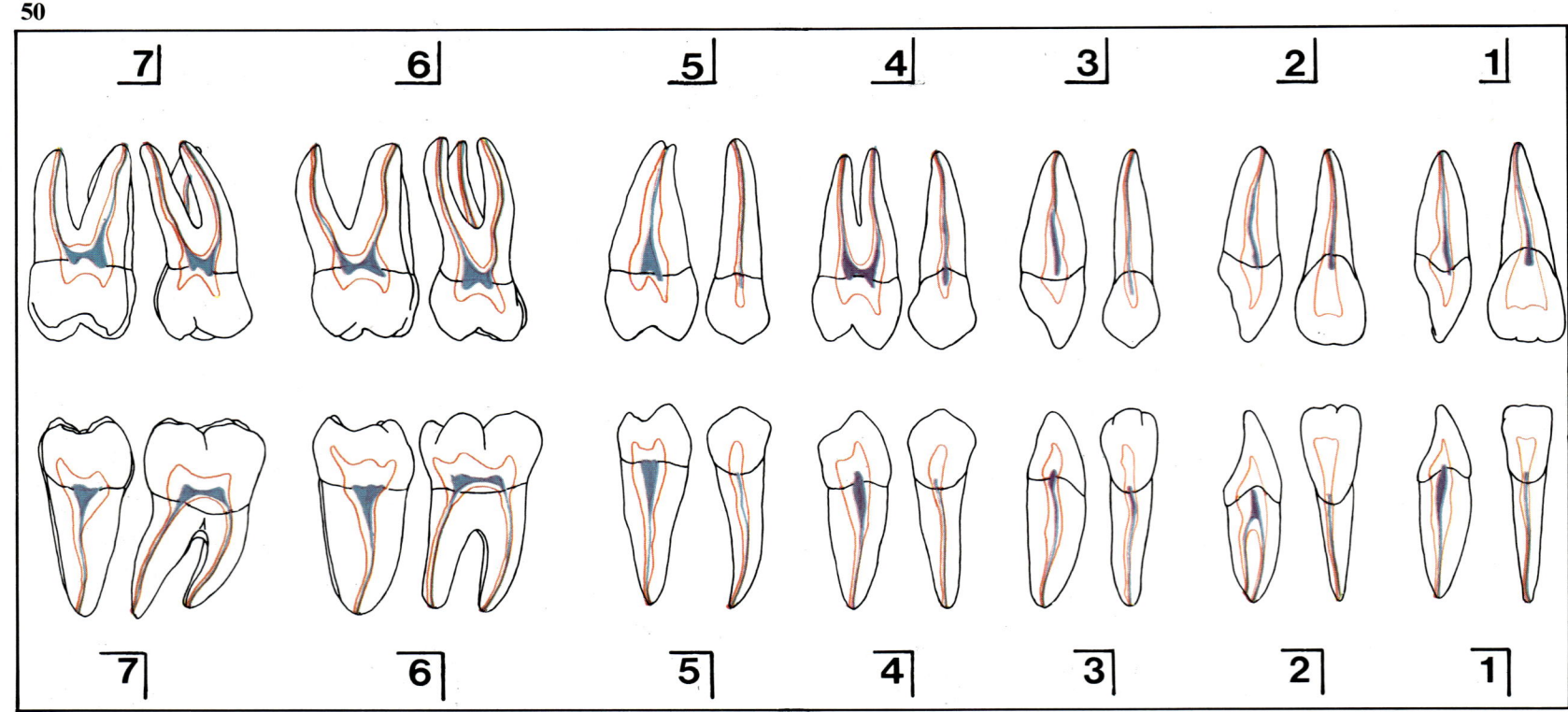

50 Pulp morphology in teeth of the permanent dentition. The teeth are identified numerically according to the Zsigmond system. The red outline shows the pulp cavity in the young tooth, the blue outline, the pulp in the old tooth. Buccal and distal views of the teeth are shown. The descriptions of the pulp cavities are not always borne out in detail in individual teeth, there being much variation. As a general rule, in anterior teeth the pulp chambers merge imperceptibly into the root canals. In the cheek teeth, the pulp chambers and root canals are morphologically distinct. Pulp horns or cornua extend from the pulp chambers to the mesial and distal angles of the incisor teeth and towards the cusps of cheek teeth. Each root generally contains one root canal. However, the mandibular molars have two root canals in their mesial roots. Where roots are fused, the tooth still maintains the usual number of root canals. The size of the pulp cavity decreases significantly with age. When the tooth first erupts into the oral cavity, the apical foramen is wide. However, with subsequent development of the root the apical foramen narrows.

The morphology of the pulp cavities of deciduous teeth is extremely variable, especially once root resorption has begun. The pulp cavities of deciduous teeth are proportionately larger than those of permanent teeth, and pulp horns may extend some way into the cusps.

The alignment and occlusion of the permanent teeth

Tooth alignment may be defined as the arrangement of the teeth within the dental arches, occlusion as the relationship of the dental arches when tooth contact is made.

Traditionally, textbooks describe a standard set of tooth relationships which is called 'normal'. Normal is a term which is generally used to describe states or situations which are the ordinary or most frequent. Alternatively, normal may define an authoritative standard or ideal which, in medical terms, is the healthy state. In these terms, malocclusions could be regarded as normal for they are more commonly found in the population than 'normal occlusion', they rarely predispose to dental disease and, in most cases, are not associated with masticatory dysfunction. Our knowledge of the relationship between the structure and function of the dental arches during mastication is not yet sufficient to provide an authoritative standard for tooth relationships, in structural terms the ideal occlusion being a rather subjective concept. If there is an ideal occlusion, at present it can only be defined in broad functional terms. We believe that the characteristics of an ideal occlusion are those:

1 where the teeth are aligned such that the masticatory loads are within physiological range and act through the long axes of as many teeth in the arch as possible;
2 where lateral jaw movements occur without undue mechanical interference;
3 where, in the rest position of the jaw, the gap between teeth, the freeway space, is adequate for the individual concerned;
4 where the tooth alignment is aesthetically pleasing to their possessor.

Despite these criticisms, the traditional descriptions of 'normal' tooth relationships provide a convenient *type* for the classification of malocclusions in clinical situations. In order to avoid the difficulties of defining normality with respect to tooth relationships, we have chosen to use the terms anatomical alignment and anatomical occlusion instead of normal alignment and normal occlusion.

The anatomical alignment of teeth

51 The dental arches. The size and shape of the arches vary considerably between individuals, though generally they take the form of catenary curves. The dental arches may be divided into three segments. A curved line in the coronal plane (A) describes the anterior segment which extends across the midline from canine to canine. A straight line describes the middle segments (B) which extend from the distal edge of the canines to the mesiobuccal cusps of the first molars. The posterior segments (C) extend from the mesiobuccal cusps of the first molars backwards. Both the middle and posterior segments lie in the sagittal plane, the posterior segments being more nearly parallel to this plane than the middle segments.

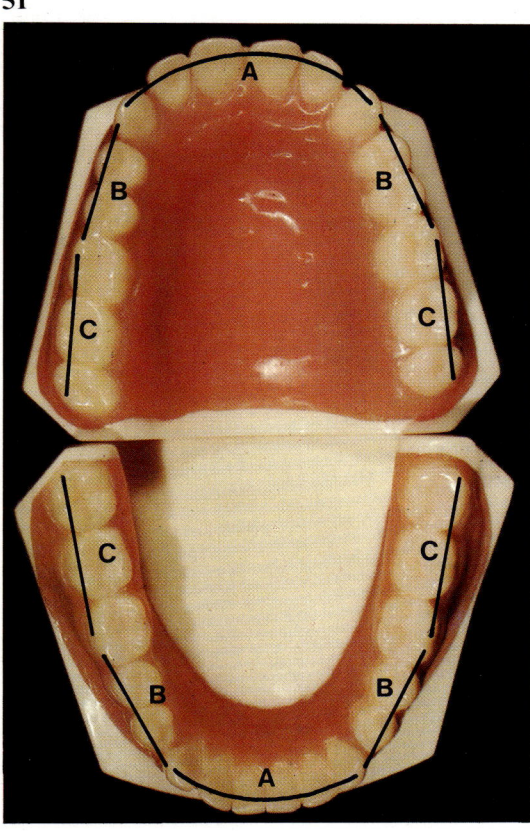

52 The neutral zone. The spatial configuration of the arches is dependent upon an interaction between the eruptive movements carrying the teeth into their functional positions and, once erupted, the forces brought to bear upon each tooth. The term neutral zone is used to describe that space in which there is an equilibrium of forces such that the teeth attain a position of relative stability. Imbalance in this system, such as that produced by abnormal tongue thrusting behaviour during swallowing, can result in malalignment of the teeth. The diagram shows the configuration of the neutral zone (the stippled area) in the *incisor region* (A) and the *molar region* (B). The tongue is labelled 1, the lips 2, and the cheek 3.

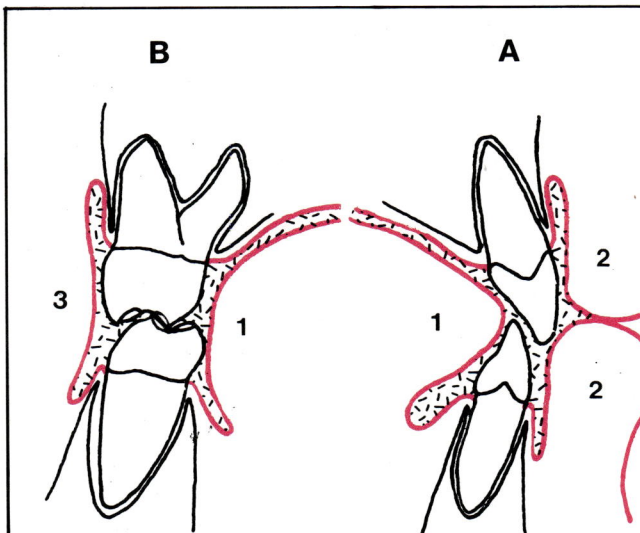

The angulation or axial positioning of individual teeth within the alveolus relative to perpendiculars dropped from a hypothetically flat occlusal plane

In the following series of diagrams, the angles quoted are average figures though variation is considerable. The teeth are not drawn to scale and the numerical dental shorthand is used to identify the tooth (M = mesial).

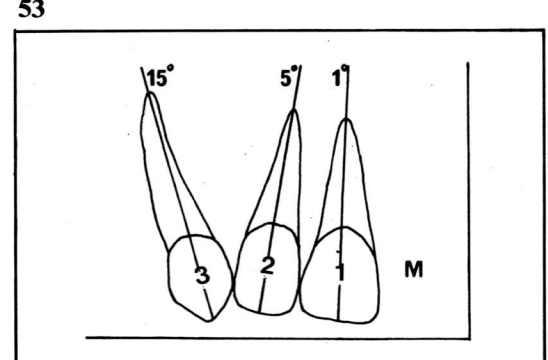

53 Alignment of the maxillary incisors and canine viewed buccally.

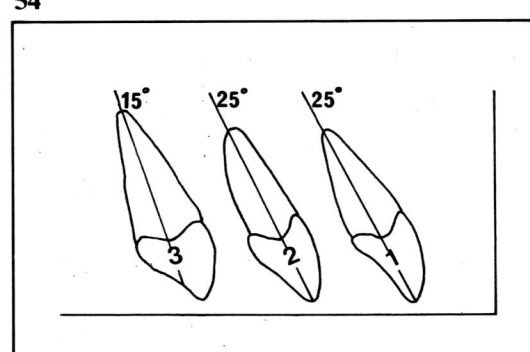

54 Alignment of the maxillary incisors and canine viewed distally.

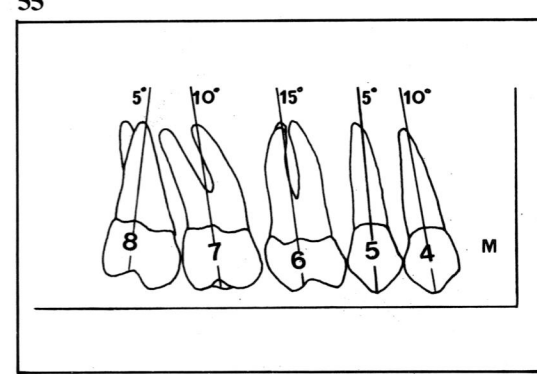

55 Alignment of the maxillary premolars and molars viewed buccally.

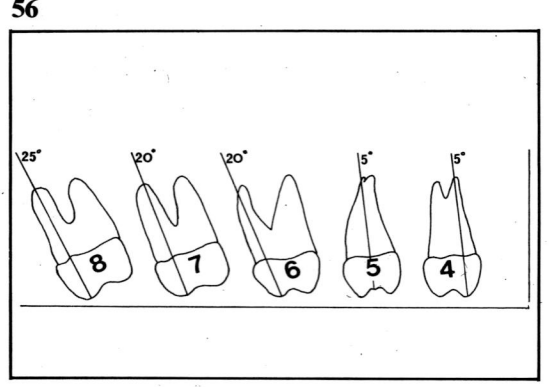

56 Alignment of the maxillary premolars and molars viewed distally.

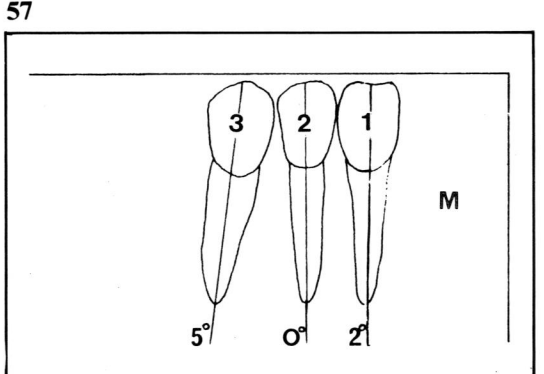

57 Alignment of the mandibular incisors and canine viewed buccally.

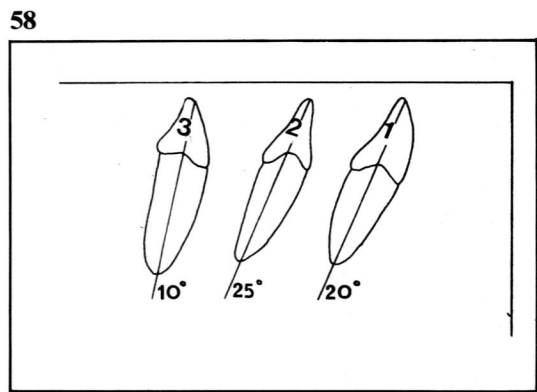

58 Alignment of the mandibular incisors and canine viewed distally.

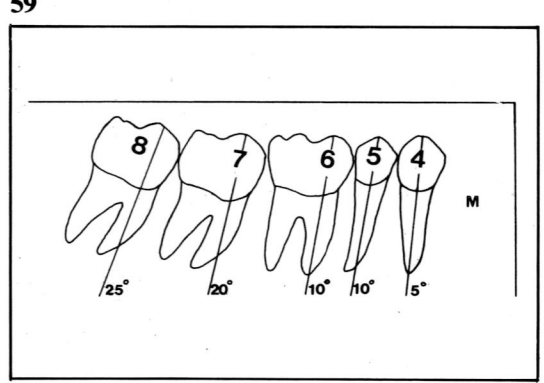

59 Alignment of the mandibular premolars and molars viewed buccally.

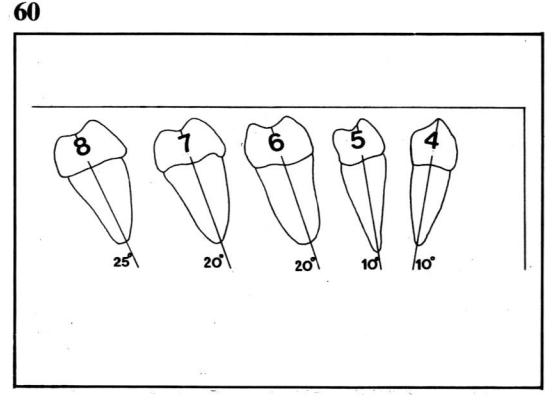

60 Alignment of the mandibular premolars and molars viewed distally.

The curvatures of the teeth and arches

61 The curvatures of the teeth and their functional significance. Figures **53** to **60** may give the impression that the axes of the teeth are straight and run perpendicular to a horizontal, flat, occlusal plane. However, as shown in these dissected specimens of the jaws, neither the axes of the teeth nor the occlusal planes are straight but are curved in all directions. The curved axes of the teeth have a tendency to parallelism and are inclined mesially. It is often thought, mistakenly so, that the forces of mastication are at right angles to the occlusal surfaces of the teeth. If this were so and if the occlusal plane and axes of the teeth were not curved, the arches might not be stable and the masticatory loads might be at an unfavourable angle to the teeth. It has been suggested that during mastication, the loads strike the teeth such that the components of force tend to produce drifting of the teeth mesially and this may be related to the mesial inclination of the curved axes of the teeth.

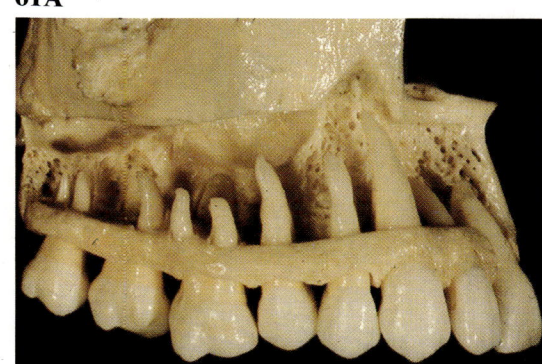

61A

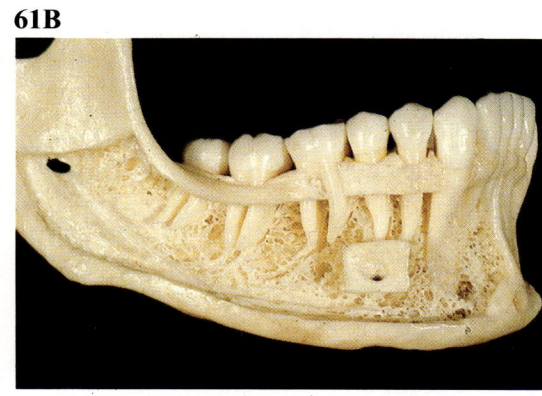

61B

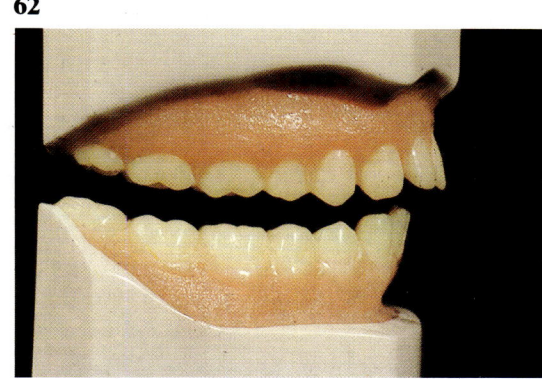

62

62 Curvatures of the occlusal plane – the curve of Spee. The teeth align themselves such that the occlusal plane is not flat but describes a relatively linear curve in the anteroposterior direction, the curve of Spee. The mandibular curve of Spee is concave, the maxillary curve, convex. An appreciation of the contribution of each tooth to the curve of Spee may be gained from analysis of the alignment of the long axes of the teeth (figures **55** and **59**). It has been suggested that the curves of Spee help the achievement of occlusal balance during mastication by encouraging simultaneous contact in more than one area of the dental arches.

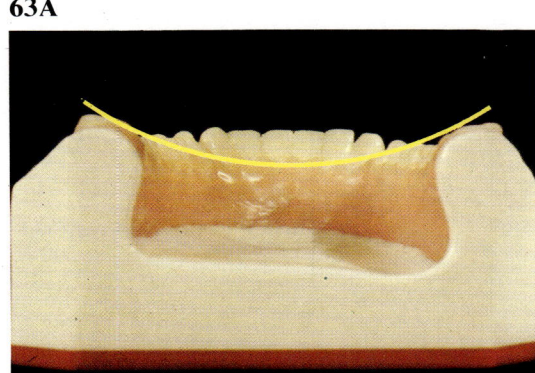

63A

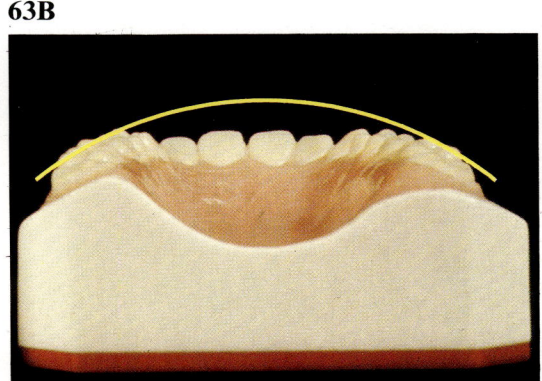

63B

63 Curvatures of the occlusal plane – the curves of Wilson. The occlusal curves of Wilson are aligned in the transverse plane. Analysis of the alignment of the long axes of the posterior teeth (figures **56** and **60**) shows that the curves of Wilson are such that the occlusal surfaces of the mandibular molars are directed lingually, while those of the maxillary molars are directed buccally. The curves of Spee and Wilson were once thought to be related 3-dimensionally, the occlusal surfaces of the teeth being aligned on the curved surface of a segment of a sphere having a radius of about 10cm. However, attempts to demonstrate and then measure the spherical curves (of Monson) have been unsuccessful.

The anatomical occlusion of teeth

The relationships of the jaws in function are so variable that our understanding of the functional articulation of teeth remains poor. To simplify analysis, several occlusal positions have been strictly defined. These positions may be classified into those which are symmetric and those which are asymmetric. This corresponds with the classification of mandibular movements into symmetric and asymmetric movements (see pages 44–45). The symmetric occlusal positions include centric occlusion and bilaterally protrusive position. The asymmetric occlusal positions are those associated with lateral gliding movements.

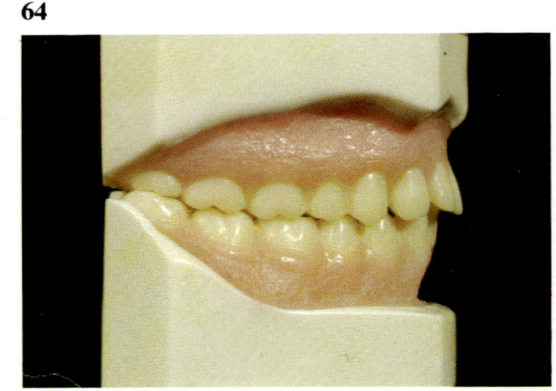

64 Lateral view of the arrangement of teeth in anatomical centric occlusal position. Centric position has been defined as the terminal position of physiological jaw movements. It is the relationship between the two arches when the teeth are brought into contact with the mandibular condyles centrally positioned at rest in the glenoid fossae. According to Angle, the key to the intercuspal relationships between the teeth in centric position is to be found in the relative positions of the maxillary and mandibular first permanent molars. In the 'normal' or anatomical condition, each arch is bilaterally symmetrical. Since the anterior maxillary segment is slightly larger than the corresponding mandibular segment, each maxillary tooth will contact its corresponding mandibular antagonist and its distal neighbour. Thus, the maxillary first permanent molar will contact the distal part of the mandibular first permanent molar and the mesial part of the mandibular second permanent molar.

65 The relationships between maxillary and mandibular permanent teeth in anatomical centric occlusal position. The teeth are identified according to the Zsigmond numerical system (see page 18).

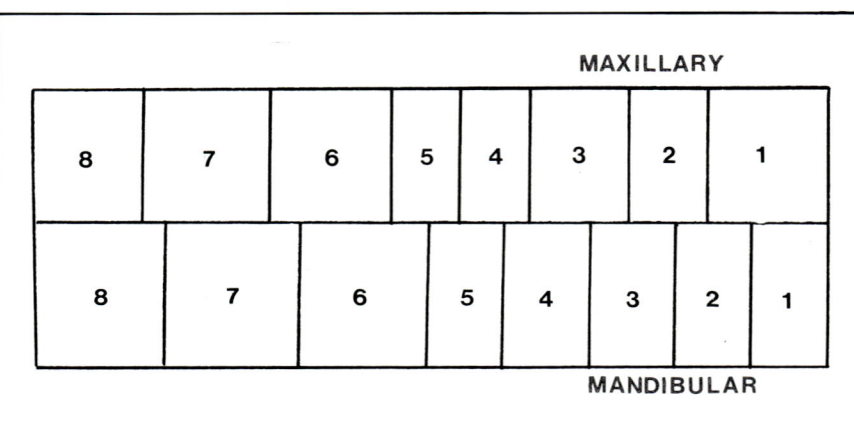

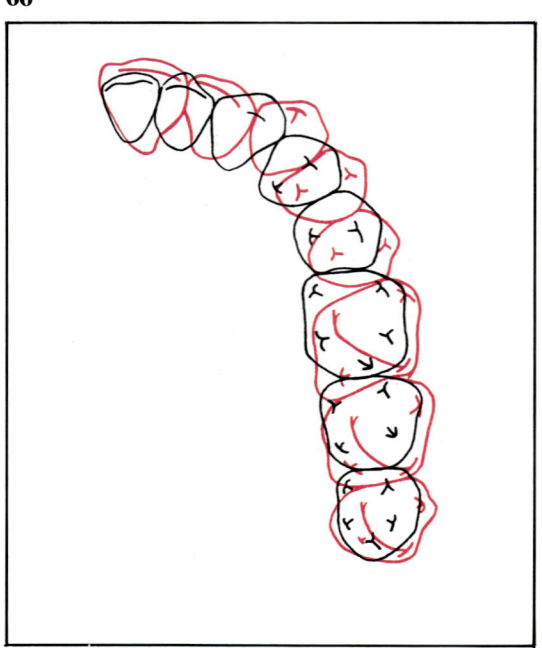

66 The relationships between the maxillary and mandibular permanent teeth in anatomical centric occlusion shown by the superimposition of the occlusal surfaces of the teeth in the maxillary arch (red) on those of the mandibular arch (black). This diagram not only illustrates the general anteroposterior relationships of the maxillary teeth and their antagonists, but also the buccolingual relationships of the arches. Since the maxillary arch is a little larger and broader than the mandibular arch, there is a slight overlap of the mandibular arch by the maxillary arch such that the buccal cusps of the maxillary teeth extend a few millimetres beyond the buccal occlusal edge of the mandibular teeth. This overlap is termed overjet.

67 The buccolingual incisor relationships in anatomical centric occlusion. The maxillary incisors overlap the mandibular incisors in two planes. The overlap in the horizontal plane, overjet, is approximately 1 to 2mm. The vertical overlap, peculiar to the incisors and canines, is termed overbite. The overbite in anatomical centric occlusion is such that the palatal surfaces of the maxillary incisors overlap the incisal third of the labial surfaces of the mandibular incisors.

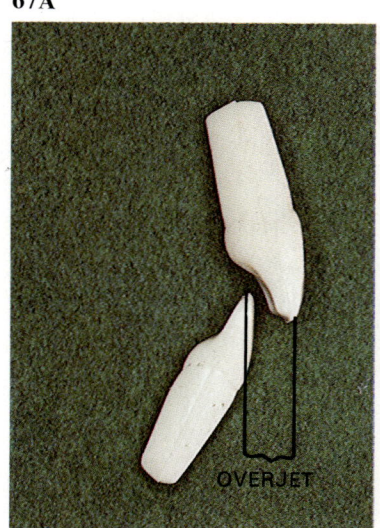
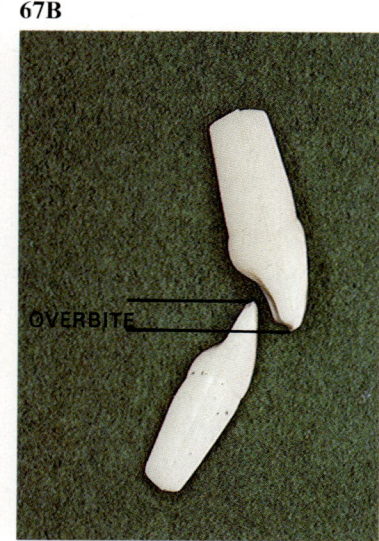

68 The occlusal surfaces of the permanent dentition marked to show the positions of hard contact in anatomical centric occlusion (centric stops). The black marks represent the intercuspal contact positions. While the major markings register on the occlusal surfaces of the posterior teeth, note the labioincisal and palatoincisal markings of the mandibular and maxillary incisors. As befits the anatomical overjet relationships, the tips of the maxillary buccal cusps and the mandibular lingual cusps remain relatively unmarked. Similar marks can be made *in vivo* by interposing articulating paper between the teeth and then instructing the patient to go into centric position.

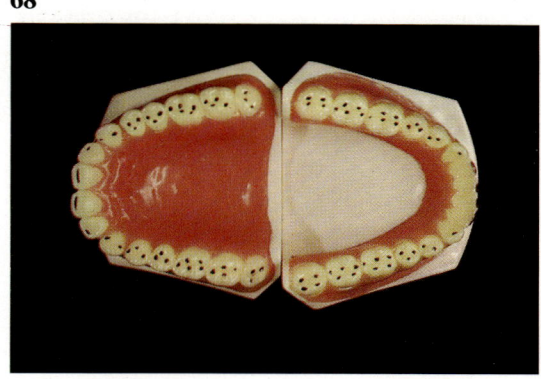

Variations in the relationships of the dental arches in centric position

Malocclusions should be regarded as anatomical variations rather than as abnormalities, for while they may be aesthetically displeasing, they are rarely involved in masticatory dysfunction. Our lack of understanding of the relationships between masticatory efficiency and tooth and arch form is responsible for the classification of malocclusion in terms of variations in the anatomical centric position and not in more functional terms.

Malocclusions result from malposition of individual teeth, malrelationship of the dental arches and/or with variation in skeletal morphology of the jaws. Techniques for determining the skeletal relationships of the jaws are described on page 69. Two classifications describing malposition of teeth and malrelationship of the arches are in general use. One, Angle's classification, relies upon the relationship of the arches in the anteroposterior plane using the first permanent molars as key teeth. The other classification relates malocclusion to the position of the incisors.

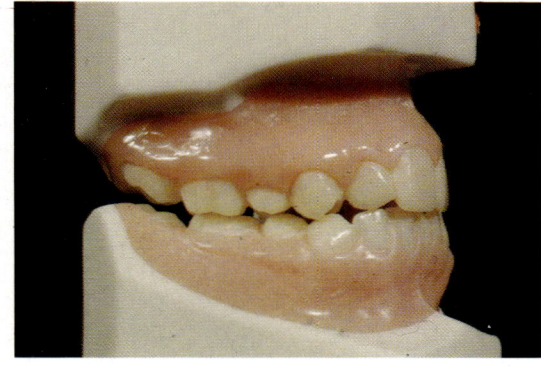

69 Angle's Class I malocclusion. Though one or more of the teeth are malpositioned, this does not affect the standard anatomical relationship of the first permanent molars (see figures **64** and **65**). In the models shown the maxillary canine is missing and the premolars are malaligned.

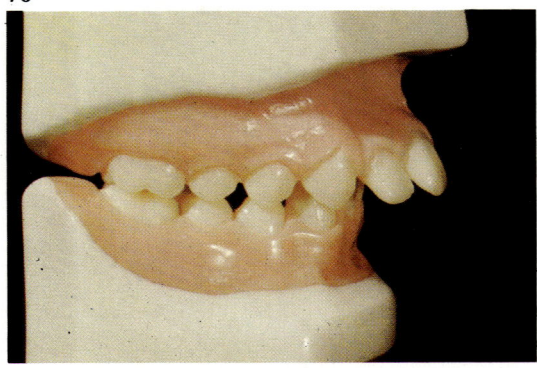

70 Angle's Class II malocclusion. Division 1. Angle's Class II malocclusion is characterised by a 'prenormal' maxillary arch relationship, the maxillary first permanent molars occluding at least half a cusp more mesial to the mandibular first permanent molars than the standard anatomical position. The division 1 indicates that the maxillary incisors are proclined.

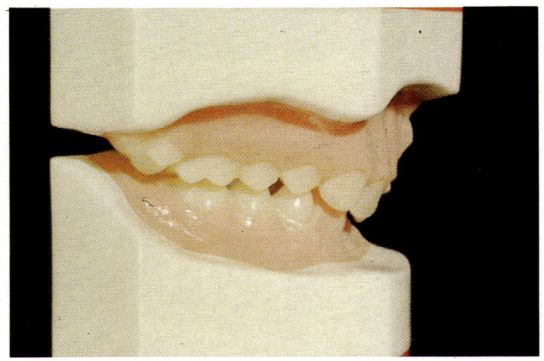

71 Angle's Class II malocclusion. Division 2. The molar relationship is 'prenormal': the 'division 2' indicates that the maxillary incisors are retroclined. Frequently, however, only the central incisors are retroclined, the lateral incisors being proclined.

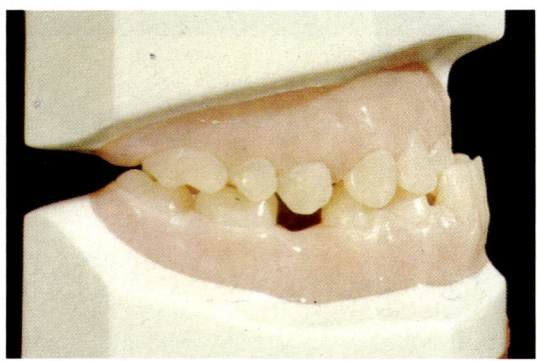

72 Angle's Class III malocclusion. This malocclusion is characterised by a 'postnormal' maxillary arch relationship, the maxillary first permanent molars occluding at least half a cusp more distal to the mandibular first permanent molars than the standard anatomical position. The incisor relationship varies from 'normal' overjet to an edge-to-edge bite to reverse overjet.

Since the permanent molars do not have a fixed relationship in the arch and may migrate following early loss of deciduous teeth, the classification of malocclusion based upon incisor relationships is often preferred to the Angle's classification. Furthermore, a classification of malocclusion related to the incisors is seen by many clinicians to be more appropriate since a major objective of orthodontic treatment is to establish an anatomical incisor relationship (patients being more concerned and aware of the aesthetics of the incisor relationship than they are of the molar relationship).

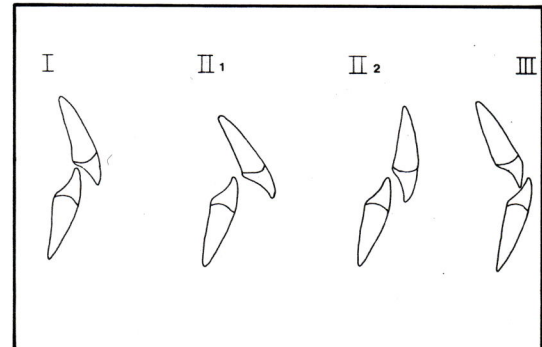

73 Classification of malocclusion using incisor relationships.
Class I. The incisal margins of the mandibular incisors occlude with, or lie directly below, the middle of the palatal surfaces of the maxillary incisors (i.e. on the cingulum shelf).
Class II. The incisal margins of the mandibular incisors lie behind the middle part of the palatal surfaces of the maxillary incisors. Class II division 1 indicates that the upper central incisors are proclined; Class II division 2 indicates that the upper central incisors are retroclined.
Class III. The incisal margins of the mandibular incisors lie in front of the middle part of the palatal surfaces of the maxillary incisors.

It must be emphasised that although Angle's terms are used in classifying incisor relationships, it is not the same as Angle's classification.

Tooth contacts in protrusive and lateral occlusal positions

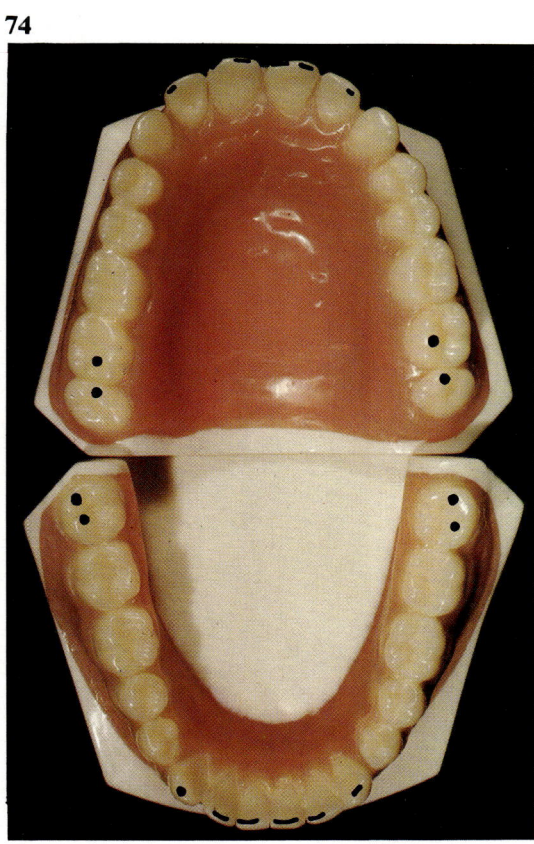

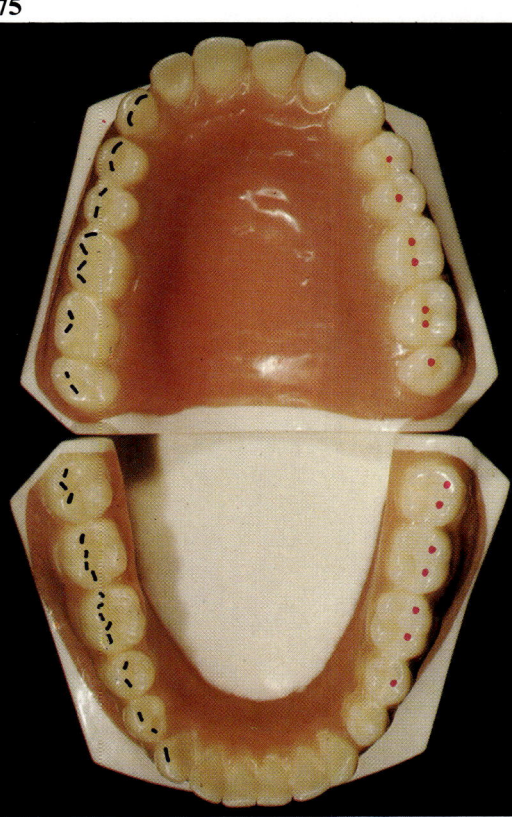

74 Protrusive occlusal relationships of the arches shown by the marking of tooth contacts on the occlusal surfaces of the teeth. During protrusive movement, the mandible is depressed and then moved directly forward so that the anterior teeth are brought together in an edge-to-edge bite. In this situation, the mandibular arch is brought forward by only a few millimetres from its centric relationship with the maxillary arch.

75 Lateral occlusal relationships of the arches. The models of the maxillary and mandibular arches show tooth contacts in the right lateral occlusal position. During right lateral movement, the mandible is initially depressed so that the teeth are separated. The jaw then moves to the right and the teeth behind the canines are brought into contact. On the working side (black contact markings) the teeth meet on the occlusal third of their buccal cusps. The incisors and canines are not usually in contact. The red markings on the lingual cusps of the left maxillary teeth and the buccal cusps of the left mandibular teeth represent the approximate balancing contacts. It is thought that balancing contacts on the non-working side may counteract stresses set up by torsion of the mandible during lateral movements.

Little information is available concerning tooth contacts during mandibular movements, particularly in situations such as those which occur with the intervention of a bolus of food during mastication. It is clear, however, that while displacement of the mandible may be quite extensive, the time the opposing teeth come into contact is very limited.

Mandibular posture

When the mandible is at rest, a gap of a few millimetres remains between the occlusal surfaces of the teeth, the so-called freeway space. The opinion has long been held that the position of rest is innate and unalterable throughout life. However, the concept of a fixed mandibular resting posture is an over-simplification. Indeed, psychological state, body posture and fatigue are well known short-term influences that can change the resting interocclusal distance. Furthermore, recent research shows that following speech, mastication or swallowing, the mandible appears to return to whatever position of rest it can find. In the long term, ageing and the removal of occlusal contacts affect the resting position. Although the physiological mechanisms responsible for maintaining a rest position are not fully understood, recent evidence suggests that the physical properties of the soft tissues are responsible for the rest position, not tonic activity of the elevator muscles of the jaw.

Several instruments and techniques have been devised to measure freeway space – some elaborate, some relatively simple. All suffer from inaccuracies produced by examiner bias, and to misconceptions of the nature of the mandibular resting posture. The use of measuring techniques relies upon the concept that the mandibular resting position is innate and unalterable. Consequently, the removal of teeth is deemed not to affect the rest position. Thus, when a patient has lost all natural occlusal contacts, it is considered necessary only to put a prosthesis into the mouth at a level which reproduces the freeway space and the original occlusal vertical dimension is restored.

Although most clinicians would prefer objective criteria for determining vertical jaw relationships, it is realised by many that, because of the relative instability of such relationships, at best, one has to rely upon such subjective assessments as overall facial appearance, mandibular position during deglutition, jaw posture giving greatest comfort, position allowing the development of maximum biting force, lip and tongue posture. Nevertheless, however one gauges the mandibular resting position, if one is to place prosthetic appliances into the mouth, it is necessary to ensure that the vertical dimensions of the jaws are not adversely affected.

76A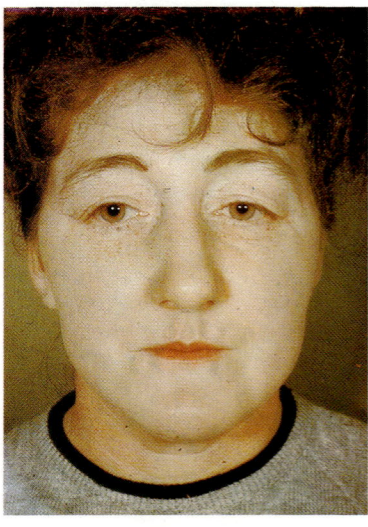

76B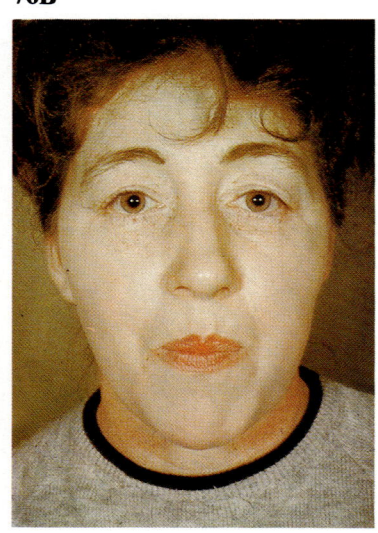

77A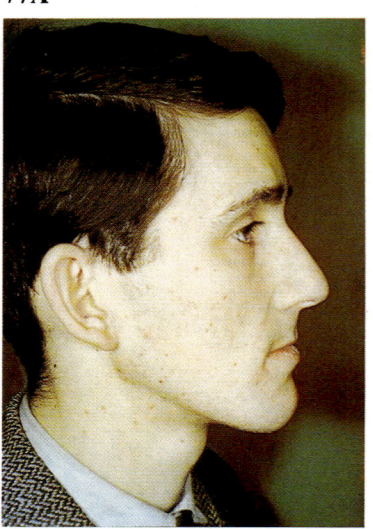

77B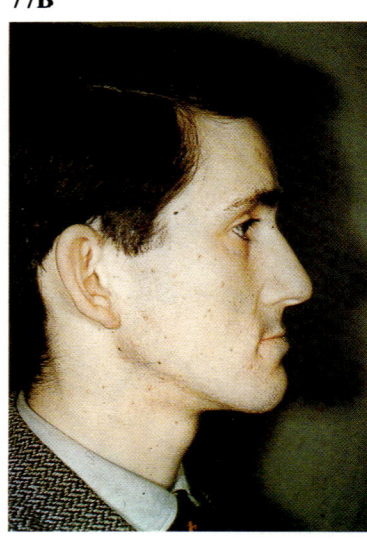

76 The appearance produced as a result of over-opening.
76A Normal resting position for patient without dentures.
76B Over-opened appearance produced typically by the wearing of dentures without the provision of adequate freeway space. Note that the result of over-opening is an elongation of the face, a parting of the lips at rest and a 'strained', facial appearance.

77 The appearance produced by over-closure.
77A Normal resting position.
77B Over-closed appearance. The general effect of over-closure on facial appearance is to produce features of increased age. There is a closer approximation of the nose and chin than normal. The greater the degree of over-closure, the more the soft tissues of the face appear to sag and fall in and the more pronounced are the lines on the face.

The temporomandibular joint

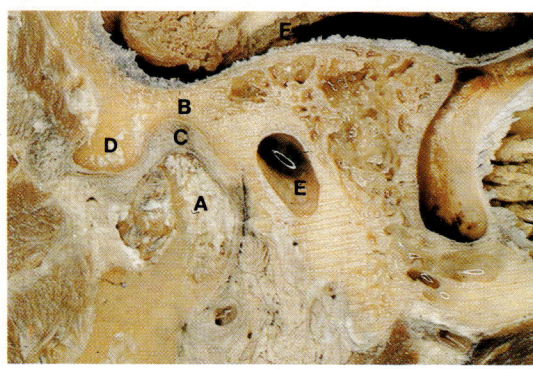

78 The temporomandibular joint (TMJ) is the synovial articulation between the mandible and the cranium. The specimen shown is a sagittal section through the joint illustrating the articulation of the head of the mandibular condyle (A) into the glenoid fossa of the temporal bone (B), with an articular disc (C) intervening. The TMJ, although basically a hinge joint, also allows some gliding movements. Movement of the condylar head occurs within the glenoid fossa and down a bony prominence immediately anterior to the glenoid fossa, the articular eminence (D).

Since the joints develop in membrane, the articular surfaces are covered with fibrous tissue. The articular disc is also fibrous and is moulded to the bony joint surfaces. It is of variable thickness, being thinnest centrally. Anteriorly, the disc covers the articular eminence and is attached to its anterior margin and to the articular margin of the condyle of the mandible. The disc is also attached anteriorly to the lateral pterygoid muscle. Medially and laterally, the disc is attached to the joint capsule. Posteriorly, the disc becomes bilaminar, the upper part attaching to the anterior margin of the squamotympanic fissure, the lower part attaching to the posterior margin of the condyle.

The joint capsule is not shown, but is attached to the neck of the condyle and the bony margins of the glenoid fossa. The capsule is thin but becomes organised laterally to form the temporomandibular ligament. Posteriorly, the capsule forms a thick, vascular, but loosely arranged connective tissue, the retrodiscal pad. Synovial membrane lines the joint capsule but not the articular disc.
E External auditory meatus.
F Floor of middle cranial fossa.

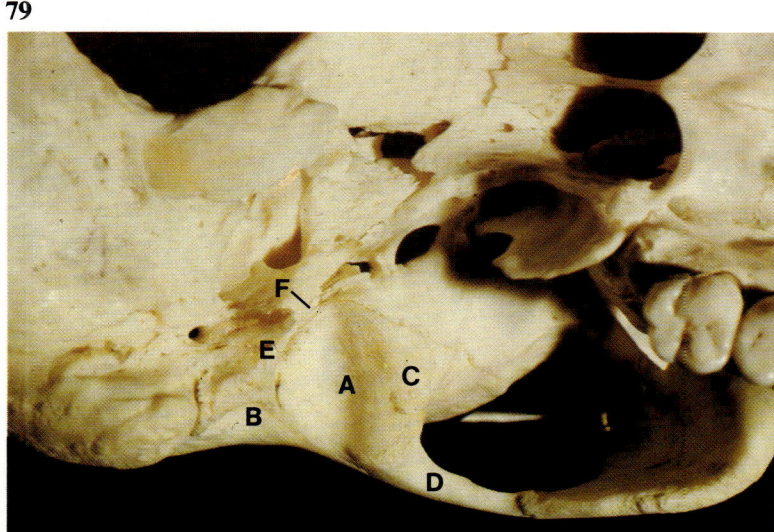

79 The glenoid fossa (A) is an oval depression in the temporal bone lying immediately anterior to the external auditory meatus (B). It is bounded anteriorly by the articular eminence (C), laterally by the zygomatic process of the temporal bone (D) and posteriorly by the tympanic plate of the temporal bone (E). The petrotympanic fissure (F) separates the glenoid fossa from the petrous part of the temporal bone and is the site at which the chorda tympani exits from the cranium into the infratemporal fossa. Occasionally, a ridge of bone, the postglenoid process, forms a prominence at the posterior boundary of the glenoid fossa immediately anterior to the external auditory meatus. The shape of the glenoid fossa does not exactly conform to the shape of the mandibular condyle, the articular disc moulding together the joint surfaces. The bone of the central part of the glenoid fossa is extremely thin and may be translucent. Masticatory loads are not dissipated through the glenoid fossa but through the teeth and thence the facial bones and base of the cranium.

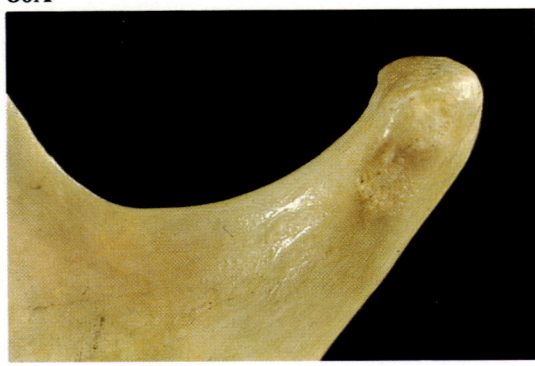
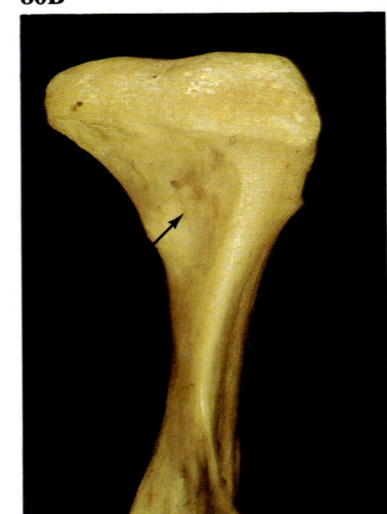
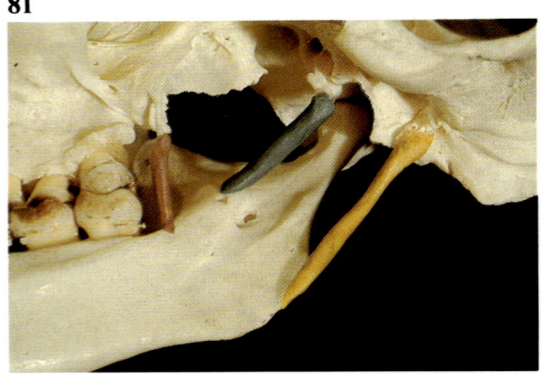

80A & 80B The mandibular condyle. The size and shape of the condyle varies considerably. The broad articular head of the condyle joins the ramus through a thin bony projection termed the neck of the condyle. The anteroposterior dimension of the condylar head is approximately half the mediolateral dimension. The long axis of the condyle is not, however, at right angles to the ramus but diverges posteriorly from a strictly coronal plane such that the long axes of the two condyles, if extended, would meet, forming an obtuse angle of approximately 150 degrees at the anterior border of the foramen magnum. The convex anterior and superior surfaces of the head of the condyle are the articular surfaces. The posterior surface of the head of the condyle is, however, broad and flat. A small depression, the pterygoid fossa (*arrow*), marks part of the attachment of the lateral pterygoid muscle and is situated on the anterior part of the neck below the articular surface of the condyle.

81 The accessory ligaments of the temporomandibular joint. The stylomandibular and sphenomandibular ligaments are described as accessory ligaments of the temporomandibular joint, though neither has any significant influence upon mandibular movements. The stylomandibular ligament (yellow) is a reinforced lamina of the deep cervical fascia as it passes medial to the parotid salivary gland. It extends from the tip of the styloid process of the temporal bone and the stylohyoid ligament to the angle of the mandible. The sphenomandibular ligament (green) is a remnant of the perichondrium of Meckel's cartilage (the cartilage of the embryonic first branchial arch) and extends from the spine of the sphenoid bone to the lingula near the mandibular foramen. Also shown is the pterygomandibular raphe (red) from which the buccinator and superior constrictor muscles arise. It extends from the pterygoid hamulus to the posterior end of the mylohyoid line in the retromolar region of the mandible.

Movements of the mandible at the temporomandibular joint

Mandibular movements may be classified either as bilaterally symmetrical or bilaterally asymmetrical. Since the mandible is a single bone, movement through one temporomandibular joint cannot occur without a similar coordinating or dissimilar reactive movement in the other joint. Depression, elevation, protrusion and retraction of the mandible are bilaterally symmetrical movements since they require similar coordinating movements through both temporomandibular joints. Lateral excursions of the mandible are bilaterally asymmetrical movements during which there are dissimilar activities through the joints.

Opening of the mouth is accomplished by a hinge movement within the glenoid fossa or, more commonly, by a hinge movement accompanied by protrusion of the mandible down the posterior slope of the articular eminence of the temporal bone.

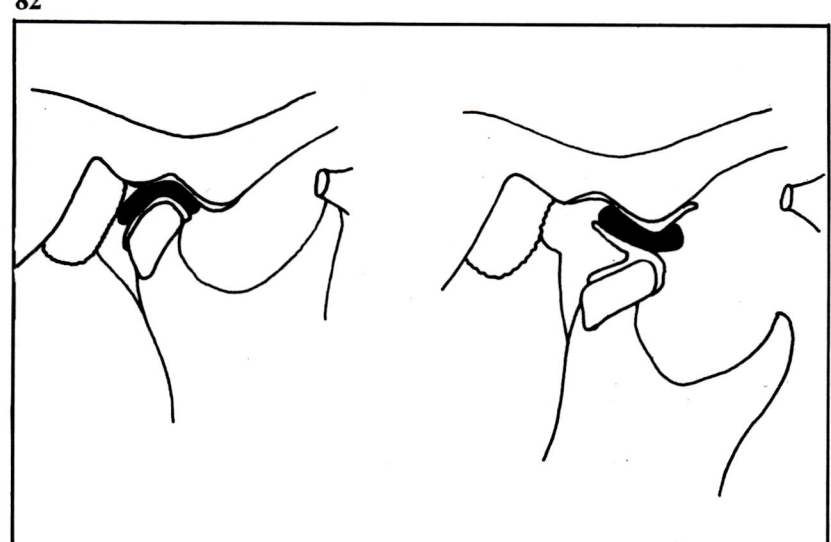

82 The changing relationships between the mandibular condyle, articular disc and temporal bone when the mouth is opened. It is said that the joint space above the disc is associated with anterior gliding movements, while the joint space below the disc is associated with hinge movements.

Retraction of the mandible takes the condyle from a position on the articular eminence back into the glenoid fossa. Little backward movement is possible from within the glenoid fossa.

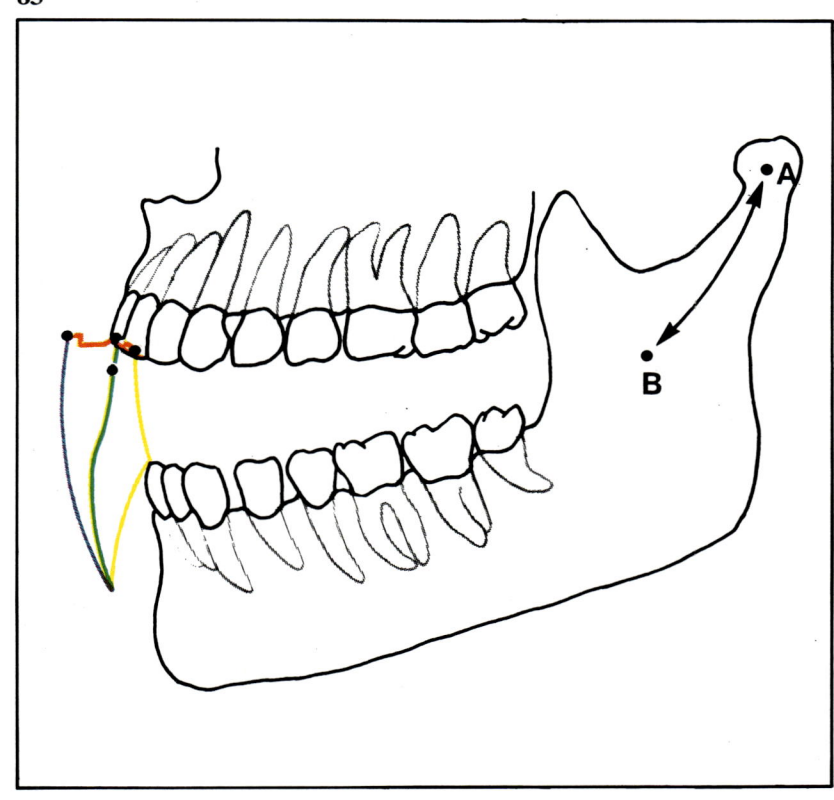

83 The envelope of motion of the contact point between the lower incisors. This view, from the left side, demonstrates symmetrical mandibular movements produced during opening and closing of the jaw. The term envelope of motion is used to describe specific patterns or paths traced by a fixed point on the mandible. The envelope describes both conscious and reflex motions and the patterns so produced are said to be species specific. The paths produced during opening and closing of the jaw describe curved trajectories. The yellow trajectory depicts a conscious movement from rest position to a fully opened position, which takes place in two phases. The first phase is a hinge-like movement during which the condyles are maximally retruded within the glenoid fossae. When the teeth are opened by approximately 25mm, the second phase of opening occurs by anterior movement or protrusion of the condyle down the articular eminences. The blue and red trajectories describe a biphasic path of closure from a fully opened mandibular position, which can only be performed with conscious effort. The first phase (the blue trajectory) takes the mandible up to a protruded, closed position, while the second phase (the red trajectory) takes the mandible from this protruded contact position to a retruded contact position. The green trajectory describes the free, habitual, unconscious, reflex movement during both mandibular opening and closing. The points on the ramus represent the centres of rotation during opening and closure. Point A is the fulcrum associated with simple hinge movements. The path described between Point A and Point B represents the shifting fulcrum of movement during opening and closure involving hinge movements and protrusion or retrusion of the mandible.

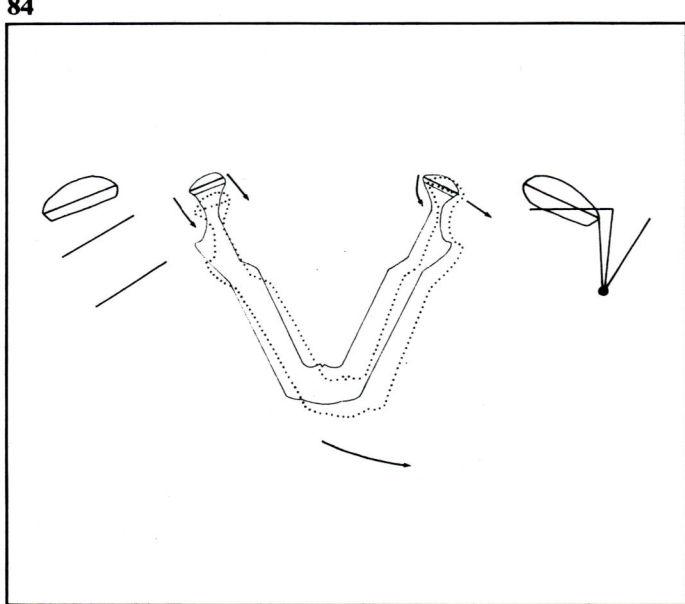

84 Bilaterally asymmetrical motion of the mandible produced during side-to-side movements. Lateral movements are produced by protrusion of the condyle down the articular eminence on one side with reactive movements of the other condyle (rotation around a laterally shifting axis). The solid outline indicates the position of the mandible in centric position; the broken outline indicates the position associated with lateral movement of the mandible to the left. Drawings of the condyles are also given to illustrate the changing positions of the long axes of the condyles during this lateral movement.

Oro-facial soft tissues

The muscles of mastication

Although many muscles, both in the head and neck, are involved in mastication, the muscles of mastication is a collective term reserved for the masseter, temporalis and medial and lateral pterygoid muscles.

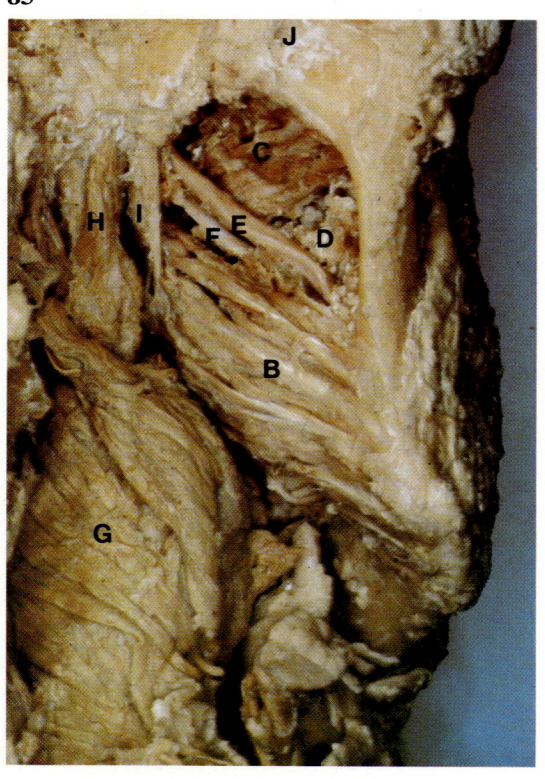

85 Dissection of the masseter (A), medial pterygoid (B) and lateral pterygoid (C) muscles viewed from behind the posterior border of the mandibular ramus. The pterygomandibular space (D) lies between the ramus and the medial pterygoid muscle, the two nerves passing through it being the inferior dental (E) and lingual (F) nerves. Also shown are the constrictor muscles of the pharynx (G) (the infratemporal fossa being the space between the superior constrictor and the ramus); the levator palati (H) and tensor palati (I) muscles and the posterior aspect of the temporomandibular joint (J).

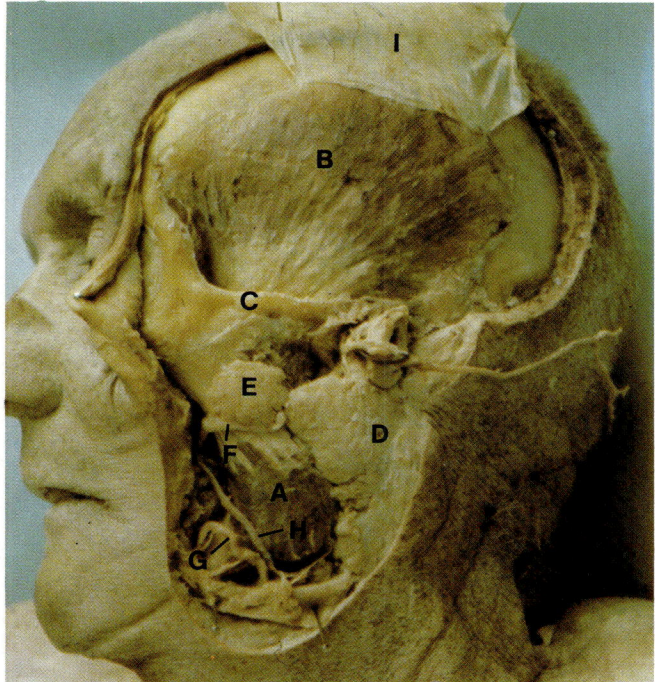

86 Lateral view of head, dissected to show the masseter (A) and temporalis (B) muscles. Also shown in this dissection are the zygoma (C), parotid gland (D), accessory parotid gland (E), parotid duct (F), facial artery (G), facial vein (H) and temporal fascia (I).

The appearance of the pterygoid muscles in the infratemporal fossa is shown in figure **110**.

Attachments of the muscles of mastication

The masseter muscle may be divided into superficial and deep parts. The superficial part arises from tendinous fibres attached to the lower border of the zygomatic arch and passes downwards and backwards to be inserted into the lower half of the lateral surface of the mandibular ramus. The deep part is most distinct in the posterior part of the muscle. It arises from the inner surface and lower border of the zygomatic arch and passes vertically downwards to be inserted into the mandibular ramus above the insertion of the superficial part of the muscle.

The temporalis muscle has a wide origin across the lateral surface of the skull, in the temporal fossa below the inferior temporal line. The muscle fibres converge towards their tendinous insertion on the tip and temporal crest of the mandibular coronoid process, deep to the zygomatic arch. The posterior fibres pass horizontally forwards, the anterior fibres pass vertically down on to the coronoid process.

The medial pterygoid muscle, being situated on the medial side of the mandibular ramus, lies within the infratemporal fossa. It originates as two heads. A small, anterior head arises from the pyramidal process of the palatine bone and the tuberosity of the maxilla. The posterior head forms the bulk of the muscle and arises from the medial surface of the lateral pterygoid plate. The fibres from both heads run downwards and backwards to be inserted on to the medial side of the angle of the mandible.

The lateral pterygoid muscle also lies within the infratemporal fossa and arises by two heads. The larger, inferior head arises from the lateral surface of the lateral pterygoid plate. The smaller, superior head arises from the infratemporal surface of the greater wing of the sphenoid. The fibres run backwards in a more or less horizontal plane across the infratemporal fossa to be inserted into the neck of the mandibular condyle and the disc and capsule of the temporomandibular joint.

Movements of the mandible produced by the muscles of mastication

Elevation Produced by masseter, medial pterygoid and anterior fibres of temporalis.
 Depression Produced by lateral pterygoid.
 Protrusion Produced by lateral and medial pterygoid.
 Retraction Produced by posterior fibres of temporalis.

Lateral excursions Produced by medial and lateral pterygoids of both sides acting alternately.

(All the muscles of mastication receive their motor innervation from the mandibular division of the trigeminal nerve.)

The circum-oral muscles of facial expression

The muscles of facial expression are characterised by their superficial arrangement in the face, by their activities on the skin (brought about directly by their attachment to the facial integument), and by their common motor innervation, the facial nerve. They are all derived embryologically from mesenchyme of the second branchial arch. Functionally, the muscles of facial expression are grouped around the orifices of the face (i.e. the orbit, nose, ear and mouth) and should be considered primarily as muscles controlling the degree of opening and closing of these apertures. The expressive functions of the muscles have developed secondarily. The muscles of facial expression vary considerably between individuals in terms of size, shape and strength.

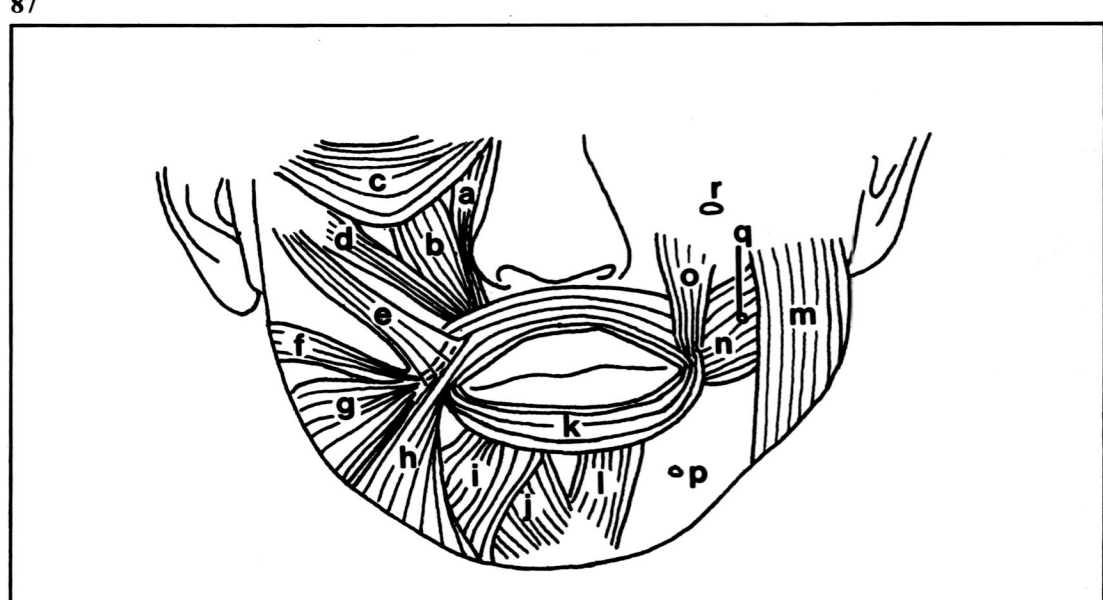

87 The superficial muscles around the lips and cheeks. These may be subdivided into two groups: the various parts of the orbicularis oris muscle and muscles which are radially arranged from the orbicularis oris muscle. The fibres of the orbicularis oris muscle (k) pass around the lips. It is divided into four parts, each part corresponding to a quadrant of the lips. Its muscle fibres do not gain attachment directly to bone but occupy a central part of the lip. Muscle fibres in the philtrum insert on to the nasal septum. The range of movement produced by the orbicularis oris muscle includes lip closure, protrusion and pursing. The radial muscles can be divided into superficial and deep muscles of the upper and lower lips. The levator labii superioris (b), levator labii superioris alaeque nasi (a), and zygomaticus major (e) and minor (d) are superficial muscles of the upper lip. The levator anguli oris (o) is a deep muscle of the upper lip. The depressor anguli oris (h) is a superficial muscle of the lower lip and the depressor labii inferioris (i), and mentalis muscles (j) are deep muscles of the lower lip. As their names suggest, the levator labii superioris elevates the upper lip, the depressor labii inferioris depresses the lower lip, and the corners of the mouth are raised and lowered by the levator and depressor anguli oris muscles. Two muscles extend to the corner of the mouth, the risorius and buccinator muscles. The risorius muscle lies superficial to the buccinator muscle. The risorius muscle stretches the angles of the mouth laterally. The buccinator arises from the pterygomandibular raphe and from the buccal side of the maxillary and mandibular alveoli above the molar teeth. Most of the fibres insert into mucous membrane covering the cheek, other fibres intercalate with the orbicularis oris muscle in the lips. As its fibres converge towards the angle of the mouth, the central fibres decussate. The main function of the buccinator muscle is to maintain the tension of the cheek against the teeth during mastication. Also shown on the diagram are the inferior fibres of the orbicularis oculi muscle (c), the platysma muscle (g), the masseter muscle (m), the infraorbital foramen (r), the mental foramen (p) and the passage of the parotid duct through the buccinator muscle (q). Some of the circum-oral facial muscles are shown in dissection in figure **106**.

Muscles of the tongue

The intrinsic muscles of the tongue can be divided into three fibre groups, the transverse, longitudinal and vertical groups. Rarely can these three groups be distinguished in dissections but their interlacing gives the tongue its characteristic appearance in cross section. The transverse fibres arise from a sheet of connective tissue running longitudinally through the midline of the tongue, the lingual septum. The transverse fibres pass laterally from the septum to intercalate with fibres of the other groups of intrinsic muscles. The longitudinal fibres may be subdivided into upper and lower groups, the superior and inferior longitudinal muscles of the tongue. The vertical fibres pass directly between the upper and lower surfaces particularly at the lateral borders of the tongue. The function of the intrinsic muscles is to change the shape of the tongue. They receive their motor innervation from the hypoglossal cranial nerve.

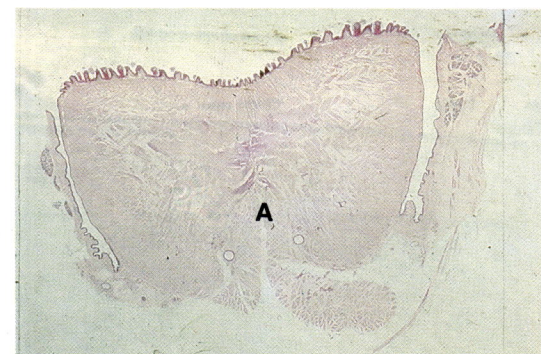

88 Cross-section through tongue. This illustrates the interlacing of the fibres of the intrinsic muscles. A, lingual septum.

The extrinsic muscles of the tongue arise from the skull and hyoid bone and thence spread into the body of the tongue. The extrinsic musculature is composed of four groups of muscles, genioglossus, hyoglossus, styloglossus and palatoglossus.

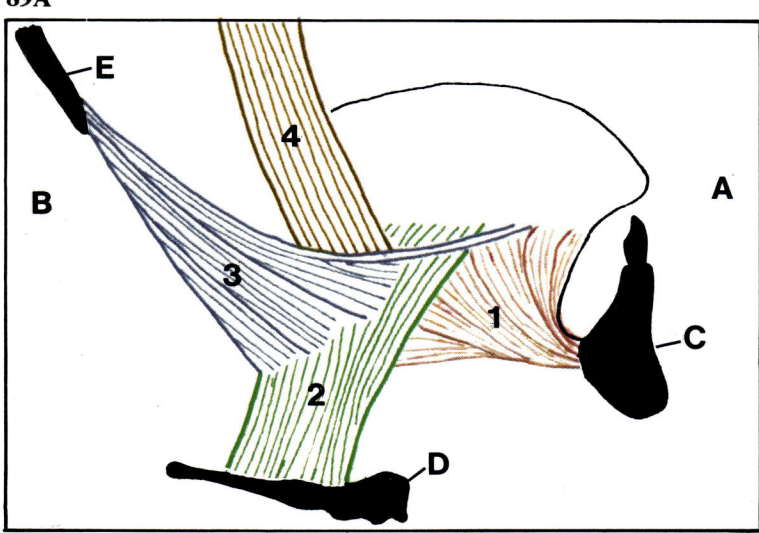

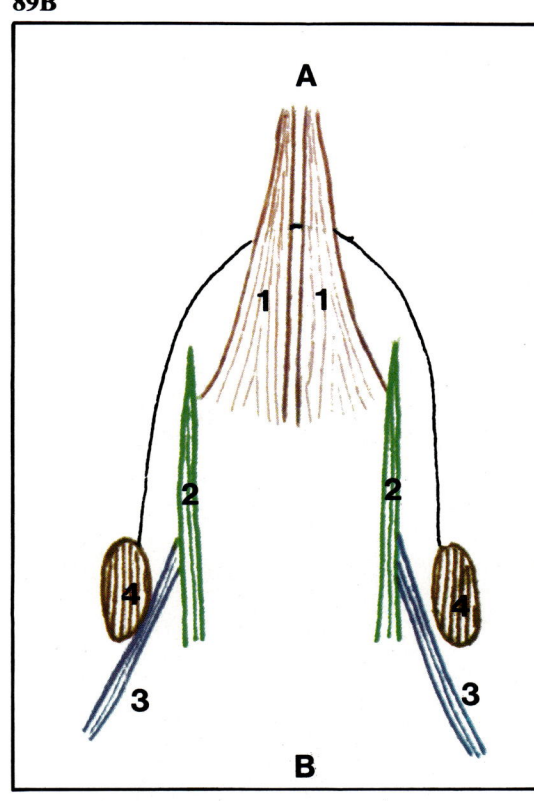

89A & 89B The relationships of the extrinsic muscles to the tongue. The first diagram is a lateral view, the second one an inferior view of the tongue. A, anterior; B, posterior; C, mandible; D, hyoid bone; E, styloid process. The *genioglossus muscles* (1) arise from the superior genial tubercles on the medial surface of the body of the mandible. At this level the two muscles cannot be readily separated. As the muscles enter the tongue, a thin strip of connective tissue intervenes between the right and left genioglossus muscles. The bulk of the fibres fan out into the body of the tongue; but its superior fibres pass upwards and anteriorly to the tip of the tongue and some of its inferior fibres insert on to the body of the hyoid bone. The genioglossus is mainly a protractor and depressor of the tongue. The *hyoglossus muscles* (2) originate from the superior border of the greater horns of the hyoid bone and pass vertically upwards into the tongue. Their function is to depress the tongue. Each *styloglossus muscle* (3) arises from the anterior surface of the styloid process of the temporal bone from which the muscle runs downwards and forwards to enter the tongue below the insertion of the palatoglossus muscle. At this point, its fibres intercalate with the fibres of the hyoglossus before continuing forwards towards the tip of the tongue. The styloglossus muscle is a retractor of the tongue. Each *palatoglossus muscle* (4) arises from the aponeurosis of the soft palate and descends to the tongue as the anterior pillar of the fauces, whence its fibres intercalate with the transverse fibres of the tongue. Its action is to raise the tongue in order to narrow the transverse diameter of the oropharyngeal isthmus. The extrinsic muscles of the tongue are innervated by the hypoglossal nerve excepting palatoglossus which is innervated by the cranial part of the accessory nerve via the pharyngeal plexus. Some of the extrinsic muscles of the tongue may be seen in dissection in figure **109**.

Muscles of the soft palate

90 The palatal muscles viewed from below. Functionally, the soft palate is a fibrous aponeurosis whose shape and position is altered by the *tensor palati muscles* (A), the *levator palati muscles* (B), the *palatoglossus muscles* (C) and the *palatopharyngeus muscles* (D).

The tensor palati muscle arises from the scaphoid fossa of the sphenoid bone at the root of the pterygoid plates and from the lateral side of the cartilaginous part of the Eustachian tube. From its origin, the fibres converge towards the pterygoid hamulus whence the muscle becomes tendinous, the tendon bending at right angles around the hamulus to become the palatine aponeurosis. The anterior border of the aponeurosis is attached to the posterior border of the hard palate. Medially, it merges with the aponeurosis of the other side. Posteriorly, it becomes indistinct, merging with submucosa at the posterior edge of the soft palate. When the tensor palati muscle contracts, the aponeurosis becomes a taut, horizontal plate of tissue upon which other palatine muscles may act to change its position. The motor innervation of the tensor palati muscles is derived from the mandibular division of the trigeminal nerve via the nerve to the medial pterygoid muscle and the otic ganglion. The levator palati muscle originates from the base of the skull at the apex of the petrous part of the temporal bone, anterior to the opening of the carotid canal and from the medial side of the cartilaginous part of the Eustachian tube. The muscle curves downwards, medially and forwards to enter the palate immediately below the opening of the Eustachian tube.

The levator muscles of the palate form a U-shaped muscular sling. When the palatine aponeurosis is stiffened by the tensor muscles, contraction of the levator muscles produces an upwards and backwards movement of the soft palate. In this way, the nasopharynx is shut off from the oropharynx by the apposition of the soft palate on to the posterior wall of the pharynx. The nerve supply to the levator palati muscles is derived from the cranial part of the accessory nerve via the pharyngeal plexus.

The palatopharyngeus muscle arises from two heads, one from the posterior border of the hard palate, the other from the upper surface of the palatine aponeurosis. The two heads unite after arching over the lateral edge of the palatine aponeurosis where the muscle passes downwards beneath the mucous membrane of the lateral wall of the oropharynx as the posterior pillar of the fauces (palatopharyngeal arch). The muscle is inserted into the posterior border of the thyroid cartilage of the larynx. The main action of the palatopharyngeus muscle is to elevate the larynx and pharynx, but it may also arch the relaxed palate and depress the tensed palate. Its nerve supply is derived from the accessory nerve via the pharyngeal plexus.

Passavant's muscle is said to be a sphincter-like muscle which encircles the pharynx at the level of the palate, inside the fibres of the superior constrictor muscles. It is formed by fibres arising from the anterior and lateral part of the upper surface of the palatine aponeurosis. Contraction of this muscle forms a ridge, Passavant's ridge, against which the soft palate is elevated.

The salpingopharyngeus muscle (not shown) is a slip of muscle which arises from the cartilage of the Eustachian tube and which passes downwards to converge with the palatopharyngeus muscle.

The palatoglossus muscle has previously been described (see figure **89**). E = buccinator muscle. F = musculus uvulae.

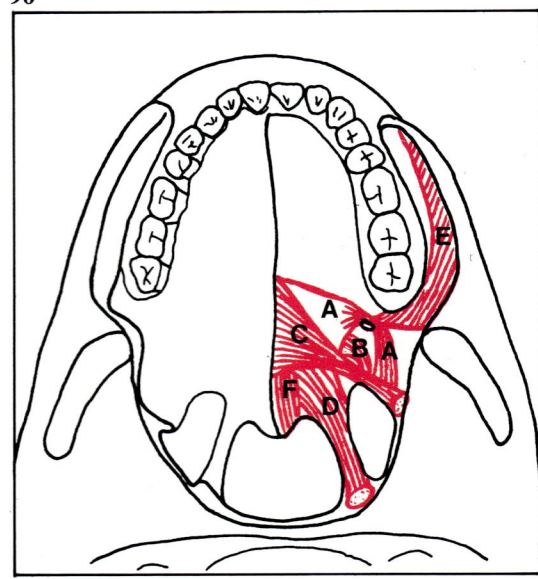

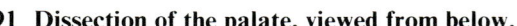

91 Dissection of the palate, viewed from below.
A Anterior palatine nerves and vessels crossing lateral margin of hard palate.
B Palatoglossus muscle.
C Palatopharyngeus muscle.
D Aponeurosis from tensor palati.
E Muscle fibres in the uvula (musculus uvulae).
F Pterygoid hamulus.
The levator and tensor palati muscles are also shown in figure **85**.

92 Muscles at the oropharyngeal isthmus. In this diagram, the palatal tonsil and mucous membrane have been removed to reveal the muscles bounding the tonsillar crypt i.e. the palatoglossus muscle (A), the palatopharyngeus muscle (B) and the superior constrictor muscle of the pharynx (C). Also shown are the tonsillar blood vessels, the dorsum of the tongue (D), the soft palate (E), the Eustachian (auditory) tube (F), the tensor palati muscle (G) and the levator palati muscle (H).

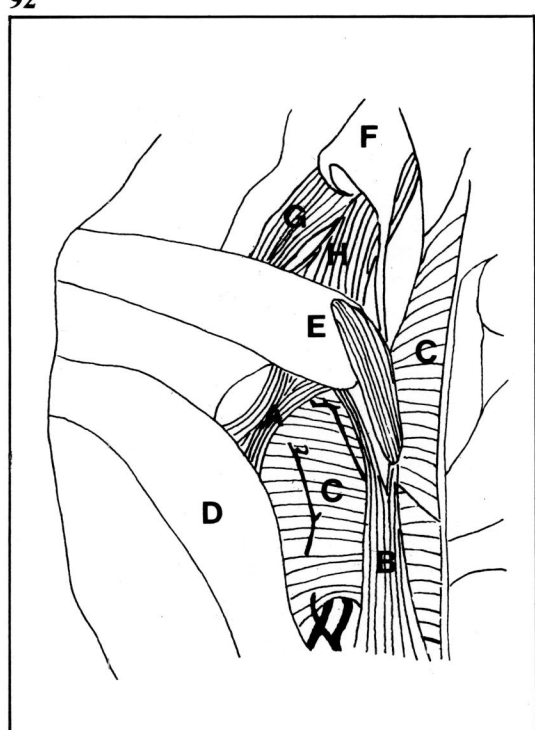

Innervation of oro-dental tissues

Excepting regions around the oropharyngeal isthmus, the mucous membrane lining the vestibule and oral cavity proper receives sensory innervation from the maxillary and mandibular divisions of the trigeminal nerve. The trigeminal nerve also supplies the teeth and their supporting tissues. Both the major and minor salivary glands are supplied by secretomotor, parasympathetic fibres from the facial and glossopharyngeal nerves. The motor innervation of the muscles related to the jaws and oral cavity has been described previously.

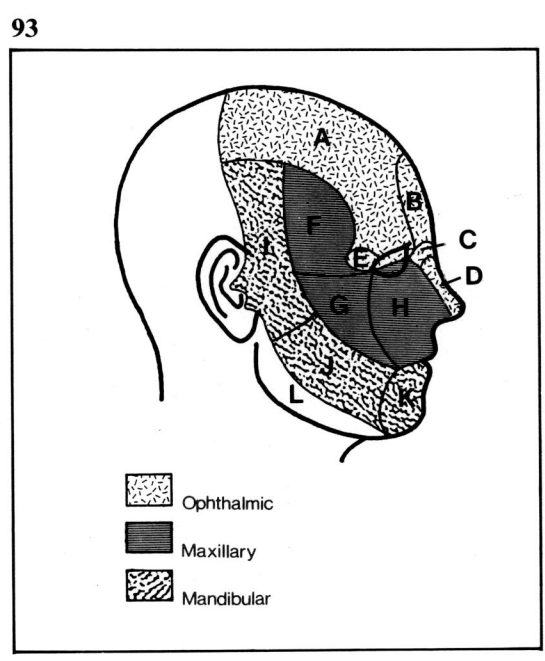

93 Cutaneous innervation of the face.
A Peripheral nerve field associated with supraorbital nerve.
B Peripheral nerve field associated with supratrochlear nerve.
C Peripheral nerve field associated with infratrochlear nerve.
D Peripheral nerve field associated with external nasal nerve.
E Peripheral nerve field associated with lacrimal nerve.
F Peripheral nerve field associated with zygomaticotemporal nerve.
G Peripheral nerve field associated with zygomaticofacial nerve.
H Peripheral nerve field associated with infraorbital nerve.
I Peripheral nerve field associated with auriculotemporal nerve.
J Peripheral nerve field associated with buccal nerve.
K Peripheral nerve field associated with mental nerve.
L Peripheral nerve field associated with great auricular nerve.

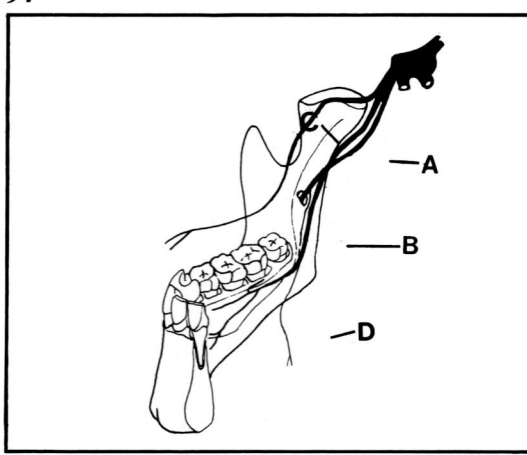

94 The relationships of the inferior dental (A), lingual (B), buccal (C) and mylohyoid (D) nerves. The inferior dental nerve, the terminal branch of the posterior column of the mandibular division of the trigeminal, arises in the infratemporal fossa deep to the lower head of the lateral pterygoid muscle. On emerging from behind this muscle, it lies within the pterygomandibular space (see figures **85** and **110**). Here it gives off a mylohyoid branch which is a motor nerve to the anterior belly of the digastric and mylohyoid muscles. It may also have a sensory twig which enters the mandible in the mental region to participate in the nerve supply to the lower incisors. The inferior dental nerve enters the ramus through the mandibular foramen. This foramen is centrally positioned in the ramus. The buccal nerve, the terminal branch of the anterior column of the mandibular nerve, arises behind the upper head of the lateral pterygoid and, passing between the two heads of this muscle, crosses the anterior border of the ramus at or slightly below the level of the occlusal plane. The nerve crosses the upper part of the retromolar fossa and breaks up into a number of branches within the buccinator muscle. Like the inferior dental nerve, the lingual nerve is derived from the posterior column of the mandibular nerve behind the lateral pterygoid muscle. Here it receives the chorda tympani nerve. At the level of the mandibular foramen, the lingual nerve lies on the medial pterygoid muscle anterior to the inferior dental nerve (see figure **110**). It leaves the pterygomandibular space, passing downwards and anteriorly to lie close to the lingual alveolar plate of the third mandibular molar tooth. At this point, the nerve lies immediately beneath the oral mucosa and thus may easily be damaged during surgical procedures in this region. Before curving forwards into the tongue, the nerve lies above the origin of the mylohyoid muscle and lateral to the hyoglossus (see figure **109**).

Nerve supply to the teeth and gingivae

	Nasopalatine nerve	Anterior palatine nerve			Palatal gingiva
Maxilla	Anterior superior dental nerve	Middle superior dental nerve	Posterior superior dental nerve		Teeth
	Infraorbital nerve	Posterior superior dental nerve & buccal nerve			Buccal gingiva
	1 2 3	4	5 6	7 8	
Mandible	Mental nerve		Buccal nerve & perforating branches of inferior dental nerve		Buccal gingiva
	Incisive nerve	Inferior dental nerve			Teeth
	Lingual nerve & perforating branches of inferior dental nerve				Lingual gingiva

The numbers represent tooth positions according to the Zsigmond System.

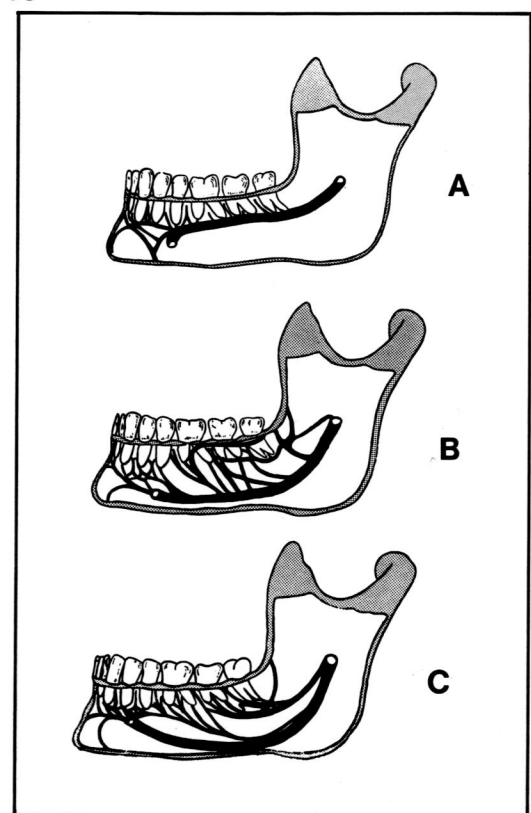

95 The course of the inferior dental nerve through the mandible. The distribution of nerves to the premolars and molars is variable, dental branches either coming directly from the inferior dental nerve by short (A) or long (B) branches or indirectly through alveolar branches (C). In rare instances, the nerve to the mandibular third molar may arise from the inferior dental nerve before it enters the mandibular canal. Communications between the inferior dental nerve and nerves from the temporalis and lateral pterygoid muscles have been described, the nerves penetrating the mandible through foraminae in the region of muscle attachments. It has been suggested that such nervous connections might explain why, in approximately 5 per cent of patients, the teeth may not be anaesthetised after the main trunk of the inferior dental nerve has been blocked at the mandibular foramen by the injection of local anaesthetic solution.

It is said that, in any one individual, the mandibular canal remains in a relatively fixed position with respect to the lower border of the mandible. The canal is often closely related to the roots of the mandibular molars. Indeed, the roots of lower third molars may even be perforated by the mandibular canal.

In the premolar region, the main trunk of the inferior dental nerve divides into mental and incisive nerves. The mental nerve runs for a short distance in a mental canal before leaving the body of the mandible at the mental foramen to emerge on to the face. In about 50 per cent of cases the mental foramen lies on a vertical line passing through the mandibular second premolar. However, in negroid races the mental foramen may be situated slightly more posteriorly midway between the roots of the second premolar and first permanent molar. In an adult with a full dentition, the mental foramen usually lies midway between the upper and lower borders of the mandible. During the first and second years of life as the prominence of the chin develops, the opening of the mental foramen alters in direction from facing forwards to facing upwards and backwards. As well as supplying the skin of the lower lip, the mental nerve provides fibres to an incisor plexus which innervates the labial periodontium of the mandibular incisors. The incisive nerve runs forwards in an intraosseous incisive canal. This nerve primarily supplies the incisors and canine teeth but may also supply the first premolar. In some instances, the canine may be supplied directly from the inferior dental nerve.

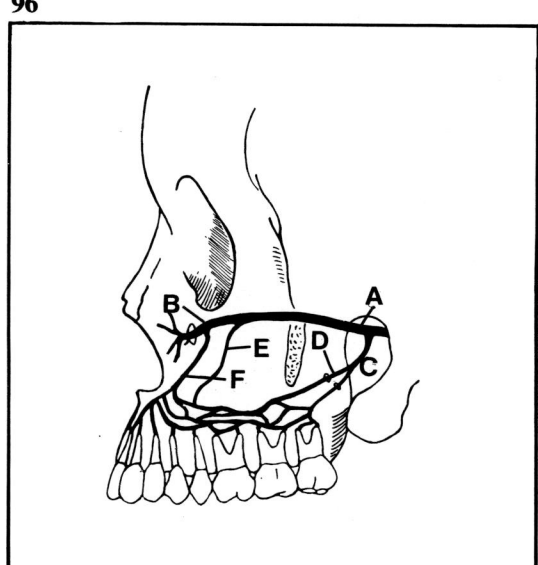

96 The superior dental nerves and associated dental plexuses. A, maxillary nerve. B, infraorbital nerve. C, pterygopalatine fossa. D, E, and F, posterior, middle and anterior superior dental nerves respectively.

The posterior superior dental nerve arises from the maxillary nerve in the pterygopalatine fossa whence they descend to the posterior wall of the maxilla. The dental branches of the nerve enter the maxilla and run in narrow, posterior superior dental canals above the roots of the molar teeth. The gingival branch does not enter the bone, however, but runs downward and forward along the outer surface of the maxillary tuberosity.

The middle superior dental nerve is found in about 70 per cent of subjects. The nerve generally arises from the infraorbital nerve in the floor of the orbit though alternatively, it may arise from the maxillary nerve in the pterygopalatine fossa. The nerve may run in the posterior, lateral or anterior walls of the maxillary antrum. It terminates above the roots of the premolar teeth.

The anterior superior dental nerve arises from the infraorbital nerve within the infraorbital canal, generally as a single nerve but occasionally as two or three small branches. The nerve leaves the infraorbital canal near its termination and then, diverging laterally from the infraorbital nerve, it runs in the anterior wall of the maxillary sinus. It terminates near the anterior nasal spine after giving off a small nasal branch.

The superior dental nerve forms a plexus above the root apices of the maxillary teeth. From this plexus nerves pass to the teeth though it is difficult to trace the precise innervation of the teeth from specific superior dental nerves. As a general rule, however, the incisors and canine are supplied by the anterior nerve, the molars by the posterior nerve and intermediate areas by the middle nerve.

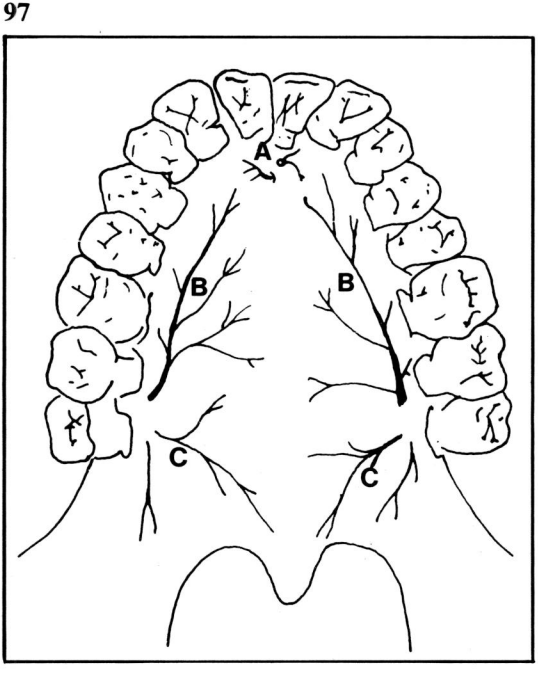

97 The sensory nerve supply to the palate is derived from branches of the pterygopalatine ganglion. A small area behind the incisor teeth is supplied by terminal branches of the nasopalatine nerves (A). These nerves emerge on to the palate at the incisive foramen. The remainder of the hard palate is supplied by the anterior palatine nerves (B), emerging on to the palate at the greater palatine foraminae. The soft palate is supplied by the posterior palatine nerves (C), emerging on to the palate via the lesser palatine foraminae. Thus, the maxillary division of the trigeminal nerve supplies most of the palate. However, there is evidence to suggest that some areas supplied by the posterior palatine nerves may also be innervated by fibres from the facial nerve. The posterior part of the soft palate and the uvula may be supplied by the glossopharyngeal nerve.

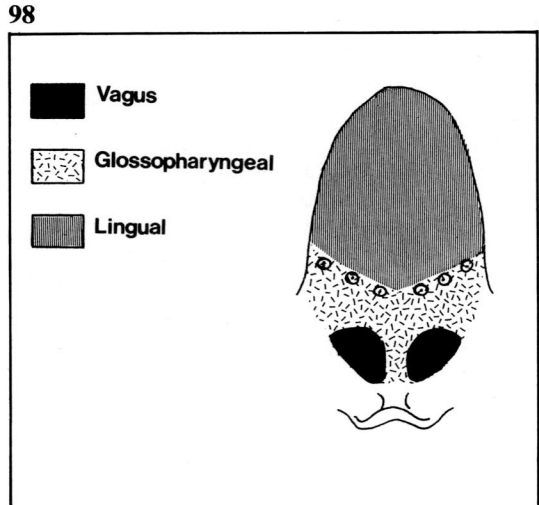

98 Sensory innervation of the tongue. Three distinct nerve fields can be recognised on the dorsum of the tongue. The anterior part of the tongue in front of the circumvallate papillae is supplied by the lingual nerve, though its accompanying chorda tympani fibres are those associated with the perception of taste. Behind, and including, the circumvallate papillae, the tongue is supplied primarily by the glossopharyngeal nerve, both general sensation and taste. A small area on the posterior part of the tongue around the epiglottis is supplied by the vagus nerve via its superior laryngeal branch. The mucosa on the ventral surface of the tongue is supplied by the lingual nerve.

The mucosa of the upper lip is supplied by the infraorbital branch of the maxillary division of the trigeminal nerve, that of the lower lip by the mental branch of the mandibular division of the trigeminal nerve.

The mucosa of the cheeks is supplied by the buccal branch of the mandibular division of the trigeminal.

The mucosa on the floor of the mouth is supplied by the lingual nerve.

The mucosa over the pillars of the fauces is supplied by the glossopharyngeal nerve.

The chorda tympani nerve provides secretomotor fibres via the submandibular parasympathetic ganglion to the submandibular and sublingual salivary glands, and probably also to minor salivary glands in the lips, cheeks and tongue. The lesser superficial petrosal branch of the glossopharyngeal nerve supplies the parotid gland via the otic parasympathetic ganglion. The greater superficial petrosal branch of the facial nerve probably supplies palatal and pharyngeal glands via the pterygopalatine parasympathetic ganglion.

Blood supply to oro-dental tissues

The face is supplied mainly through the facial artery. This artery first appears on the face as it hooks round the lower border of the mandible at the anterior edge of the masseter. It then runs a tortuous course between the facial muscles towards the medial angle of the eye (figure 106). There is a rich anastomoses with the artery of the opposite side and with additional vessels supplying the face (transverse facial branches of the superficial temporal artery, infraorbital and mental branches of the maxillary artery and the dorsal nasal branch of the ophthalmic artery).

The main arteries to the teeth and jaws are derived from the maxillary artery, a terminal branch of the external carotid. The dental arteries roughly follow the same course as the dental nerves.

Mandibular teeth and periodontium. The inferior dental artery which supplies the mandibular teeth is derived from the maxillary artery before it crosses the lateral pterygoid muscle in the infratemporal fossa. A mylohyoid branch is given off before the inferior dental artery enters the mandibular foramen. The inferior dental artery passes through the mandibular foramen to enter the mandibular canal and terminates as the mental and incisive arteries.

Posteriorly, the buccal gingiva is supplied by the buccal artery (a branch of the maxillary artery as it crosses the lateral pterygoid muscle) and by perforating branches from the inferior dental artery. Anteriorly, the buccal gingiva is supplied by the mental artery and by perforating branches of the incisive artery. The lingual gingiva is supplied by perforating branches from the inferior dental artery and by the lingual artery of the external carotid.

Maxillary teeth and periodontium. The posterior superior dental artery arises from the maxillary artery in the pterygopalatine fossa. Occasionally, it is derived from the buccal artery. It courses tortuously over the maxillary tuberosity before entering bony canals to supply molar and premolar teeth. The artery also gives off branches to the adjacent buccal gingiva, maxillary sinus and cheek.

The middle superior dental artery, when present, arises from the infraorbital artery which is itself a branch of the third part of the maxillary artery in the pterygopalatine fossa. The middle superior dental artery runs in the lateral wall of the maxillary sinus, terminating near the canine tooth where it anastomoses with the anterior and posterior superior dental arteries. The anterior superior dental artery also arises from the infraorbital artery and runs downwards in the anterior wall of the maxillary sinus to supply the anterior teeth. Like the superior dental nerves, the dental arteries form plexuses.

The buccal gingiva around the posterior maxillary teeth is supplied by gingival and perforating branches from the posterior superior dental artery and by the buccal artery. The labial gingiva of anterior teeth is supplied by labial branches of the infraorbital artery and by perforating branches of the anterior superior dental artery.

The palatal gingiva is supplied primarily by branches of the greater palatine artery, a branch of the third part of the maxillary artery in the pterygopalatine fossa.

The palate, the cheek, the lips

The palate derives its blood supply from the greater and lesser palatine branches of the maxillary artery. The greater palatine artery passes through the incisive foramen where it anastomoses with the nasopalatine artery.

The cheek is supplied by the buccal branch of the maxillary artery, the floor of the mouth and tongue by the lingual arteries. The lips are mainly supplied by superior and inferior labial branches of the facial arteries.

Venous drainage of oro-dental tissues

The venous drainage of this region is extremely variable. The facial vein is the main vein draining the face. It begins at the medial corner of the eye by confluence of the supraorbital and supratrochlear veins and passes across the face behind the facial artery. Below the mandible, it joins with the anterior branch of the retromandibular vein to form the common facial vein.

Small veins from the teeth and alveolar bone pass into larger veins which surround the apex of each tooth or into veins running in the interdental septa. In the mandible, the veins are then collected into one or more inferior dental veins which themselves may drain anteriorly through the mental foramen to join the facial veins or posteriorly through the mandibular foramen to join the pterygoid plexus of veins in the infratemporal fossa. In the maxilla, the veins may drain anteriorly into the facial vein or posteriorly into the pterygoid plexus.

No accurate description is available concerning the venous drainage of the gingiva, though it may be assumed that the buccal, lingual, anterior palatine and nasopalatine veins are involved; apart from the lingual veins which pass directly into the internal jugular veins, these veins run into the pterygoid plexuses.

The veins of the palate are rather diffuse and variable. However, those of the hard palate generally pass into the pterygoid plexus, those of the soft palate into the pharyngeal plexus.

Venous blood from the lips drains into the facial veins via superior and inferior labial veins. The veins of the tongue follow two different routes. Those of the dorsum and sides of the tongue form the lingual veins which, accompanying the lingual arteries, empty into the internal jugular veins. Those of the ventral surface form the deep lingual veins which ultimately join the facial, internal jugular or lingual veins.

Lymphatic drainage of oro-dental tissues

As the venous system, the lymphatic drainage is extremely variable.

Lymphatics from the lower part of the face generally pass through or around buccal lymph nodes to reach submandibular lymph nodes. Lymphatics from the medial portion of the lower lip drain into the submental nodes.

99 Regional lymphatic drainage of the oral structures. A, jugulo-digastric nodes. B, submandibular nodes. C, submental nodes.

The lymph vessels draining the pulp and periodontal ligament have a common outlet. As a rule, those vessels draining the incisors and canines pass anteriorly, those draining the molars run posteriorly, while the vessels from the premolars may pass anteriorly or posteriorly. The lymph vessels of all teeth, except for the lower incisors, pass directly into the submandibular lymph nodes on the same side. Lymph from the lower incisors, however, drains into the submental lymph nodes. Occasionally lymph from the molars may pass directly into the jugulo-digastric group of nodes.

The lymph vessels of the labial and buccal gingivae of the upper and lower teeth unite to drain into the submandibular nodes, though in the labial region of the lower incisors they may drain into the submental lymph nodes. The lingual and palatal gingivae of the teeth drain into the jugulo-digastric group of nodes either directly or indirectly through the submandibular nodes.

Lymphatics from the palate terminate in the jugulo-digastric group of nodes though those from the posterior part of the soft palate terminate in pharyngeal lymph nodes.

Lymphatics from the anterior two-thirds of the tongue may be subdivided into two groups of vessels, marginal and central vessels. The marginal lymphatics drain the lateral third of the upper surface of the tongue and the lateral margin of its lower surface. The remaining regions drain into the central vessels. The marginal vessels drain into the submandibular lymph nodes of the same side. The central vessels at the tip of the tongue drain into the submental lymph nodes. Central vessels behind the tip drain into ipsilateral and contralateral submandibular lymph nodes. Occasionally, both marginal and central lymph vessels pass directly into the jugulo-digastric group of nodes. Lymphatics from the posterior third of the tongue drain directly into the jugulo-digastric group of nodes.

From the regional submandibular and submental lymph nodes, lymph vessels pass respectively to the jugulo-digastric and paratracheal lymph nodes.

At the junction between the oral cavity and oropharynx lie the lingual tonsils on the pharyngeal surface of the tongue and the palatal tonsils between the pillars of the fauces. These tonsils, together with adenoid tissue in the nasopharynx, form a ring of lymphoid tissue known as Waldeyer's tonsillar ring.

Regional topography of the oral cavity and related areas

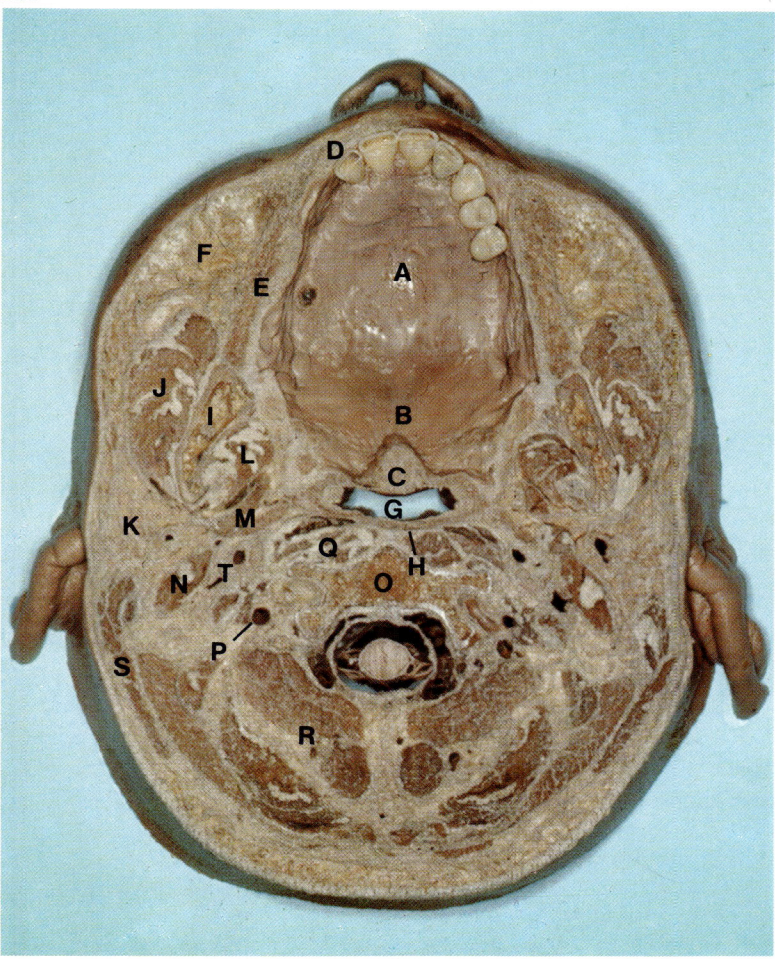

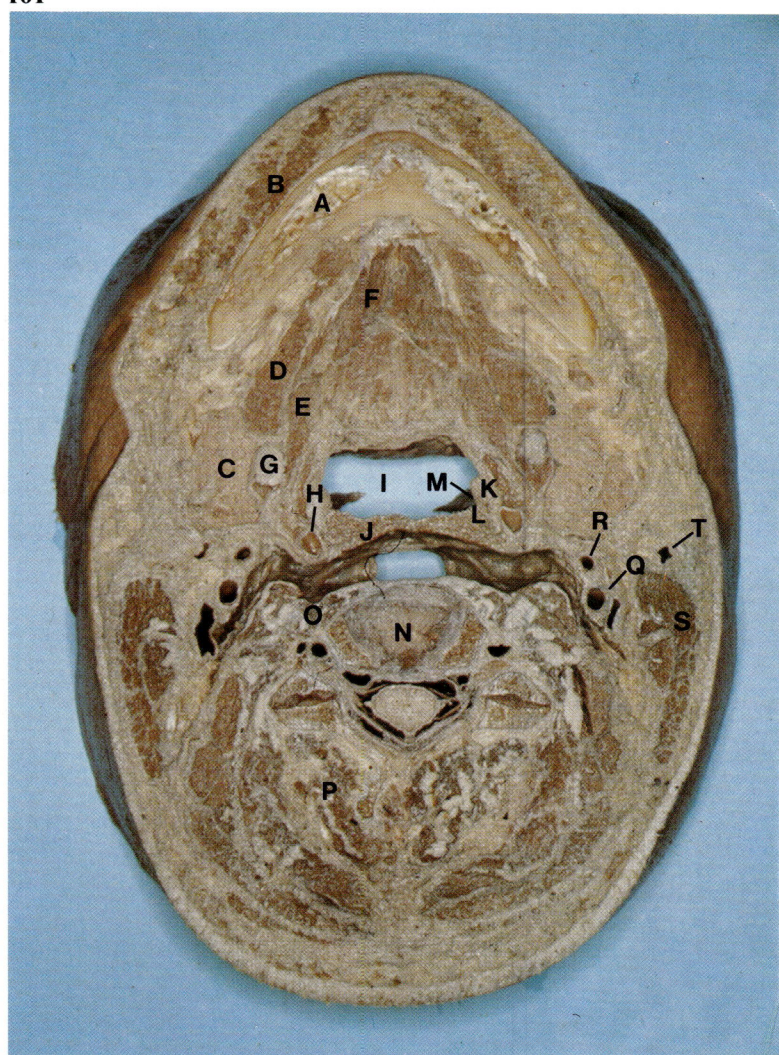

100 Transverse section through the head to show the palate and its topographic relationships.
A Hard palate.
B Soft palate.
C Uvula.
D Upper lip.
E Buccinator muscle.
F Buccal pad of fat.
G Nasopharynx.
H Superior constrictor muscle of pharynx.
I Ramus of mandible.
J Masseter muscle.
K Parotid gland.
L Medial pterygoid muscle.
M Styloid group of muscles: stylopharyngeus, stylohyoideus, styloglossus.
N Posterior belly of digastric muscle.
O Axis (second cervical vertebra).
P Vertebral artery.
Q Prevertebral muscles.
R Postvertebral muscles.
S Sternocleidomastoid muscle.
T Internal carotid artery and internal jugular vein.

101 Transverse section through the head to show the floor of the mouth and its topographic relationships.
A Body of mandible.
B Depressor labii superioris and depressor anguli oris muscles.
C Submandibular gland.
D Mylohyoid muscle.
E Hyoglossus muscle.
F Genioglossus muscle.
G Tendon of digastric muscle.
H Tip of greater horn of hyoid bone.
I Oropharynx.
J Middle constrictor muscle of pharynx.
K Palatoglossal arch ⎫ Pillars of
L Palatopharyngeal arch ⎭ the fauces.
M Tonsillar crypt.
N Cervical vertebra.
O Prevertebral group of muscles.
P Postvertebral group of muscles.
Q Carotid sheath containing internal carotid artery, internal jugular vein and vagus nerve.
R External carotid artery.
S Sternocleidomastoid muscle.
T External jugular vein.

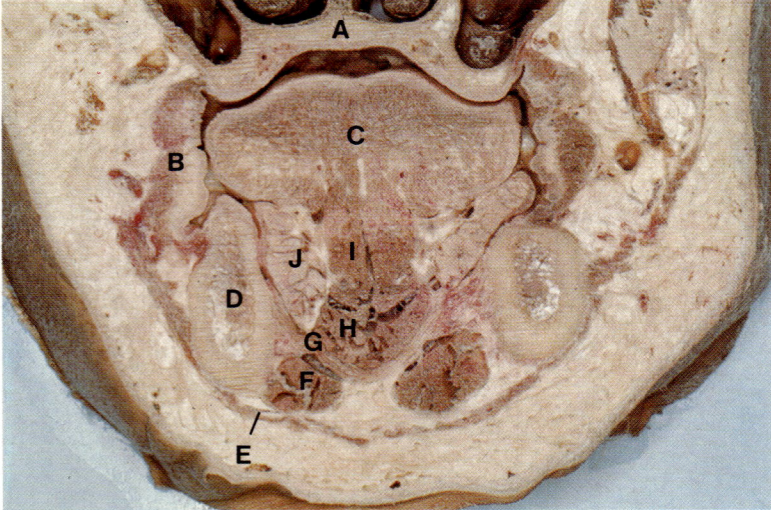

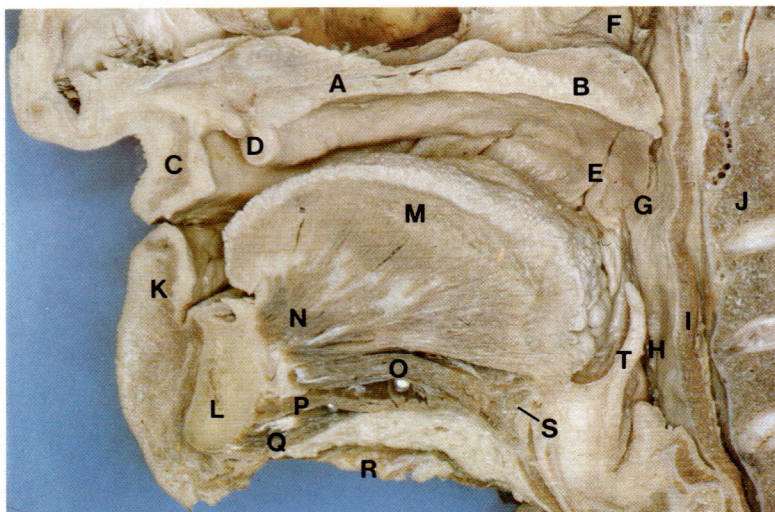

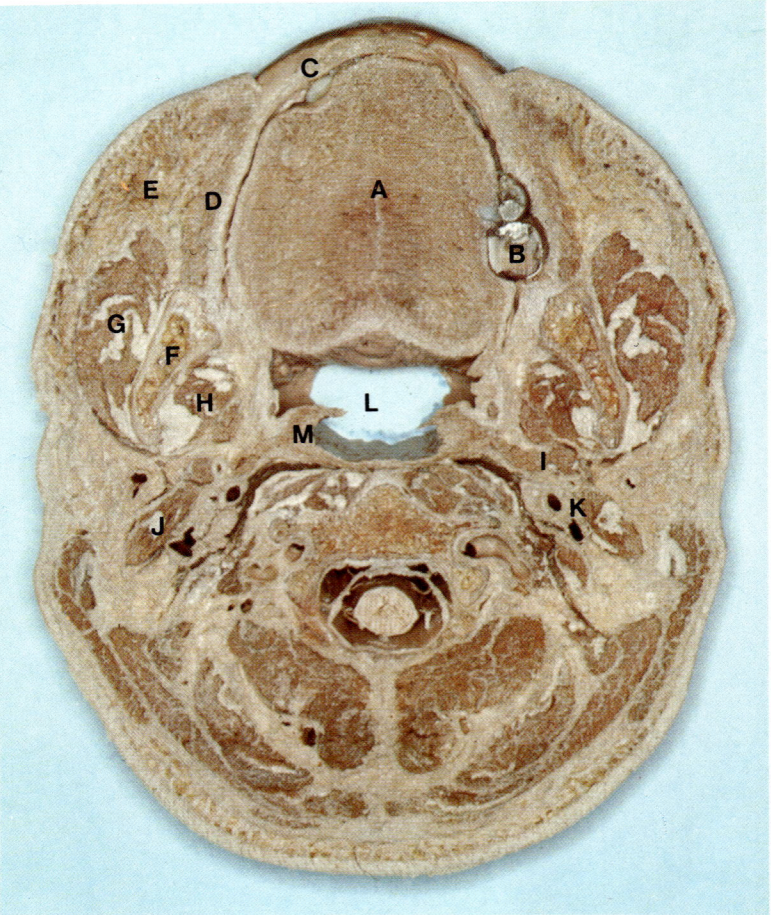

102 Coronal section through the head to show the tongue and its topographic relationships.
A Hard palate.
B Buccinator muscle.
C Tongue.
D Body of mandible.
E Platysma muscle.
F Anterior belly of digastric muscle.
G Mylohyoid muscle.
H Geniohyoid muscle.
I Genioglossus muscle.
J Sublingual salivary glands.

103 Transverse section through the head at the level of the palatine tonsil to show the tongue and its topographic relationships.
A Tongue.
B Mandibular molar.
C Lower lip.
D Buccinator muscle.
E Buccal pad of fat.
F Ramus of mandible.
G Masseter muscle.
H Medial pterygoid muscle.
I Styloid group of muscles.
J Posterior belly of digastric muscle.
K Carotid sheath containing internal carotid artery, internal jugular vein and vagus nerve.
L Oropharynx.
M Palatopharyngeus muscle.

104 Median sagittal section through the head to show the tongue and floor of mouth.
A Hard palate.
B Soft palate.
C Upper lip and superior part of orbicularis oris muscle.
D Edentulous maxillary alveolar ridge.
E Pillars of fauces.
F Nasopharynx.
G Oropharynx.
H Laryngopharynx.
I Constrictor muscles of pharynx.
J Vertebral column.
K Lower lip with inferior part of orbicularis oris muscle.
L Body of mandible.
M Tongue.
N Genioglossus muscle.
O Geniohyoid muscle.
P Mylohyoid muscle.
Q Anterior belly of the digastric muscle.
R Platysma muscle.
S Hyoid bone.
T Epiglottis.

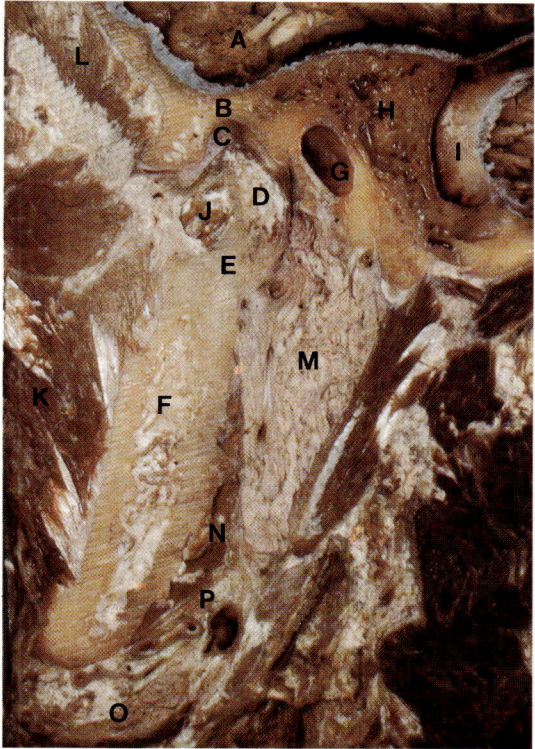
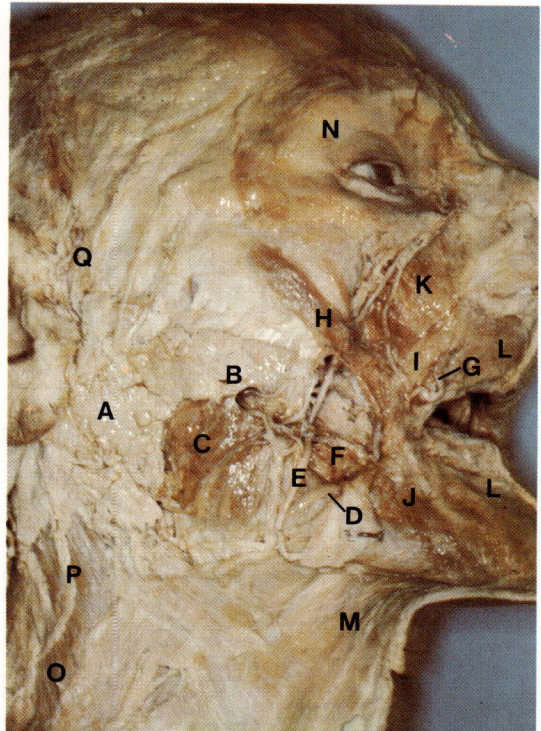
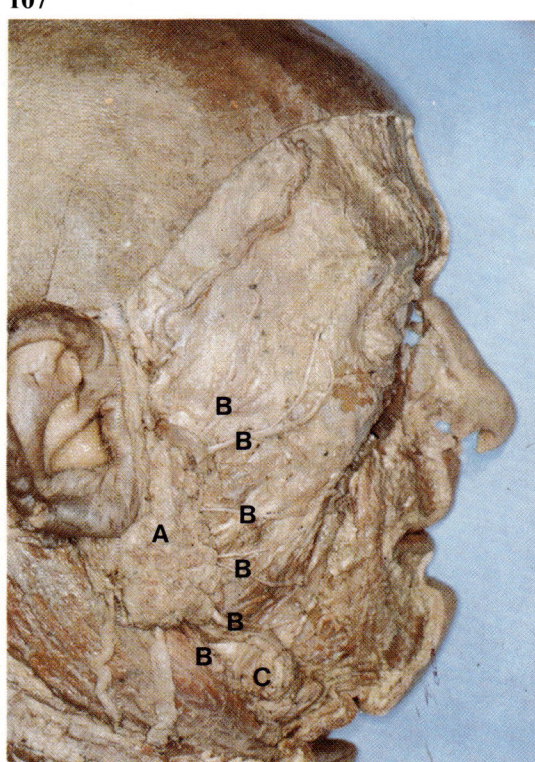

105 Section through ramus of the mandible to show the temporomandibular joint and its relationships.
A   Middle cranial fossa and temporal lobe of a cerebral hemisphere.
B   Glenoid fossa.
C   Disc of temporomandibular joint.
D   Head of condyle.
E   Neck of condyle.
F   Ramus of mandible.
G   External auditory meatus.
H   Mastoid air cells.
I   Sigmoid venous sinus.
J   Lateral pterygoid muscle.
K   Medial pterygoid muscle.
L   Temporalis muscle.
M   Parotid gland.
N   Masseter muscle.
O   Submandibular gland.
P   Facial artery and vein.

106 Superficial dissection of the face.
A   Parotid gland.
B   Accessory parotid gland and parotid duct.
C   Masseter muscle.
D   Facial artery.
E   Facial vein.
F   Buccinator muscle.
G   Superior labial artery.
H   Zygomaticus major muscle.
I   Levator anguli oris muscle.
J   Depressor anguli oris muscle.
K   Levator labii superioris muscle.
L   Orbicularis oris muscle.
M   Platysma muscle.
N   Orbicularis oculi muscle.
O   Sternocleidomastoid muscle.
P   Great auricular nerve.
Q   Superficial temporal vessels.

107 The parotid gland and submandibular gland (superficial view).
A   Parotid gland.
B   Branches of facial nerve emanating from parotid gland.
C   Submandibular gland.

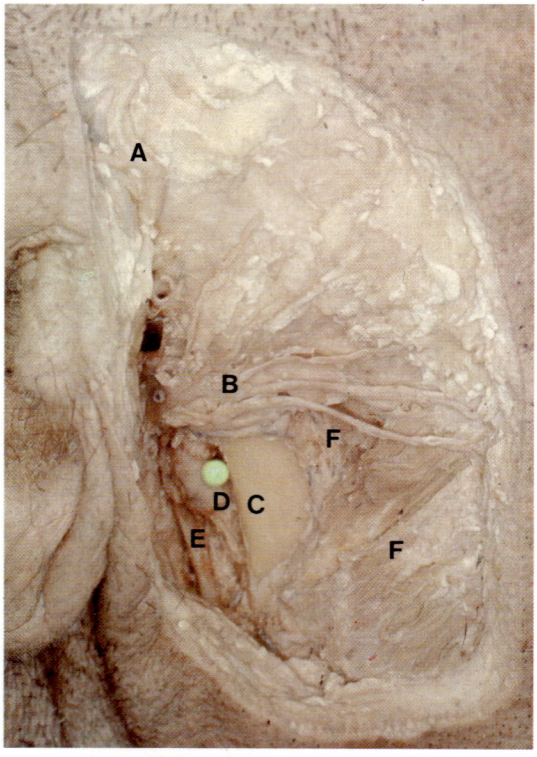

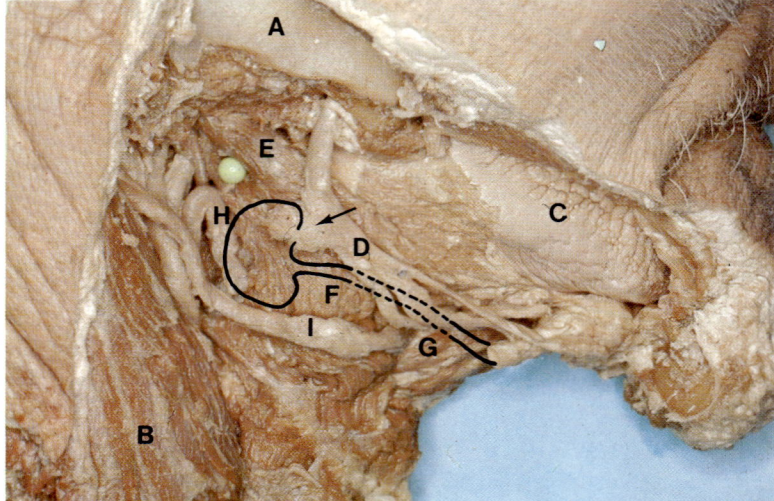

108 Deep dissection of the parotid region.
A Superficial temporal artery.
B Branches of facial nerve.
C Posterior border of ramus of mandible which is separated by a pin from:
D External carotid artery.
E Retromandibular vein.
F Masseter muscle.

109 Dissection of deep submandibular region. The body of the mandible has been removed and the position occupied by the deep part of the submandibular salivary gland and its duct is indicated by the solid black line.
A Ramus of mandible.
B Sternocleidomastoid muscle.
C Tongue.
D Lingual nerve with submandibular parasympathetic ganglion (*arrow*).
E Styloglossus muscle.
F Hyoglossus muscle.
G Genioglossus muscle.
H Lingual artery.
I Hypoglossal nerve.

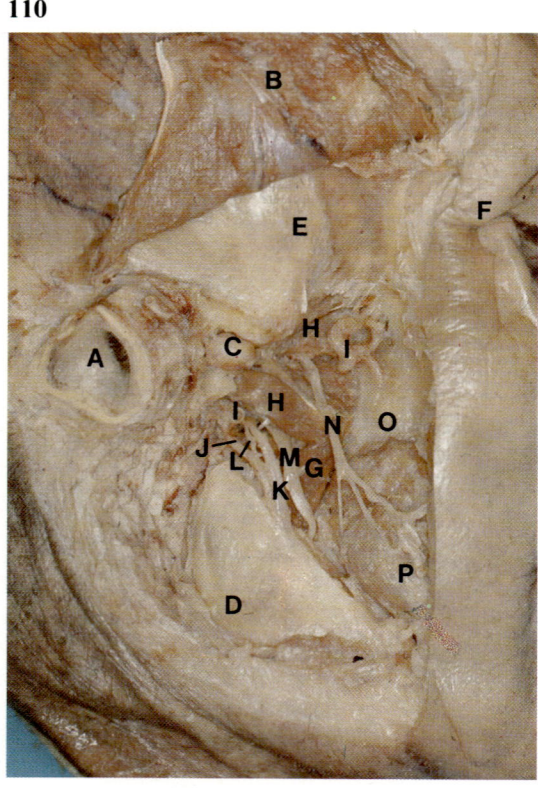

110 The infratemporal fossa is the space immediately deep to the ramus of the mandible. It is bounded medially by the superior constrictor muscle of the pharynx, anteriorly by the tuberosity of the maxilla and posteriorly by the deep part of the parotid gland and the carotid sheath and contents. The infratemporal fossa is continuous superiorly with the temporal fossa and inferiorly with the lateral pharyngeal space in the neck. The contents of the infratemporal fossa include the mandibular division of the trigeminal nerve and its branches, the maxillary artery and its branches, the medial and lateral pterygoid muscles and the pterygoid venous plexus. It is a site for injecting local anaesthetic solution around the inferior dental and lingual nerves. The dissection shows the contents of the infratemporal fossa and their relationships following removal of the ramus of the mandible and the parotid gland together with the reflection of the temporalis muscle.
A External auditory meatus.
B Reflected temporalis muscle.
C Condyle of mandible and disc at temporomandibular joint.
D External surface of angle of mandible.
E Squamous part of temporal bone.
F Outer canthus of eye.
G Medial pterygoid muscle.
H Lateral pterygoid muscle.
I Cut ends of maxillary artery.
J Inferior dental artery.
K Inferior dental nerve.
L Mylohyoid nerve.
M Lingual nerve.
N Buccal nerve.
O Tuberosity of maxilla.
P Buccinator muscle.

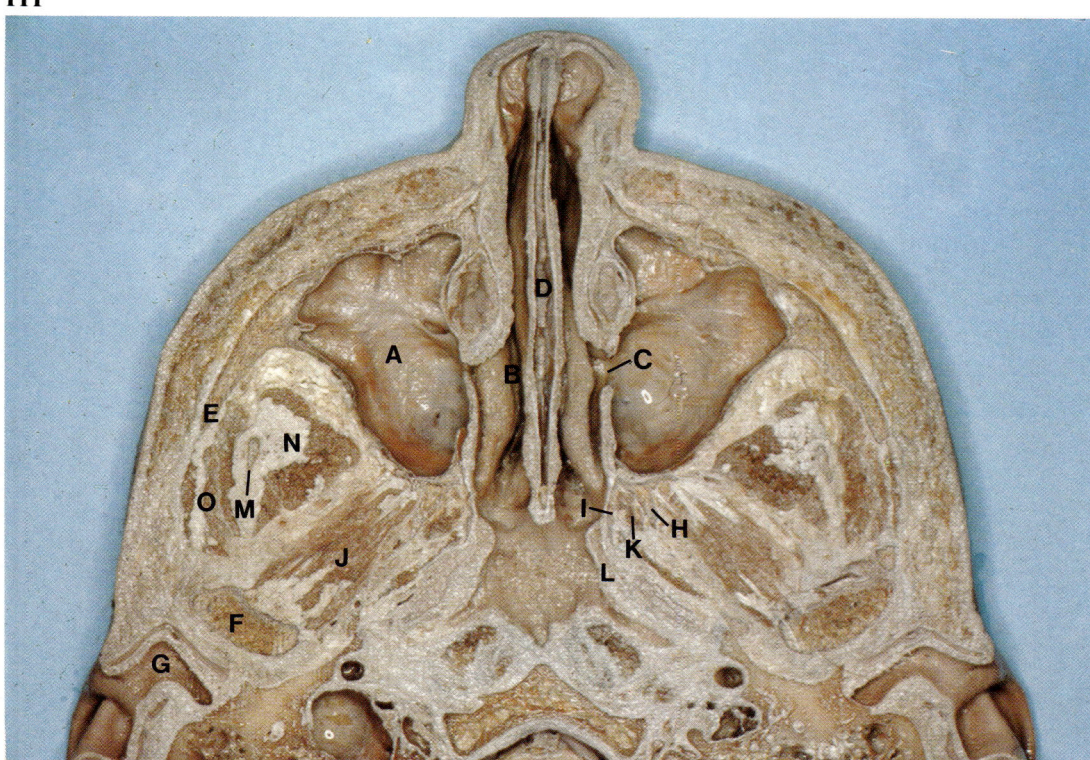

111 Transverse section through head to show the maxillary air sinuses and their topographic relationships.

A Floor of maxillary air sinus.
B Nasal fossa.
C Ostium – opening of maxillary sinus into middle meatus on the lateral wall of the nose.
D Nasal septum.
E Zygomatic arch.
F Condyle of mandible.
G External auditory meatus.
H Lateral pterygoid plate of sphenoid bone.
I Medial pterygoid plate of sphenoid bone.
J Lateral pterygoid muscle.
K Medial pterygoid muscle.
L Superior constrictor of pharynx.
M Coronoid process of mandible.
N Temporalis muscle.
O Masseter muscle.

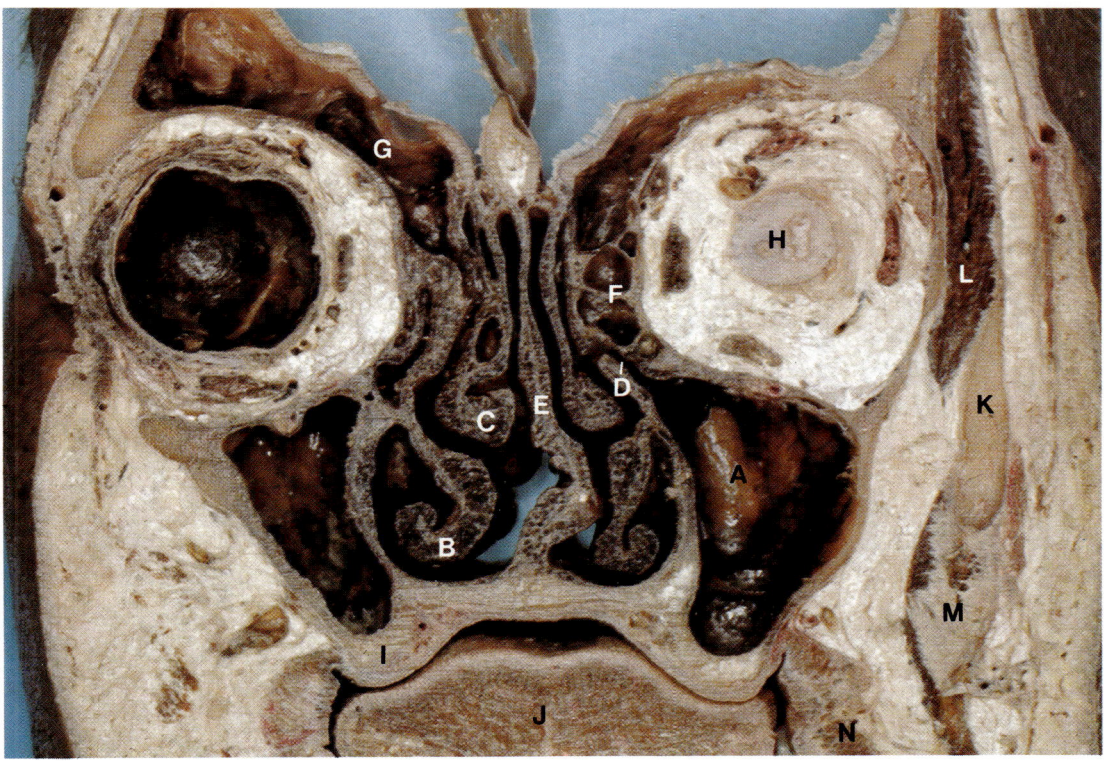

112 Coronal section through the head to show the maxillary air sinuses and their topographic relationships.

A Maxillary air sinus.
B Inferior concha on lateral wall of nose.
C Middle concha on lateral wall of nose.
D Ostium of maxillary air sinus.
E Nasal septum.
F Ethmoidal air cells.
G Frontal air sinus.
H Contents of orbit.
I Edentulous maxillary alveolus.
J Tongue.
K Zygomatic arch.
L Temporalis muscle.
M Masseter muscle.
N Buccinator muscle.

Tissue spaces around the jaws

The dissemination of infection in soft tissues is influenced by the natural barriers presented by bone, muscle and fascia. About the jaws are body compartments, the so-called tissue spaces, whose boundaries are primarily defined by the mylohyoid, buccinator, masseter, medial pterygoid, superior constrictor and orbicularis oris muscles. The fascial layers of the neck are less important in influencing the spread of infection around the jaws. None of the 'spaces' are actually empty; they are potential spaces normally occupied by loose connective tissue. It is only when inflammatory products destroy the loose connective tissue that an anatomically defined space is produced.

The most important potential spaces are:

Lower jaw
1. Submental.
2. Submandibular.
3. Sublingual.
4. Buccal.
5. Submasseteric.
6. Parotid.
7. Pterygomandibular.
8. Lateral pharyngeal.
9. Peritonsillar.

Upper jaw
10. Palatal.
11. Canine fossa.
12. Infratemporal.

113 The relationships of tissue spaces around the mandibular ramus.
1. Body of mandible bearing the molar teeth.
2. Ramus of mandible.
3. Buccinator muscle.
4. Mylohyoid muscle.
5. Buccal pad of fat.
6. Superior constrictor muscle.
7. Mucosa overlying palatal tonsil.
8. Medial pterygoid muscle.
9. Masseter muscle.
10. Parotid gland.
11. Stylomandibular ligament.
12. Base of skull.
A. Sublingual space in the floor of the mouth above the mylohyoid muscle which, over its posterior margin, leads to:
B. Submandibular space.
C. Buccal vestibule, delineated by the buccinator from:
D. Buccal space.
E. Submasseteric spaces formed by the multiple insertion of the masseter muscle on the lateral surface of the ramus.
F. Pterygomandibular space bounded by the lateral surface of the medial pterygoid muscle and the medial surface of the ramus.
G. Lateral pharyngeal space bounded by the superior constrictor of the pharynx and the medial surface of the medial pterygoid muscle.
H. Peritonsillar space bounded by the medial surface of the superior constrictor of the pharynx and its mucosa.
I. Parotid space in and around the parotid gland.

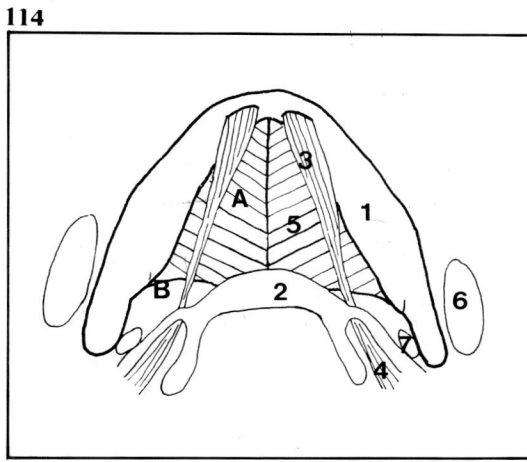

114 Inferior view of the submental and submandibular tissue spaces.
1. Body of mandible.
2. Hyoid bone.
3. Anterior belly of digastric muscle.
4. Posterior belly of digastric muscle.
5. Mylohyoid muscle.
6. Masseter muscle.
7. Medial pterygoid muscle.

A The submental space lying between the mylohyoid muscle and the investing layer of deep cervical fascia. Laterally, it is bounded by the two anterior bellies of the digastric muscles. The submental space communicates posteriorly with:
B The submandibular space.

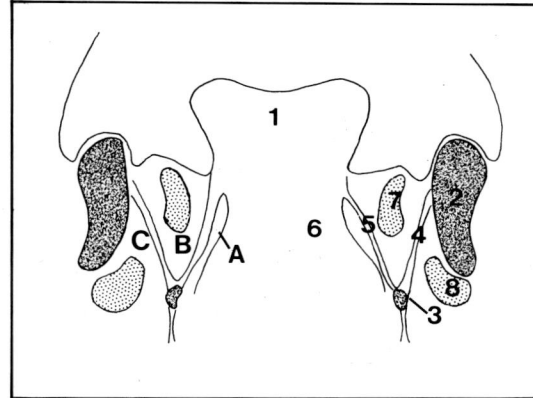

115 The relationships of a number of tissue spaces to the tongue.
1. Tongue.
2. Body of mandible.
3. Hyoid bone.
4. Mylohyoid muscle.
5. Hyoglossus.
6. Genioglossus.
7. Sublingual salivary gland.
8. Submandibular salivary gland.

A Cleft between genioglossus and hyoglossus muscles which communicates directly with the lateral pharyngeal space.
B Sublingual space between the mylohyoid and hyoglossus muscles.
C Submandibular space below the mylohyoid muscle.

In the anterior region of both the upper and lower jaws, the orbicularis oris muscle presents a barrier to pus between the vestibule on the oral side and the skin of the lip on the facial side.

In the upper jaw, pus may accumulate between the muscles of facial expression particularly in the canine fossa between the levator labii superioris and zygomaticus muscles.

The palatal space only exists when pus strips the mucoperiosteum from the underlying bone of the hard palate.

The infratemporal space is the upper extremity of the pterygomandibular space and is closely related to the maxillary tuberosity and, therefore, the upper molars.

The mode of spread of infections of dental origin through the bone of the jaws into the tissue spaces naturally depends upon the site at which the pus escapes the bone. Thus, a periapical abscess in a mandibular incisor which escapes inferior to the mylohyoid muscle will enter the submental space, while pus escaping superior to this muscle will enter the sublingual space. It should also be borne in mind that the tissue spaces are not discrete regions; they intercommunicate. Thus, a sublingual abscess may spread from the sublingual space over the posterior margin of the mylohyoid muscle into the submandibular space (see figure **113**). Furthermore, none of the muscle or fascial barriers defining the spaces are impenetrable.

The radiographic appearance of jaws and teeth

Dental radiography and radiology are concerned with the techniques of producing and interpreting photographic images of oro-dental tissues taken with X-rays. X-rays, being part of the spectrum of electromagnetic radiation, have a wavelength of approximately 10^{-8}cm compared with wavelengths around 10^{-4}cm for visible light. It is the short wavelengths which allow X-rays to penetrate materials which would otherwise absorb or reflect light. X-rays do not pass through all matter with similar ease. Materials composed of elements with low atomic numbers are readily penetrated by X-rays and are described as being radiolucent, whereas elements with high atomic numbers absorb X-rays and are termed radio-opaque. Thus, gases and soft tissues are radiolucent while calcified materials such as bone and teeth are radio-opaque. X-rays produce a photosensitisation reaction when they strike a silver-salt emulsion. When a radio-opaque structure is placed between a beam of X-rays and a photographic plate which is subsequently developed, the radio-opaque structure is 'mapped out' as a white area on the negative. It is because of the properties of tissue penetration and photosensitisation that X-rays can be used in dentistry to provide valuable information concerning underlying hard tissue structures not otherwise visible.

Because X-rays produce a shadow picture without a focus, a large object, such as a skull, does not show all its features equally distinctly on a radiograph. As a general rule, structures nearest the photographic plate appear clearer than those some distance from the plate. Superimposition may also make interpretation of radiographs difficult, for most radiographs are two-dimensional representations of three-dimensional objects. Care must be taken not to overinterpret radiographs by diagnosing pathological conditions without recourse to other diagnostic aids or clinical findings. The prime use of a radiograph is, therefore, to describe gross topographic features.

Radiographic projections describing jaws and teeth

Extra-oral

Projection/technique	Purpose
Posteroanterior skull (PA)	Survey of facial bones and mandible.
Anteroposterior skull (AP)	Survey of posterior part of cranium, mandible and temporomandibular articulation.
Reverse Towne's	Anatomy of mandibular condyles and temporomandibular articulation.
Occipitomental skull	Survey of facial bones and air sinuses.
Lateral skull	Survey of lateral regions of face, cranium and mandible. View of facial profile and covering soft tissues.
Lateral skull with cephalostat	Recording of relationships between teeth, jaws and cranial base.
Lateral oblique view of mandible	Survey of posterior regions of body of mandible and ramus.
Orthopantomogram	A tomogram to display the whole of maxilla, mandible and the dentition on a single film.
Transcranial temporomandibular joint	Movement of mandibular condyles in glenoid fossae.
Sialography	Infusion of radio-opaque material into the main salivary ducts to study their structure and distribution.
Tomography	Technique for the radiography of selected areas which under standard radiographic technique are obscured by superimposition of other structures e.g. temporomandibular joint and air sinuses.

Intra-oral

Projection/techniques	Purpose
Maxillary and mandibular occlusal views of teeth	Relationships of structures in buccolingual plane.
Periapical view of teeth	Examination of apices of teeth. Relationships of structures in mesiodistal plane.
Bitewing examination of teeth	Survey of crowns of the teeth and the alveolar crests.

Extra-oral radiographic projections of jaws and related structures

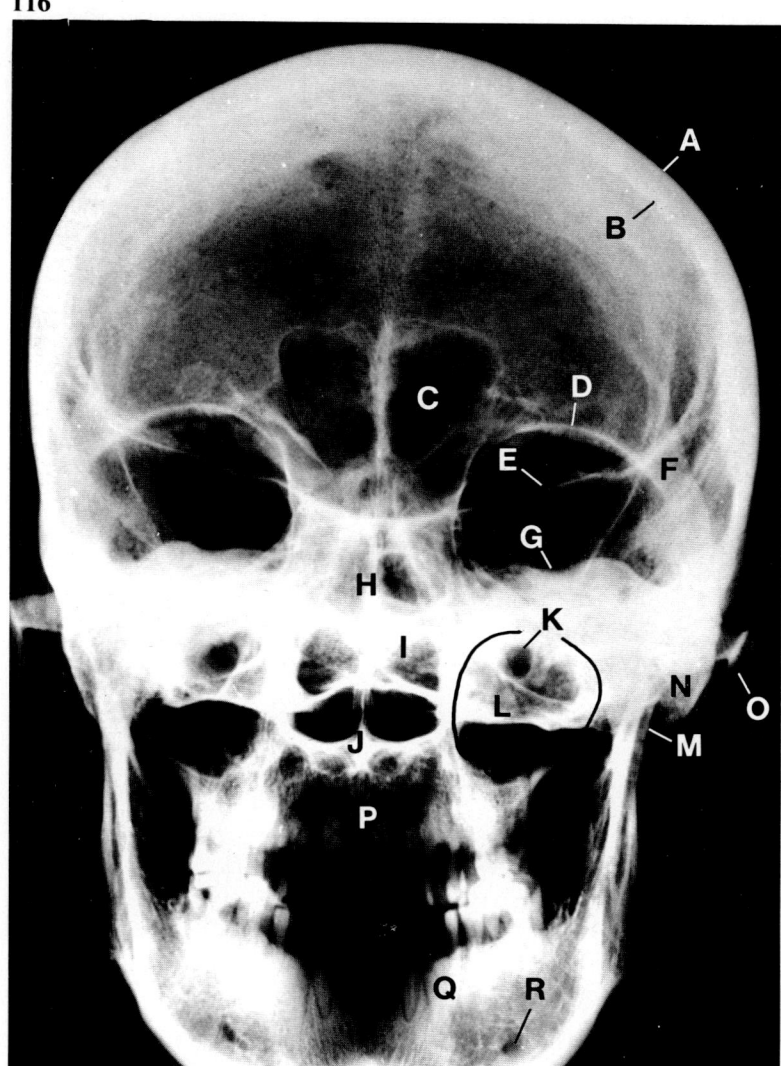

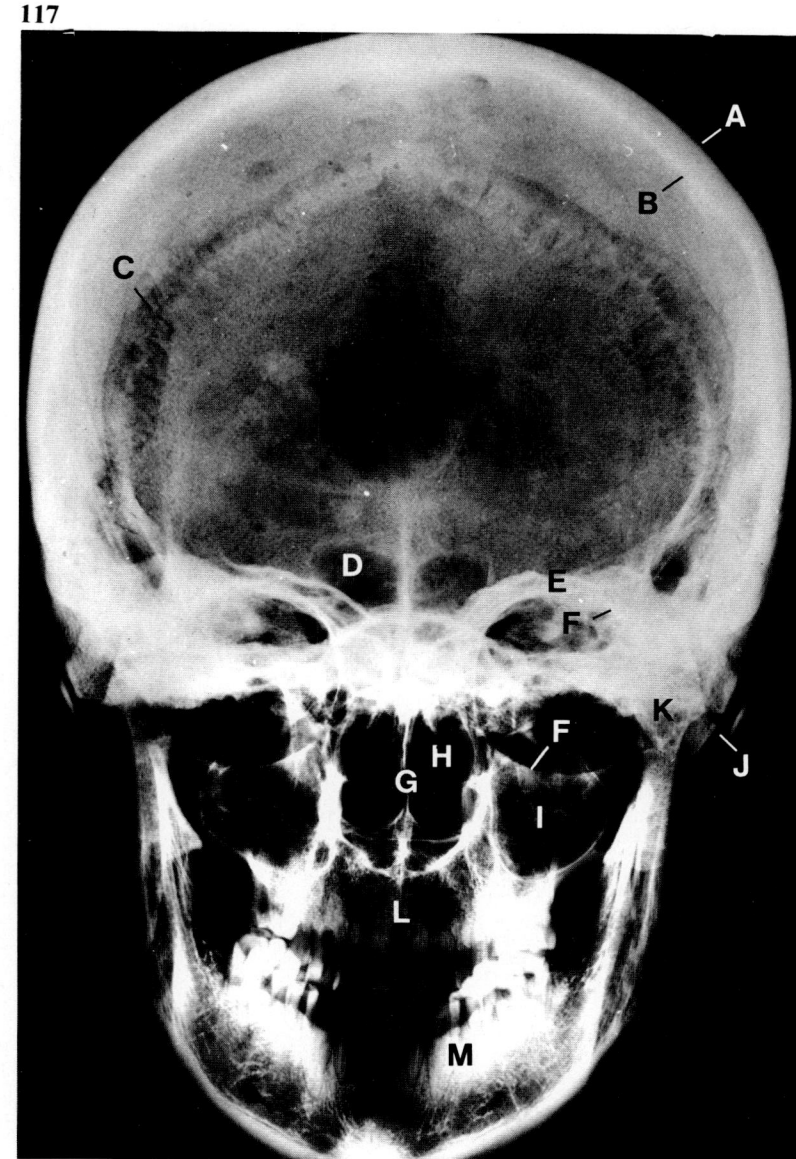

116 Posteroanterior view of skull (PA).
A Outer table of cranium.
B Inner table of cranium.
C Frontal air sinus.
D Superior rim of orbit.
E Sphenoid ridge in middle cranial fossa.
F Zygomatic process of frontal bone.
G Petrous ridge.
H Nasal septum.
I Nasal fossa.
J Anterior nasal spine.
K Infraorbital foramen.
L Maxillary air sinus.
M Neck of mandibular condyle.
N Mastoid process of temporal bone.
O Zygomatic arch.
P Maxilla and teeth.
Q Body of mandible and teeth.
R Mental foramen.

117 Anteroposterior view of skull (AP).
A Outer table of cranium.
B Inner table of cranium.
C Lambdoid suture.
D Frontal air sinus.
E Superimposed sphenoid, petrous and supraorbital ridges.
F Rim of orbit.
G Nasal septum.
H Nasal fossa.
I Maxillary air sinus.
J Zygoma.
K Condyle of mandible.
L Maxilla and teeth.
M Body of mandible and teeth.

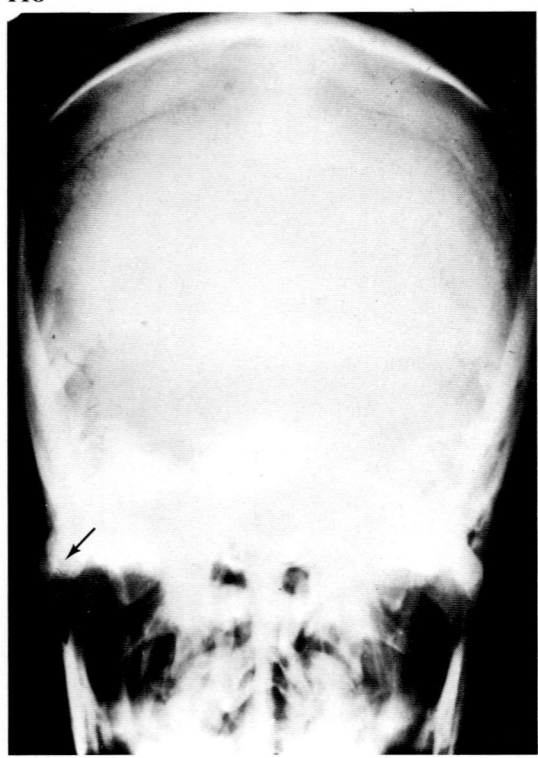

118 Reverse Towne's view showing position of mandibular condyle (*arrowed*).

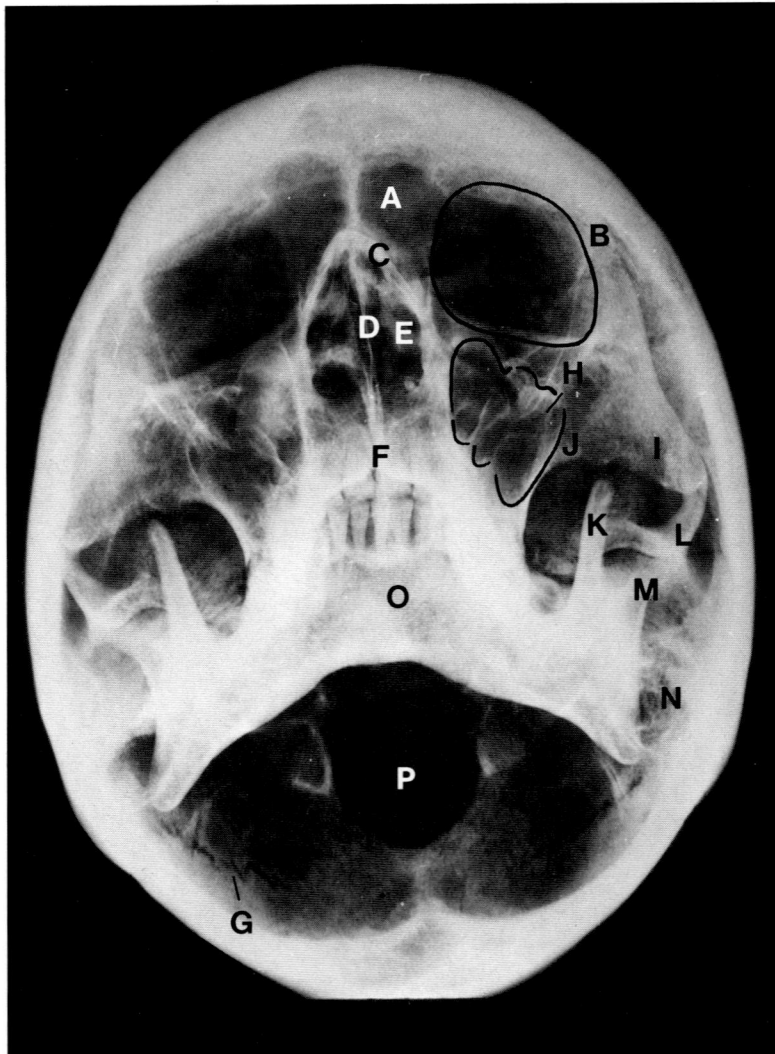

119 Occipitomental view of skull (OM 30 degrees).

A Frontal air sinus.
B Outline of orbit.
C Nasal bones.
D Nasal septum.
E Nasal fossa with superimposed shadows of ethmoidal air cells.
F Maxilla and teeth.
G Lambdoid suture.
H Malar extension of maxillary sinus.
I Zygoma.
J Outline of maxillary air sinus.
K Coronoid process of mandible.
L Zygomatic process of temporal bone.
M Condyle of mandible.
N Mastoid air cells.
O Body of mandible and teeth.
P Foramen magnum.

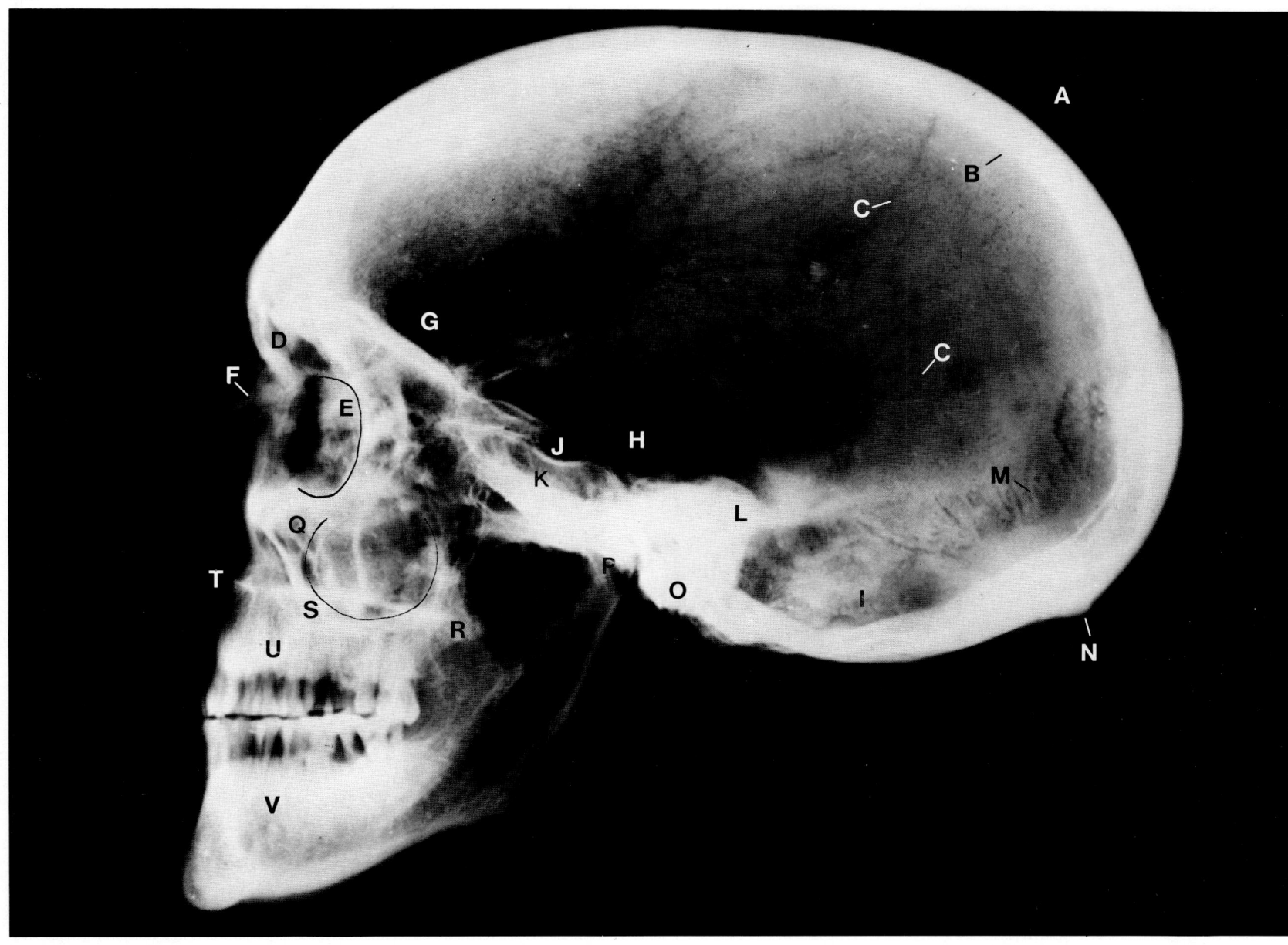

120 Lateral skull radiograph.
A Outer table of cranium.
B Inner table of cranium.
C Depressions in cranium related to middle meningeal vessels.
D Frontal air sinus.
E Margins of orbit.
F Nasal bone.
G Anterior cranial fossa.
H Middle cranial fossa.
I Posterior cranial fossa.
J Hypophyseal fossa.
K Sphenoid air sinus.
L Petrous ridge.
M Lamdboid suture.
N External occipital protuberance.
O Mastoid process.
P Condyle of mandible.
Q Margin of maxillary air sinuses.
R Coronoid process of mandible.
S Hard palate.
T Anterior nasal spine.
U Maxilla and teeth.
V Body of mandible and teeth.

Cephalometric analysis of lateral skull radiographs

Lateral skull radiographs are frequently used in dentistry to assess general skeletal morphology, particularly for recording relationships between the jaws and cranial base. Should measurements be necessary, the position of the head must be standardised using a cephalostat (headholder) so that the beam of X-rays is shot in a predetermined plane to the head from a standard distance.

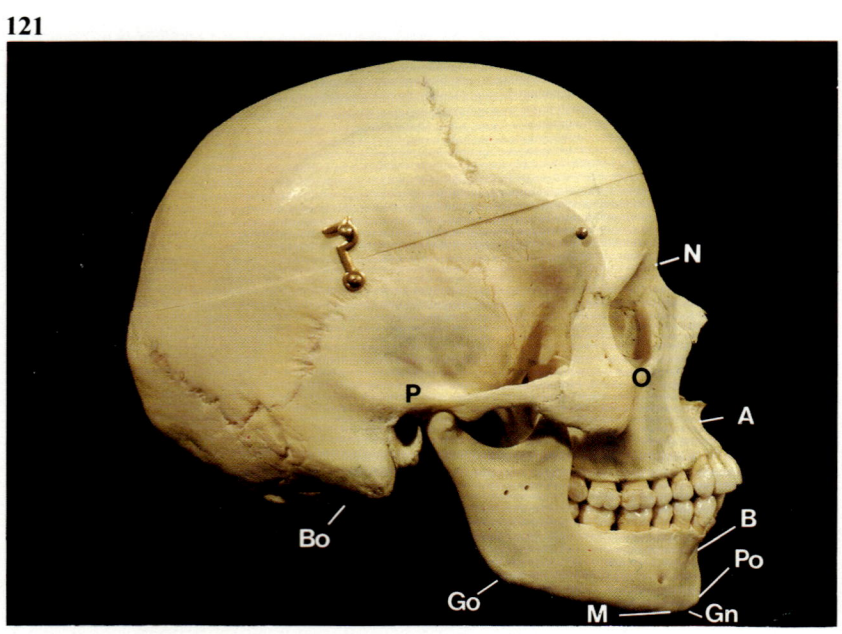

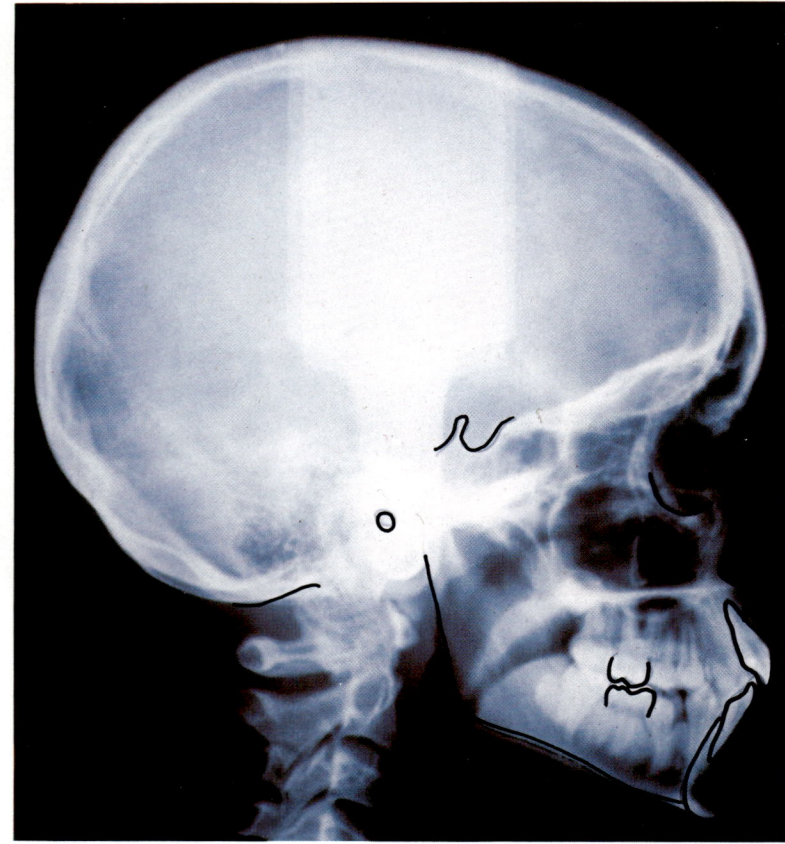

121 Lateral view of skull illustrating the more common anthropometric landmarks used in dental cephalometry.

Nasion (N)	Junction between frontal and nasal bones in midline on the frontonasal suture.
Porion (P)	Highest bony point of margin of external auditory meatus.
Orbitale (O)	The lowest point of the infraorbital margin.
Sella point (S)	Centre of shadow of sella turcica.
Bolton point (Bo)	Highest point of notch immediately posterior to occipital condyles.
Subspinale (A point)	Position of greatest concavity of maxillary alveolus in midline.
Supramentale (B point)	Position of greatest concavity of mandibular alveolus in midline.
Pogonion (Po)	Most anterior point on the chin.
Menton (M)	Lowest point of chin.
Gnathion (Gn)	Midpoint between the most anterior and inferior points of chin.
Gonion (Go)	Most inferior and posterior point at the angle of the mandible. Established by bisecting the angle formed between planes through the lower border of the mandible and posterior border of ramus.

122 Lateral skull radiograph taken using a cephalostat with tracing showing positions of anthropometric landmarks.

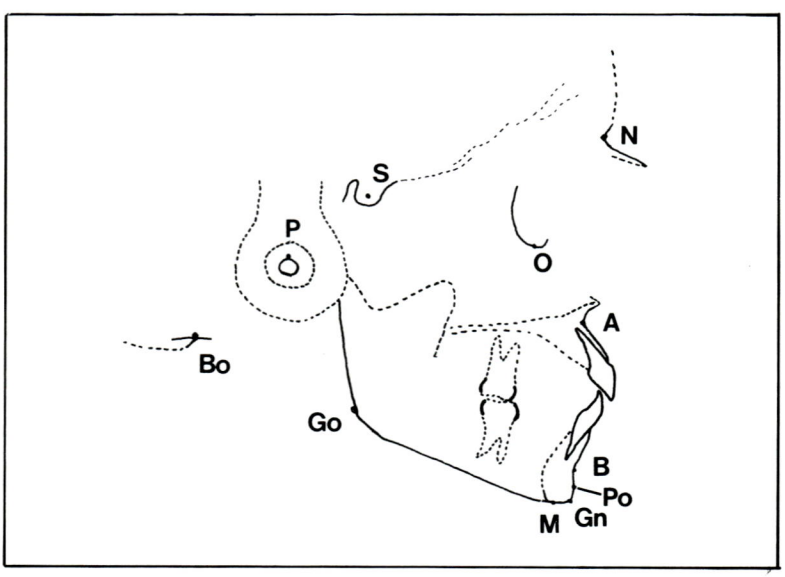

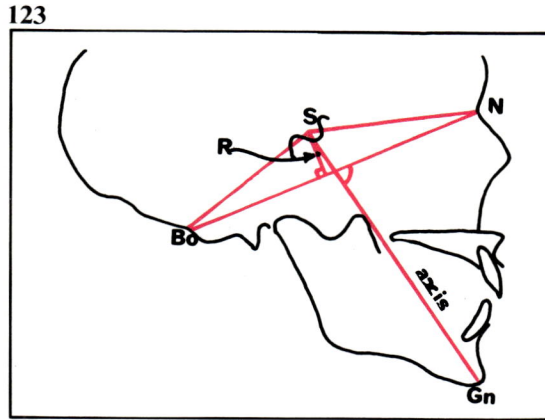

123 Planes and angles used in cephalometric growth studies. In the growing child, every bone of the skull shows some degree of growth and consequently no point can be considered 'fixed'. However, for analytical convenience several landmarks are used by convention to study the degree and direction of cranial growth.

The sella-nasion plane (S-N). This plane may be used as a baseline for growth studies.

The Bolton plane (B-N) is more commonly used as a baseline than the S-N plane and is said to delineate the cranial base.

The registration point (R) is determined by dropping a line from the sella point perpendicular to the Bolton plane. The midpoint of this line is the Registration point. It is considered by some to be a relatively fixed point at which superimposition of successive films of the same individual at differing ages can provide information concerning the pattern of growth of the individual (see figure **397**).

The Y-axis refers to a line from the sella point to gnathion which has been used to describe the general direction of facial growth. The angle between the Bolton plane and the Y-axis has been used to assess changes in growth direction.

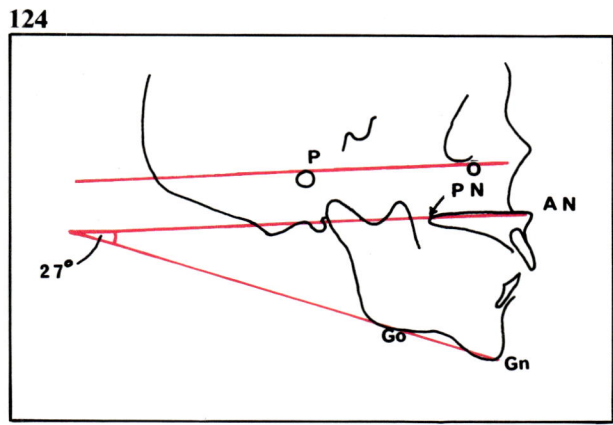

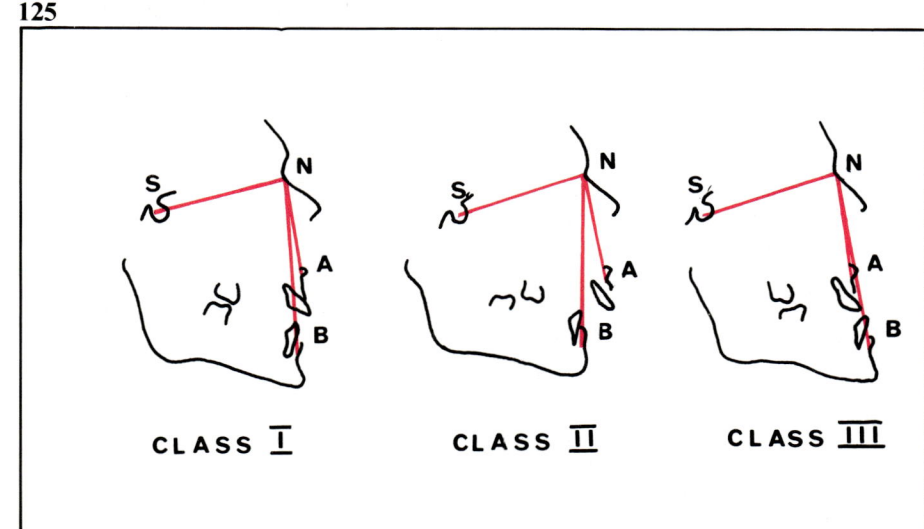

124 Cephalometric analysis of jaw relationships. The mandibular plane passes through the menton and gonion. It may be used in conjunction with the Frankfort, maxillary and S-N planes to give a measure of the vertical development of the anterior part of the face. The Frankfort plane extends from the orbitale to the porion. The Frankfort-mandibular angle in 'normal' subjects is said to be approximately 27 degrees. The maxillary plane extends from the anterior nasal spine (AN) to the posterior nasal spine (PN) and is easier to identify on a lateral skull radiograph than the Frankfort plane. Both the maxillary-mandibular plane angle and the mandibular-cranial base (B-N) angle are of the same order as the Frankfort-mandibular plane angle.

125 The use of SÑA and SÑB angles to record maxillary/mandibular skeletal relationships. Since the cranial base is said to undergo only very small degrees of change in the later years of childhood and beyond, it provides a useful basis for measuring the relationships of facial and dentoalveolar structures. The subspinale (A point) and supramentale (B point) represent the junctions of the maxillary and mandibular alveoli with their basal bone. Because of the ease of identification on lateral skull radiographs, the subspinale and supramentale are useful landmarks for recording maxillary and mandibular relationships with the S-N plane.

The angles SÑA and SÑB described the degree of prognathism relative to the cranial base. Where SÑA-SÑB difference is 2–5 degrees, the skeletal relationship between the maxilla and mandible is Class I (diagram i). Where SÑA-SÑB difference is greater than 5 degrees, the skeletal relationship is Class II (diagram ii). Where SÑB-SÑB difference is less than 2 degrees, the skeletal relationship is Class III (diagram iii). Should SNA be significantly different from 78 degrees, a correction must be made before assigning a SNA-SNB difference to a specific skeletal class.

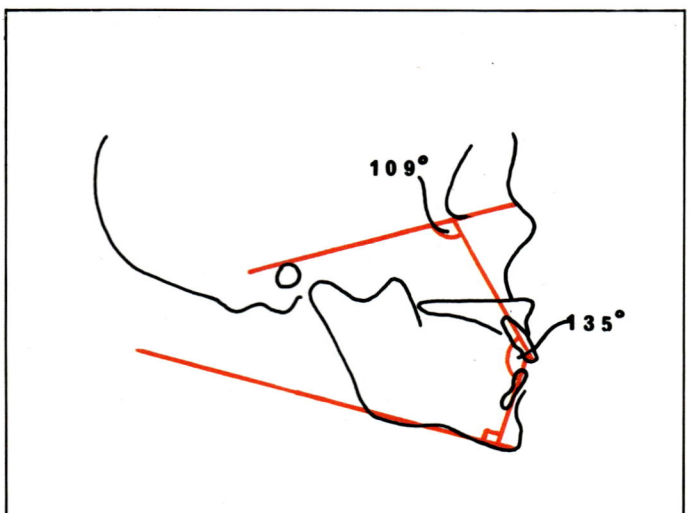

126 The inclination of the upper incisors may be determined by the angle between a line drawn through the longitudinal axis of the upper central incisors and the Frankfort plane. This angle is, on average, 109 degrees. The inclination of the lower incisors is determined as the angle formed by the longitudinal axis of the lower central incisors to the mandibular plane. It is approximately a right angle. The incisal angle formed by the junction of the longitudinal axes of the upper and lower central incisors is of the order of 135 degrees.

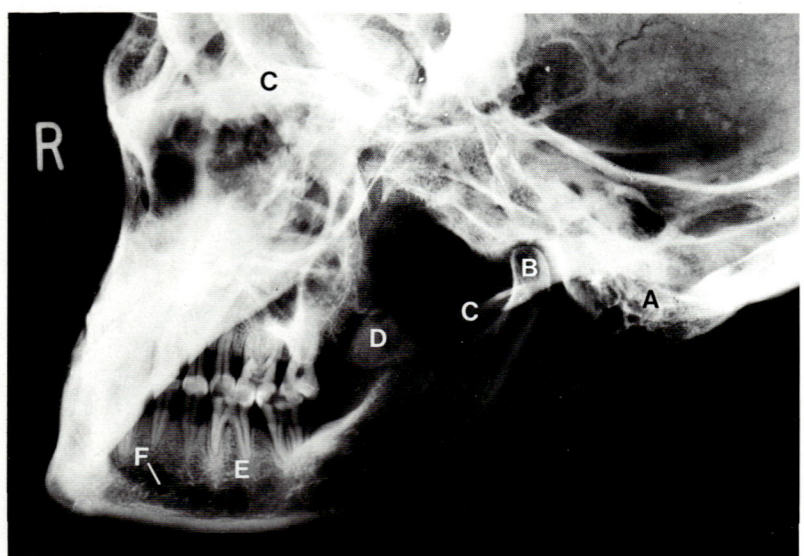

127 Lateral oblique view of mandible.
A Mastoid process of temporal bone.
B Condyle of mandible lying in glenoid fossa of temporomandibular joint.
C Zygomatic arch.
D Shadow of mandibular coronoid process on maxillary tuberosity.
E Body of mandible showing teeth posterior to premolars.
F Mental foramen.

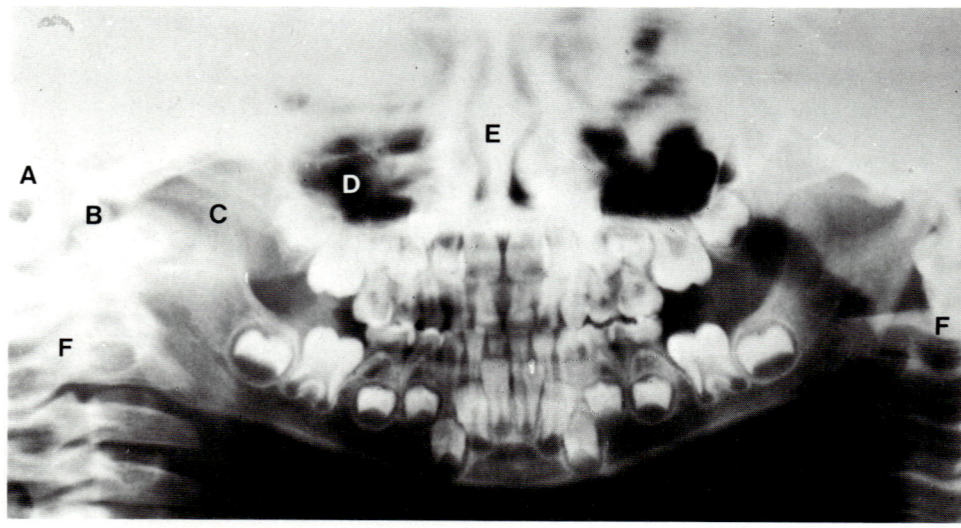

128 Orthopantomogram. A panoramic radiographic survey of the jaws and teeth. Dentition is radiographed at 6 years of age.
A External auditory meatus.
B Mandibular condyle.
C Coronoid process of mandible.
D Maxillary air sinus.
E Nasal cavity.
F Vertebral column.

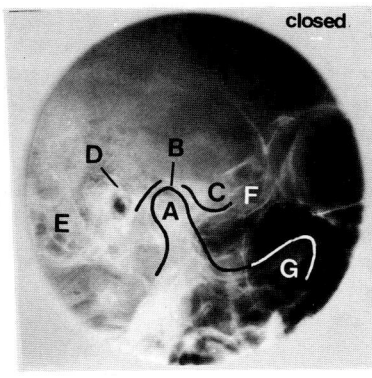

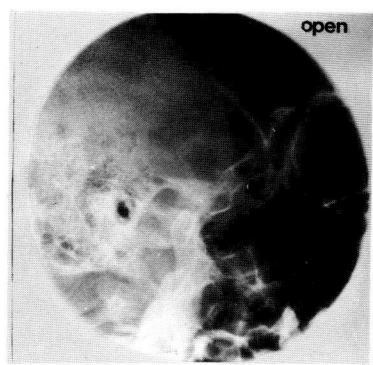

130 Sialogram. Parotid glands, lateral view. A radio-opaque oil suspension of iodine-containing compounds has been introduced bilaterally into the parotid ducts.

131 Sialogram. Right parotid gland, anteroposterior view.

129 Transcranial temporomandibular articulation (mouth closed and open).
A Mandibular condyle.
B T.M.J. cavity space.
C Articular tubercle.
D External auditory meatus.
E Mastoid air cells.
F Zygomatic arch.
G Coronoid process.

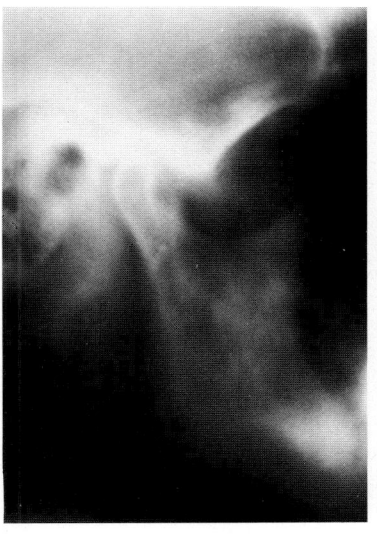

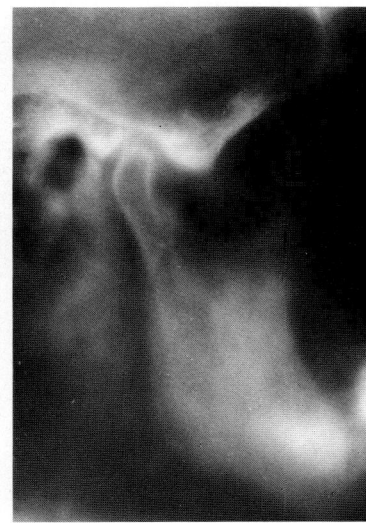

132 Tomographic examination of the temporomandibular articulation. Tomography is a radiographic technique used to study layers within a volume of tissue, in a way analogous to the examination of a single portion of bread within a whole loaf without physically slicing it. The two pictures of the temporomandibular joint illustrated here represent two layers in this region approximately 0.5cm apart.

Intra-oral radiographic projections of jaws and teeth

133 Maxillary occlusal view – nasal approach (A) and vertex approach (B). As the names suggest, the vertex and nasal occlusal views of the maxilla essentially differ in the positioning of the X-ray tube which is either to the vertex of the skull or to the nasion. Differences in the radiographic pictures obtained relate to the degree of superimposition (greater in the vertex occlusal) and the direction and proportions of the longitudinal axes of the teeth (more vertical and less distorted roots with the vertex occlusal). In addition to surveying the maxillary dentition, the maxillary occlusal views may also be used to define the nasal fossae and maxillary air sinuses.

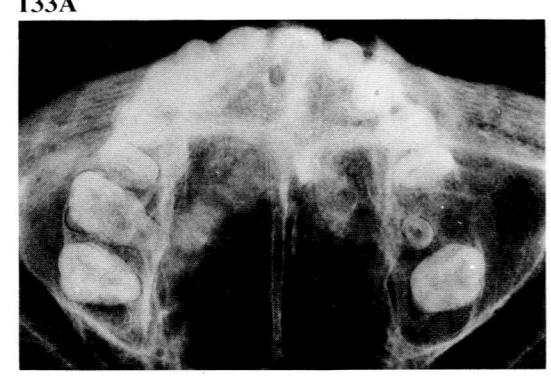
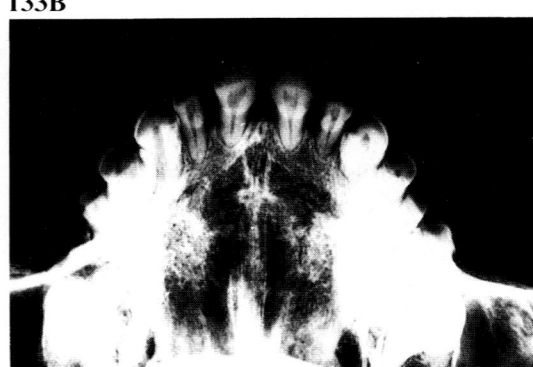
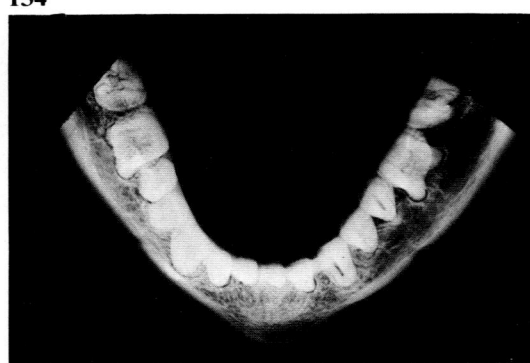
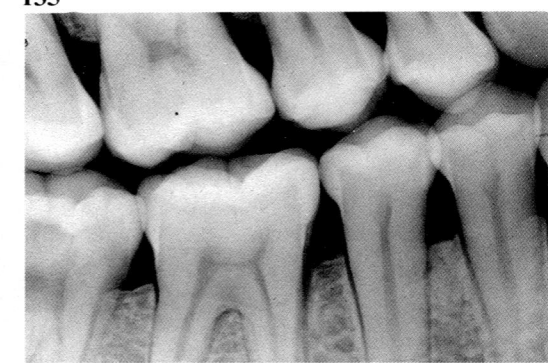

134 Mandibular occlusal view.

135 Examination of the crowns of the permanent molars and associated alveolar crests using bitewing radiographs.

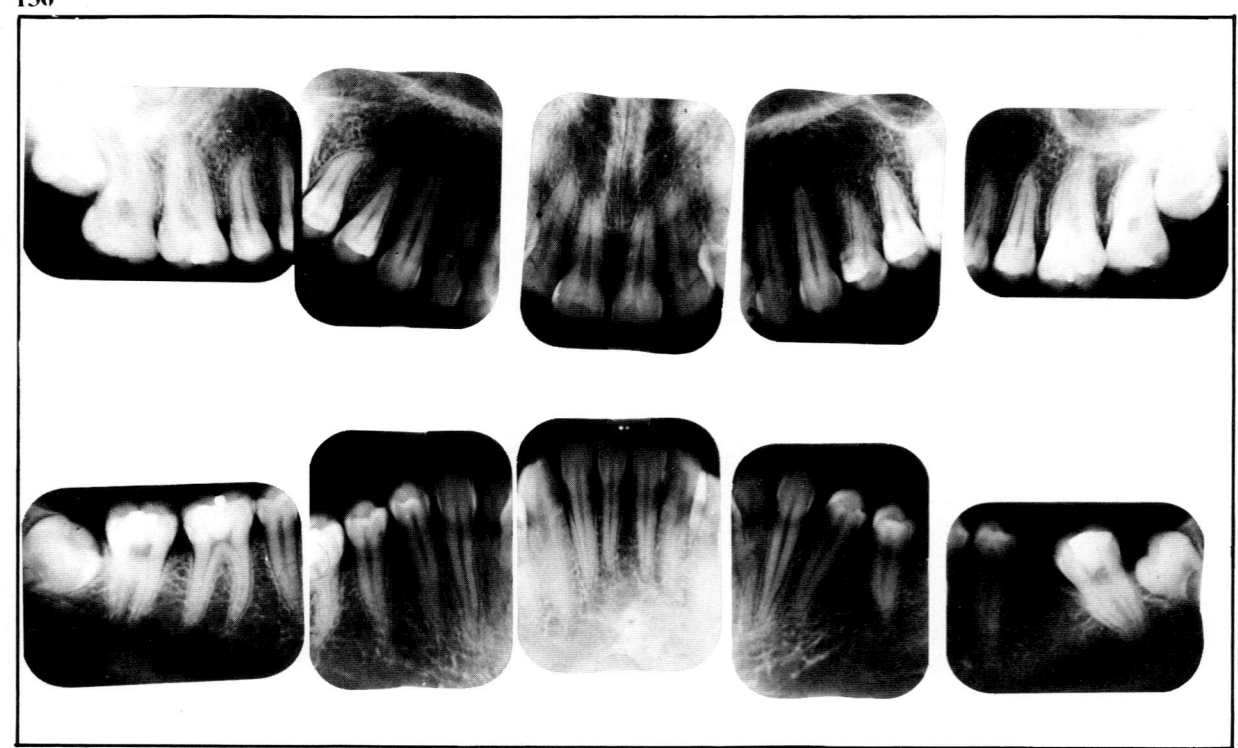

136 Intra-oral survey of the permanent dentition with periapical views of the teeth.

Anatomical features seen on intra-oral radiographs

The importance of appreciating the radiographic appearance of the teeth and their supporting tissues need hardly be emphasised. However, as essential for the interpretation of an apparent divergence from the normal is an awareness of non-dental anatomical structures which, to the unwary, may simulate pathological lesions on intra-oral radiographs.

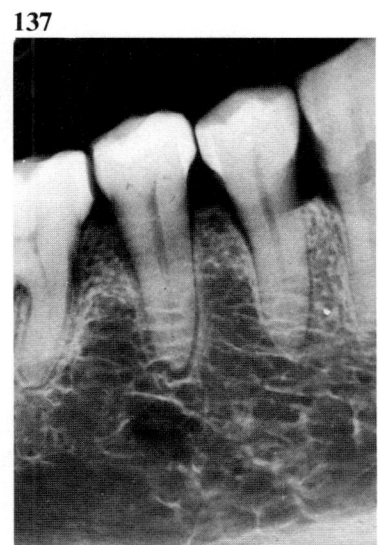

137

Radio-opacity of normal anatomical structures seen on intra-oral radiographs

Radiolucent	Radio-opaque
Dental pulp	Enamel
Gingiva and periodontal ligament	Dentine
Bone marrow	Cementum
	Cortical bony plates
	Lamina dura
Maxillary sinus	Bony walls of maxillary sinus
Nasal cavity	Bony walls of nasal cavity
Incisive foramen	Nasal septum
Median palatine suture	Anterior nasal spine
Intermaxillary suture	Maxillary tuberosity
Nasolacrimal canal	Zygomatic arch
	Coronoid process
	Pterygoid hamulus
Mandibular canal	Internal and external oblique lines of mandible
Mental foramen	Borders of mandibular canal
Mandibular symphysis	Mental and canine prominence
	Genial tubercles
Bony depressions e.g. mental and sub-mandibular fossa	
Nutrient canals	

137 Radiographic image of a tooth. Tooth substance absorbs more X-rays than any other tissue of comparable size and thickness. Enamel is the most radio-opaque and is easily distinguished, covering the anatomical crown of the tooth. In normal teeth, the enamel is of uniform density though in some areas where the enamel is thin, e.g. the cervical regions, it may appear relatively radiolucent. Such an appearance may easily be misinterpreted as dental caries. Dentine and cementum cannot be readily distinguished radiographically from each other because of their similar capacity to absorb X-rays. Owing to the lower radio-opacity of dentine, it appears comparatively 'greyer' than the enamel and the amelodental junction is clearly demarcated. The pulp of a tooth, being soft tissue, is readily penetrated by X-rays and consequently, on a radiograph, the pulp cavity is clearly defined as the central radiolucent region of the tooth. However, because of distortion, foreshortening and superimposition, care should be taken in assessing the pulpal anatomy from radiographs. The tooth is supported in the bony alveolus. In this text, the alveolus refers to the whole of the bony supporting tissue of the tooth, and the lamina dura refers to the compact bone lining the tooth socket. The morphology of the gingival margins of the alveolus (alveolar crest) is important in the diagnosis of periodontal disease. As a general rule, the width of the crest depends upon the distance the teeth are separated. Consequently, between the molars the crests are flat and horizontal while between the incisors the crests rise only as points or spines. In the healthy situation, the crest rises to the level of the cemento-enamel junction. The lamina dura is considered to be a very important structure in the radiographic interpretation of periodontal and periapical pathologies. It appears as a continuous, radio-opaque lining of the socket and usually is continuous over the alveolar crests. Discontinuity of the lamina dura in the root region is usually indicative of abnormality or disease. Between the root of the tooth and the lamina dura of the socket is the connective tissue of the periodontal ligament which appears as a thin radiolucent region.

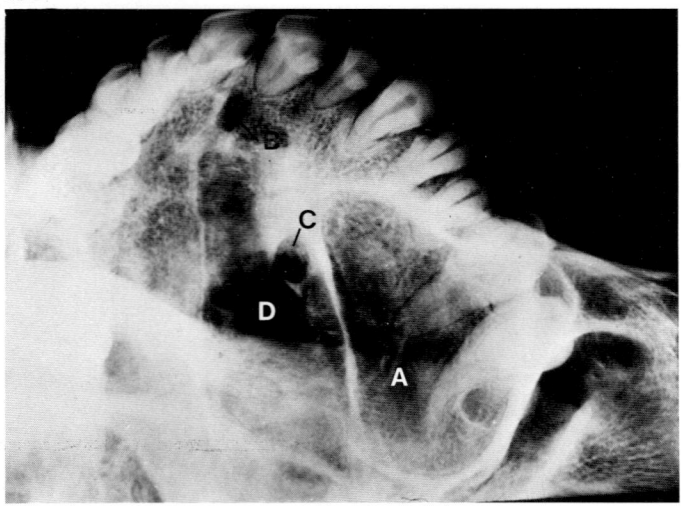

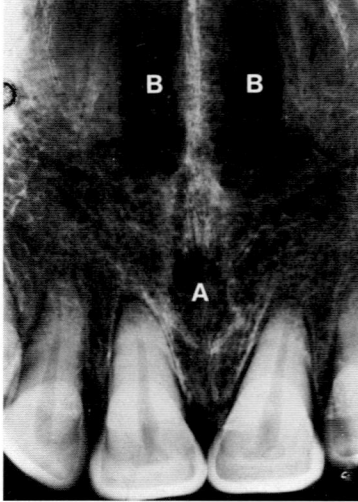

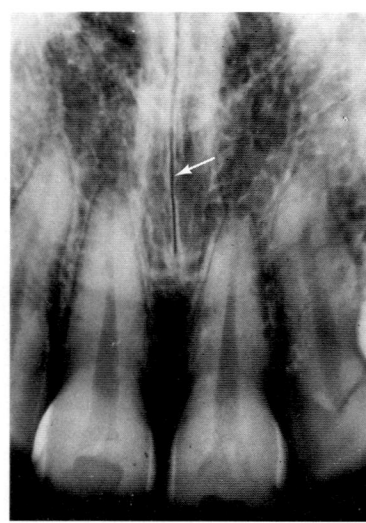

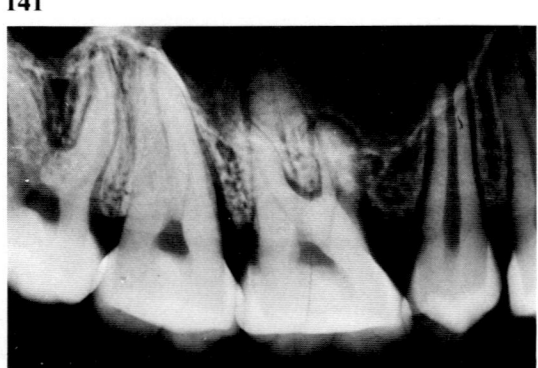

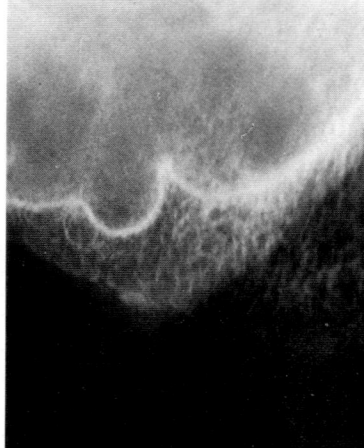

138 Radiolucent, anatomical features seen on an intra-oral, maxillary occlusal oblique view.
A Maxillary antrum.
B Incisive foramen.
C Nasolacrimal canal.
D Nasal fossa.

139 The incisive foramen (A) and nasal fossae (B) seen on an intra-oral periapical view of the maxillary central incisors.

140 The median palatine suture (*arrowed*) seen on an intra-oral periapical view of the maxillary central incisors.

141 The floor of the maxillary antrum seen on an intraoral periapical view of the maxillary premolars and molars. The maxillary antrum or sinus is an air-filled cavity of varying dimensions which appears radiographically as a dark, radiolucent shadow bounded by radio-opaque lines representing the lining layers of cortical bone. The radiolucency is not usually uniform because of superimposition of the zygomatic process and the soft tissues of the cheek. The antrum often presents not as a single sinus but as several compartments due to bony septation. It is said that the cortical lining of the antrum is not continuous but exhibits numerous, small, linear interruptions associated with nutrient canals (figure **147**). This radiographic characteristic may be important in avoiding misinterpreting the sinus as a pathological lesion. The floor of the antrum is closely related to the root apices of the maxillary teeth. It is generally stated that the sinus extends from the premolars to the tuberosity, though variations are frequent. Because of the close relationship of the teeth to the antrum, communication between the antrum and the oral cavity (oroantral fistula) following tooth extractions are unfortunately all too frequent. Because of the problems of interpreting 3-dimensional situations on a 2-dimensional radiograph, care must be taken to avoid misreading the relationship of the teeth to the antrum.

142 The maxillary antrum seen on an intra-oral view of an edentulous maxillary tuberosity.

143 The configuration termed **the Y-of-Ennis** is formed by the abutment of the anterior wall of the antrum and the floor of the nasal fossa.

144 Malar shadow. The shadow (*arrowed*) is seen on an intra-oral periapical view of the maxillary molars.

145 Radio-opaque shadow cast by a coronoid process. The shadow (*arrowed*) is superimposed on a maxillary tuberosity.

146 Shadows of the pterygoid plates (A) and pterygoid hamulus (B) near the maxillary tuberosity.

147 Nutrient canals (*arrows*) in the walls of the maxillary antrum.

148 The mandibular symphysis at birth (*arrowed*) shown on an intra-oral mandibular occlusal radiograph.

149 The genial tubercles (*arrowed*) seen on an intra-oral periapical view of the mandibular central incisors. Note the characteristic radiographic appearance of the tubercles, i.e. a radiolucent dot surrounded by a distinct radio-opaque region.

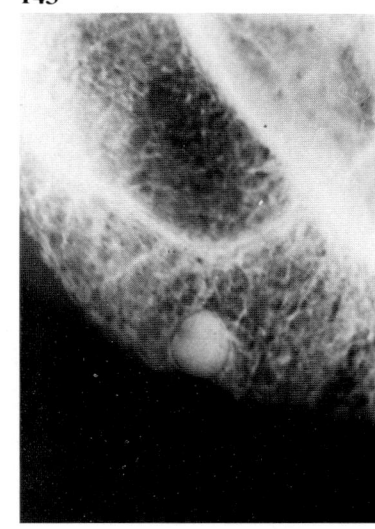
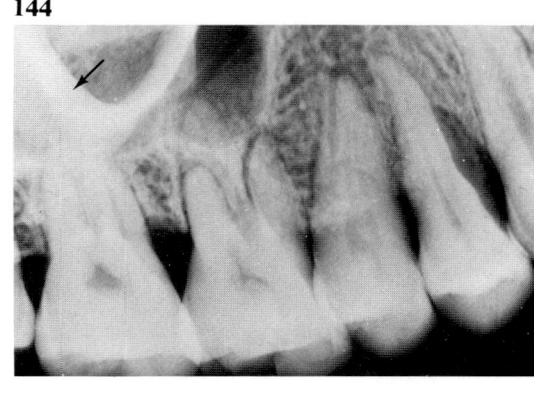
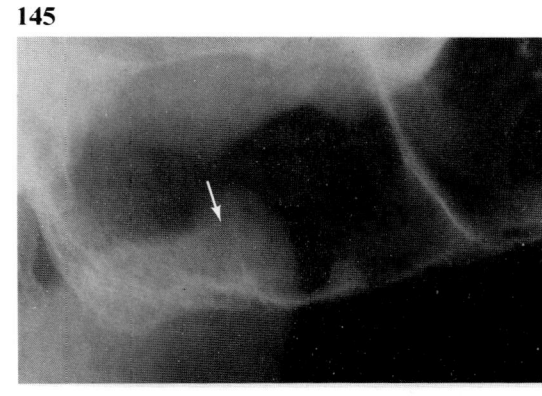
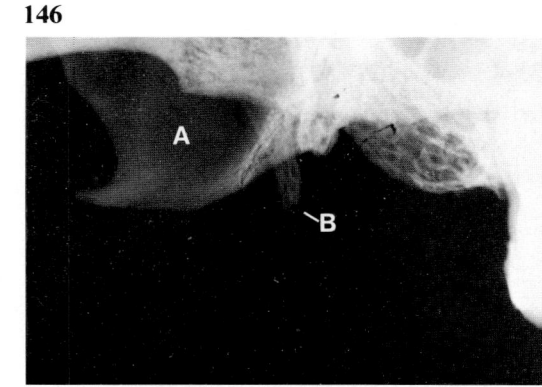
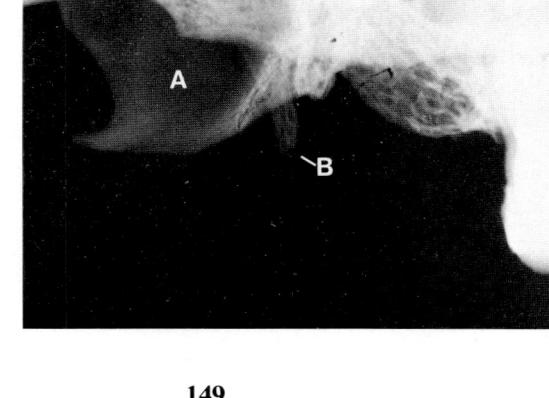
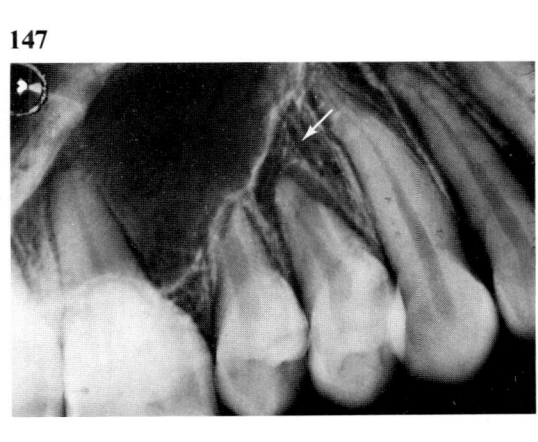
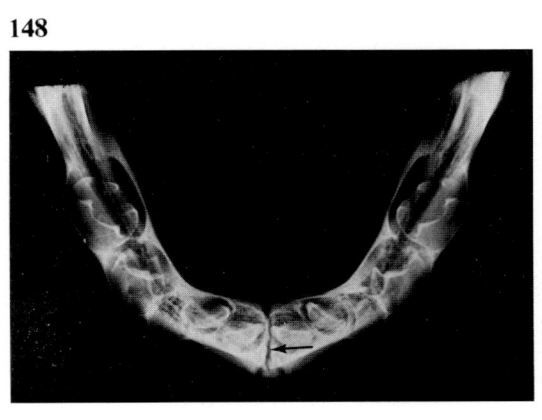
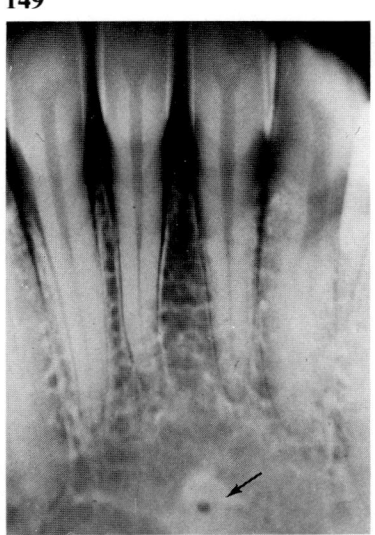

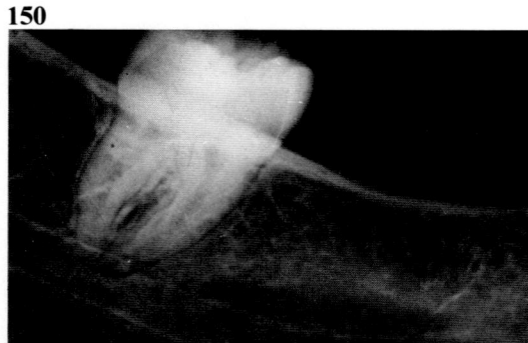

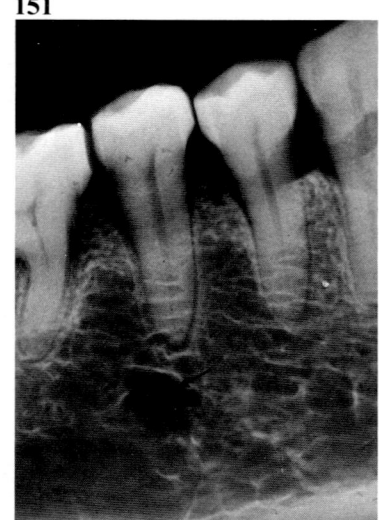

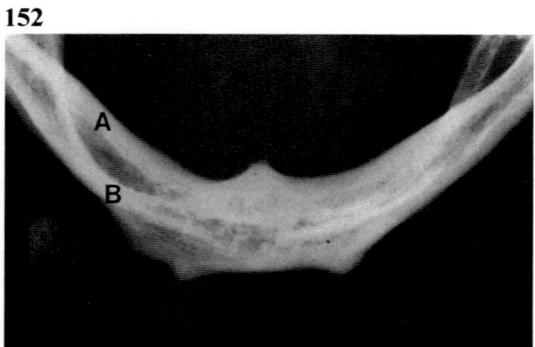

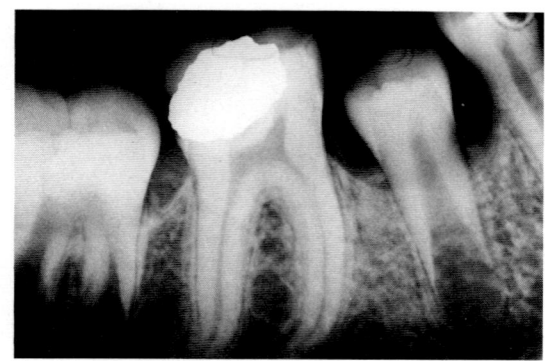

150 Mandibular canal in the region of the mandibular third molar tooth.

The inferior dental canal commences at the mandibular foramen and passes downwards and forwards from the ramus into the body of the mandible where, near the root apices of the premolars, it terminates by dividing into the mental and incisive canals. The radiographic appearance of the mandibular canal is generally that of a radiolucent shadow bounded superiorly and inferiorly by radio-opaque lines.

The width and position of the canal varies considerably. Most commonly, it is closely related to the roots of the molars though it lies some distance from the roots of the premolars. Generally, the canal lies buccal to the root apices, a feature which should be remembered when interpreting the relationship of the root apices to the canal. The precise relationship of the teeth to the canal is difficult to determine from radiographs, though some hint of a very close relationship can be obtained by reference to the densities of shadows cast by the roots and canal, the position and densities of the lamina dura and the radio-opaque margins of the canal, and the dimensions of the lumen of the canal.

151 Mental foramen (*arrowed*) near the apices of the mandibular premolars.

152 Internal (A) and external (B) oblique lines of the mandible. Occlusal view of an edentulous mandible demonstrating the prominent radio-opacities associated with these lines.

153 Radiograph of developing and erupting molars and premolars. Note the radiolucent regions associated with the emerging crowns and the developing root apices.

Microscopic appearance of oro-dental tissues

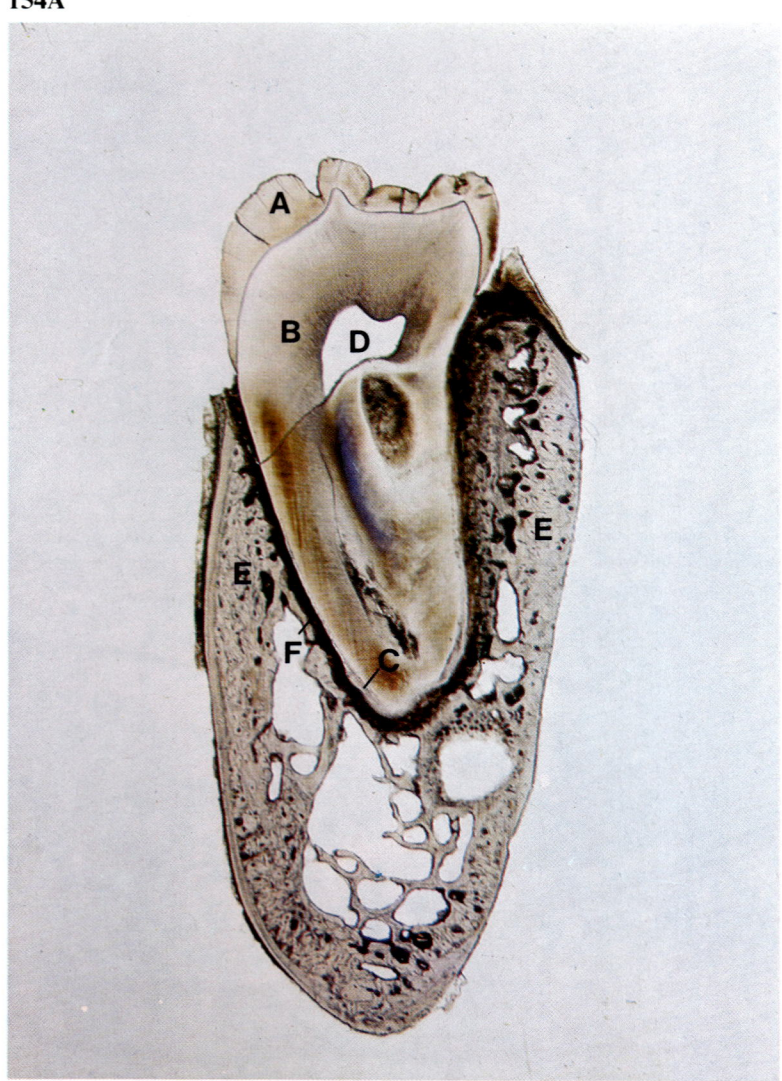
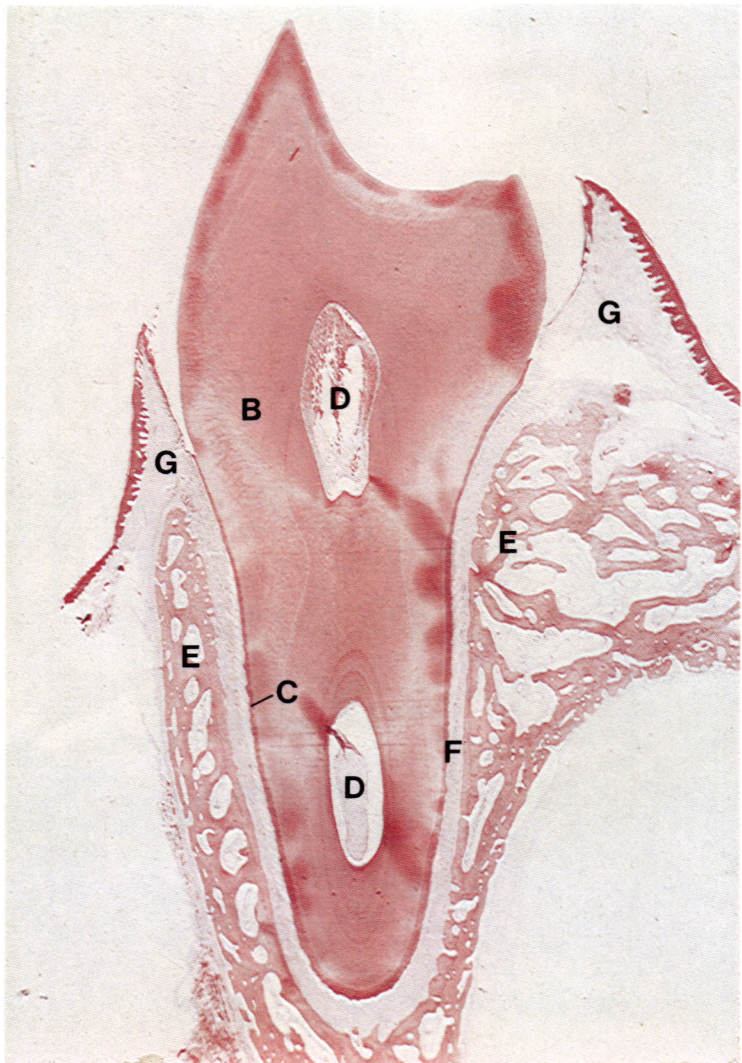

154 Ground (154A) and decalcified (154B) sections of a tooth *in situ*. The teeth are composed of three calcified tissues – enamel (A), dentine (B) and cementum (C) – surrounding an inner core of connective tissue, the dental pulp (D). Dentine forms the bulk of the tooth, being covered in the crown by enamel and in the root by cementum. The dental pulp is the sensitive, nutritive portion of the tooth which is protected from external noxious stimuli by the overlying hard tissues. Dentine, cementum and pulp are of mesenchymal origin, while enamel is derived from ectoderm.

The tissues which support the teeth in the jaws are collectively termed the periodontium and comprise the alveolar bone (E) which houses the sockets for the roots of the teeth, the periodontal ligament (F), a connective tissue which attaches the cementum to the alveolar bone, and the gingiva or gums (G).

The appearance of the dental tissues is dependent upon the method used to prepare the specimen. Thus, in ground section the soft connective tissues of the pulp, periodontal ligament and gingiva will be removed by the act of wearing away the tissues to obtain a thin section. In the ground section shown, however, the periodontal ligament has fortuitously been retained. In decalcified material, the soft connective tissues and the organic matrix of the calcified tissues are retained but, unless the decalcifying procedure is carried out under special conditions, decalcification generally results in loss of the highly mineralised enamel. (A, ×4, B, ×6)

Enamel

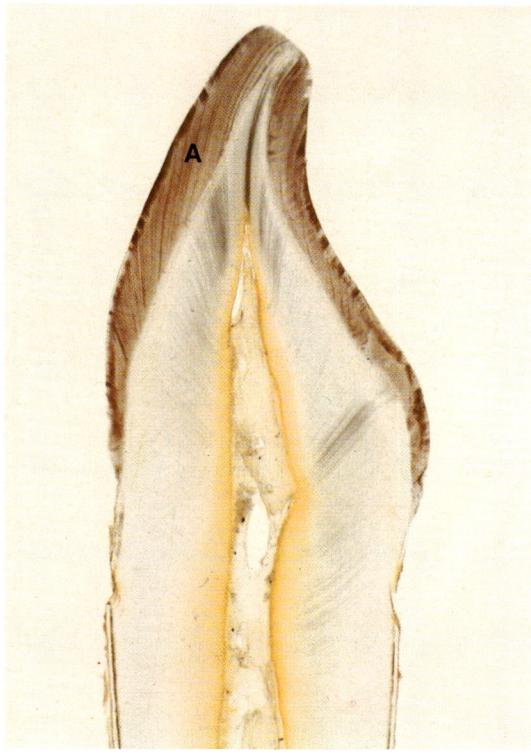

155 Longitudinal, ground section through a tooth showing distribution of enamel. Dental enamel (A) is the protective layer covering the anatomical crown of the tooth. It is thickest over the incisal edges and cusps (about 2.5mm from the amelodentinal junction to the surface) thinning down at the cemento-enamel junction to a knife edge. ($\times 8$)

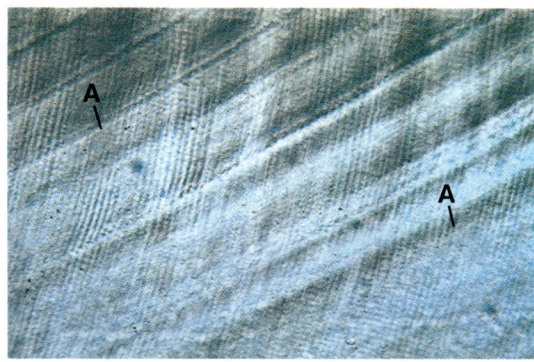

156 Ground, longitudinal section showing enamel prisms. The basic morphological unit of mammalian enamel is the prism or rod. In longitudinal section, the prisms extend approximately perpendicularly from the amelodentinal junction to the surface. Each prism is about 5μm in diameter. The lines crossing the prisms obliquely are striae of Retzius (A). ($\times 200$)

Physical properties of enamel. Enamel is semi-translucent. It is grey or bluish-white in colour. Except at the unworn biting edges of the incisors, its colour is modified by that of the underlying dentine, producing the characteristic yellowish-white appearance of the crown. In deciduous teeth where the enamel is more opaque, enamel has a whiter hue. Enamel is birefringent; its average refractive index is high (1.62). The microscopic appearance of the tissue is dependent upon the refractive index and degree of penetration of the mounting medium. For example, the brownish appearance of enamel in quinoline or Canada balsam is produced by incomplete penetration of the mounting medium into the tissue and the refraction of light by air trapped in the unpenetrated spaces. The hardness of enamel is considerable and it is this which allows enamel to withstand masticatory loads and protect the underlying dentine. Indeed, enamel is the hardest tissue in the body. The surface regions of enamel are harder than the deeper layers. Enamel has a high modulus of elasticity and is a rigid structure. It has a low tensile strength and is brittle. Permeability within enamel is somewhat limited. However, a system of pores of varying dimensions is present through which some aqueous solutions may pass (see page 81). The density of enamel is approximately 2.8–3.0g/ml. This feature is important in separating dental tissues for chemical analysis.

Chemical composition of enamel. In its mature state enamel is highly mineralised, containing by weight 96 per cent inorganic material, 1 per cent organic material and 3 per cent water. The composition of enamel by volume is approximately 89 per cent inorganic, 2 per cent organic and 9 per cent water. The inorganic component of mature enamel is mainly in the form of hydroxyapatite crystals. The organic component is difficult to analyse. It consists mainly of proteins with some carbohydrates, lactates, citrates and lipids. The protein is in two fractions of approximately equal volume, one soluble and one insoluble in dilute acids. The organic component is not fibrous but is thought to be in the form of a gel. The protein is not a type of keratin, as was once suggested, but is protein unique to enamel.

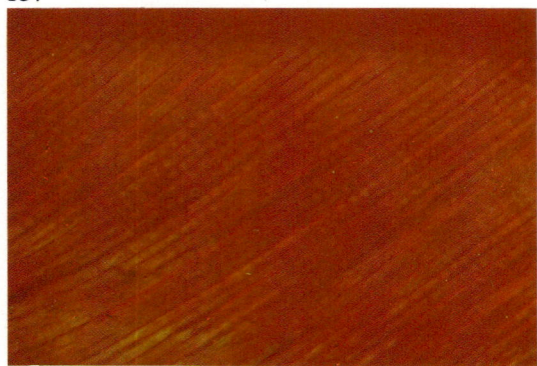

157 Decalcified, longitudinal section showing enamel prisms. Since enamel is largely composed of inorganic material, standard decalcification techniques to prepare histological sections through a tooth usually result in total loss of enamel tissue. Because of this it was once thought that mature enamel contained no organic matrix. However, demineralisation can be carried to a point where it is possible to section enamel; the surviving material retains organic and some inorganic material. The photomicrograph shows that following such procedures the prism outlines remain. (*Procyon dye*, × 300)

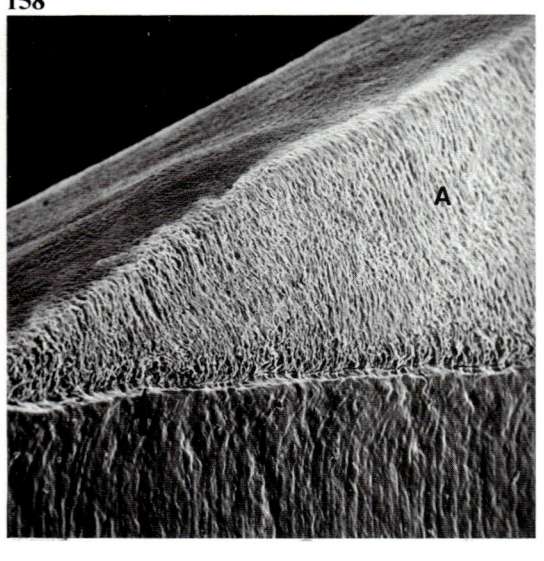

158 Longitudinal section through enamel near the cervical margin. This is a cut enamel surface which has been acid-etched in order to highlight the enamel prisms. The amelodentinal junction is indicated with an arrow. A = enamel. (*Scanning electron micrograph*, × 180)

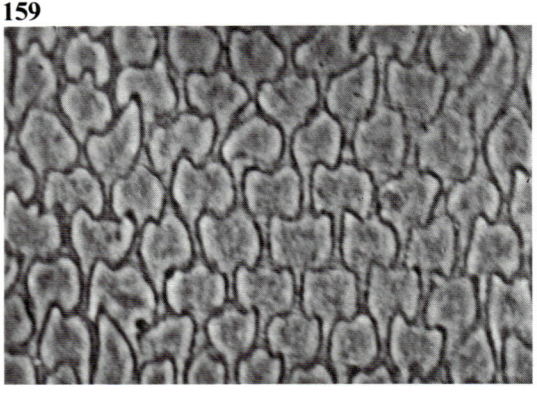

159 Ground, transverse section through enamel prisms. In the main, human enamel prisms in cross-section are keyhole-shaped. The relationships of the prisms are such that the tail of one prism lies between two heads of neighbouring prisms in the row below. The orientation of the keyhole shape is such that the tail points towards the cervical margin of the crown. Because of the close interlocking of the prisms, there is little interprismatic substance. Prism forms other than the keyhole shape have been described. In inner enamel, prisms with circular shapes may be particularly common. Variations in the appearance of prisms can be produced by varying the plane of section. (*Phase contrast*, × 1,200)

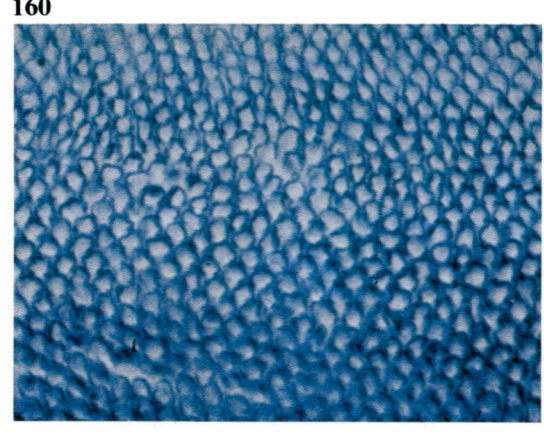

160 Decalcified, transverse section through enamel prisms. A similar prismatic pattern to that seen in ground section is observed following careful decalcification. The material outlining the prism has been called the prism sheath and is approximately 0.5μ thick. (*Stain. Light blue*, × 600)

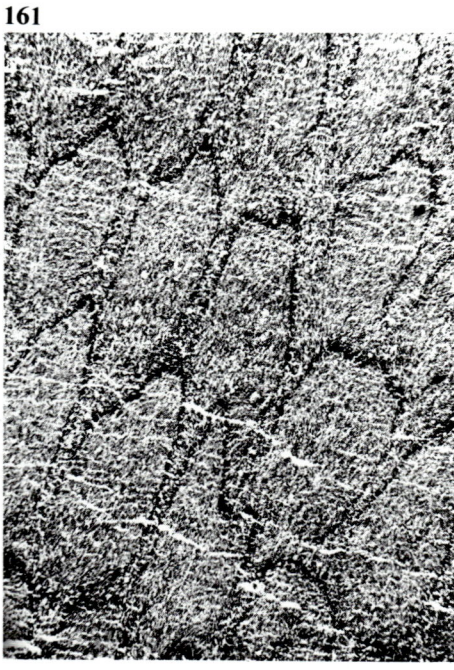

161 Transverse section through enamel showing the key-hole appearance of the prisms. The prism boundaries have been highlighted using a silver staining technique. Note that the prism sheath may be incomplete. In this preparation, elongation of the 'keyholes' results from oblique sectioning of the tissue. (*Electron micrograph*, × 2,000)

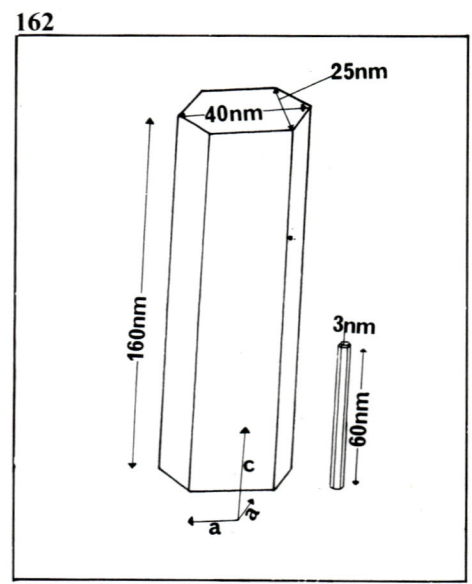

162 The hydroxyapatite crystal in enamel. Hydroxyapatite has the formula $Ca_{10}(PO_4)_6(OH)_2$. In enamel, it is in the form of large, elongated, hexagonal crystals. The long axis of the crystal corresponds to the crystallographic C-axis. The dimensions shown are those usually quoted. The smaller dentine hydroxyapatite crystal is shown for comparison.

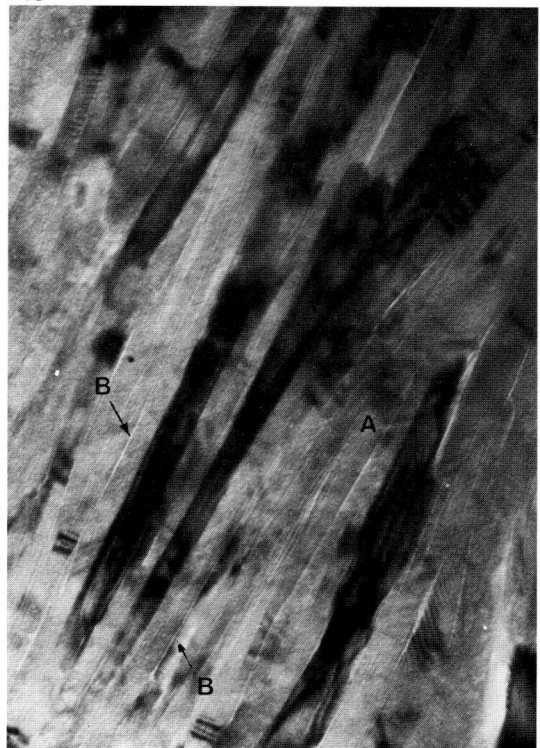

163 The appearance of enamel crystallites in longitudinal section prepared by ion-beam thinning. The dimensions of enamel crystallites (see the previous illustration) have been deduced from electron micrographs of sections of enamel prepared with a diamond knife. Such a technique may lead to shattering of the crystals with consequent artificially low measurements for their length. This view gains support from the finding that developing enamel crystals are at least 20μm long. As an alternative to the use of a diamond knife, ultra thin sections of mature enamel can be prepared using the technique of ion-beam thinning. Illustrated here is such a preparation taken from an area midway between the amelodentinal junction and the surface in the cusp of a permanent molar tooth. The enamel crystals are shown in longitudinal section with the c-axis parallel to the crystal length. The crystal length is far greater than that usually quoted; they may even extend throughout the entire length of the prism. A, enamel crystal. B, micropore. (*Electron micrograph,* × *100,000*)

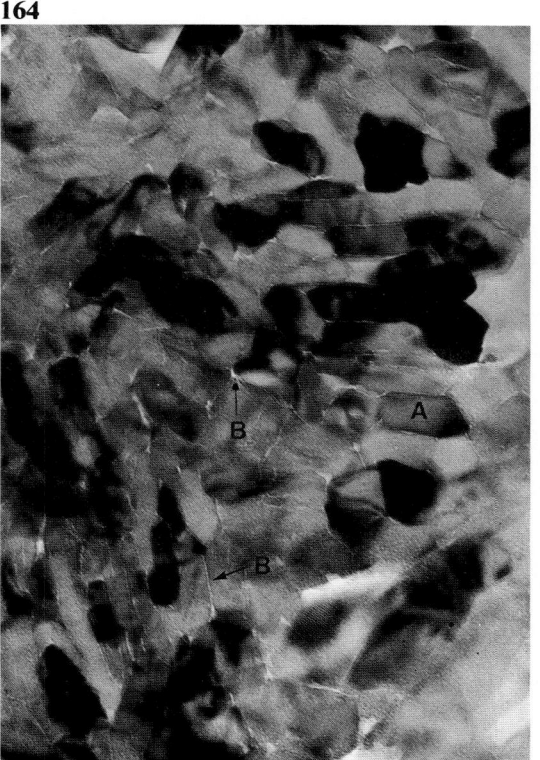

164 The appearance of enamel crystallites in cross-section prepared by ion-beam thinning. The crystallites (A) appear hexagonal. A sheath, possibly organic, may be seen around each crystal. Micropores (B) are present between crystals. (*Electron micrograph,* × *120,000*)

In vivo, the pores in enamel are water-filled spaces between the crystallites. Figures as high as 10–12 per cent have been quoted for pore volume based on thermogravimetric analysis. These values, however, may be inflated because of the release of water which is normally a structural part of the enamel crystallites. From studies based upon water absorption techniques, enamel appears to have a porosity of about 3–5 per cent by volume. Even this figure may not be a true reflection of the porosity since it may incorporate a factor related to water which is bound to the organic material. Most of the pores are only accessible to small molecules such as water, less than 0.5 per cent of the pores by volume being freely acceptable to molecules much larger than water. Polarised light studies, internal surface area measurements and etching studies suggest that many of the pores which are accessible to molecules larger than water are distributed in the prism boundaries, while the pores which are only accessible to small molecules are found throughout the enamel. The prism boundaries may be thought of as main highways through the enamel, while the rest of the porosity may be thought of as a fine network of footpaths connecting occasionally with the main highways so that access through them is slow and restricted.

165 The relationship between prism structure and crystalline orientation. This diagram represents a block of enamel cut from a mandibular tooth. The cross-sectional view shows the characteristic keyhole arrangement of the enamel prisms with the tails pointing cervically and the heads occlusally. In the head region of the prism, the long axes of the crystallites run parallel to the long axes of the prisms. In the tail region, the crystallites are orientated approximately 65–70 degrees from the long axes of the prisms.

It was once thought that prisms were bundles of enamel crystals bounded by an organic prism sheath. However, it is now generally agreed that prism boundaries result from abrupt changes in crystallite orientation, though the micropores produced by this irregular abutment may contain an excess of organic material. This organic material is thought to be relatively insoluble compared with that within the prism core, thus accounting for the persistence of prism structure in decalcified sections (see figures **157** and **160**).

166 Enamel prisms cut transversely to show variation in crystallite orientations between the head (A) and tail (B) regions of the prisms. This section comes from remineralised enamel. Because of accentuation of the crystallites, this preparation is especially useful for the demonstration of crystallite orientation. (*Electron micrograph, × 7,000*)

167 Enamel prisms cut longitudinally to show variations in crystallite orientation. This section illustrates the sudden change in crystallite orientation at the prism boundaries (*arrowed*). (*Electron micrograph, × 13,500*)

168–170 The differing reactions of the prism core and prism boundary to differing demineralising agents is evidence in favour of the view that these two regions have differing physical and/or chemical properties. Dilute acids preferentially etch the prism core. Chelating agents preferentially etch the prism boundary. However, using strong acids a variety of demineralising patterns can be produced on the same tooth surface. The following three scanning electron micrographs are taken from enamel treated with 30 per cent w/w phosphoric acid for 60 secs. Three etching patterns can be produced. Pattern 1 (figure **168**) shows preferential etching of the prism core. Pattern 2 (figure **169**) shows preferential etching of the prism boundary and Pattern 3 (figure **170**) shows an even etch which bears no relationship to enamel morphology. The absence of a common etching pattern in strong acids may indicate regional variations in prism structure and properties. (*× 1,000*)

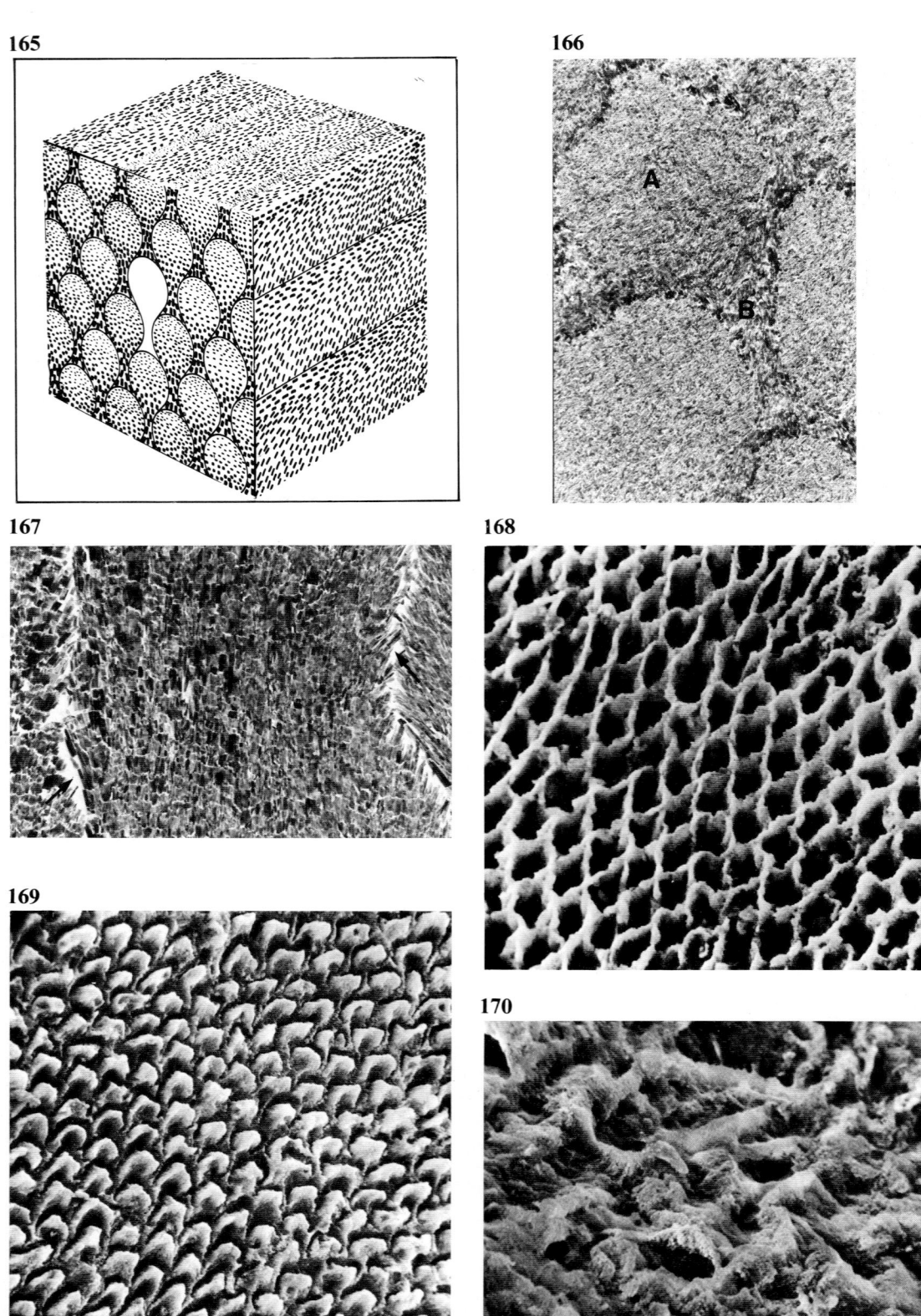

Although it has already been stated that the prisms pass perpendicularly from the amelodentinal junction to the surface in a straight direction, variations from this pattern are responsible for the appearance of Hunter-Schreger bands and gnarled enamel.

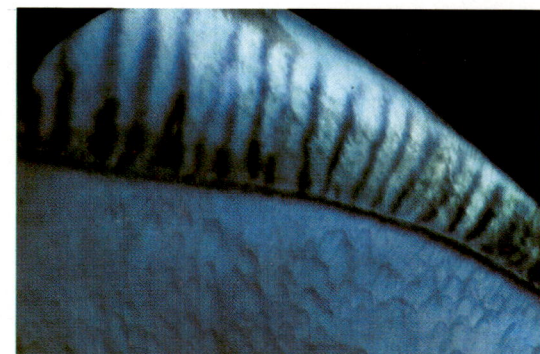

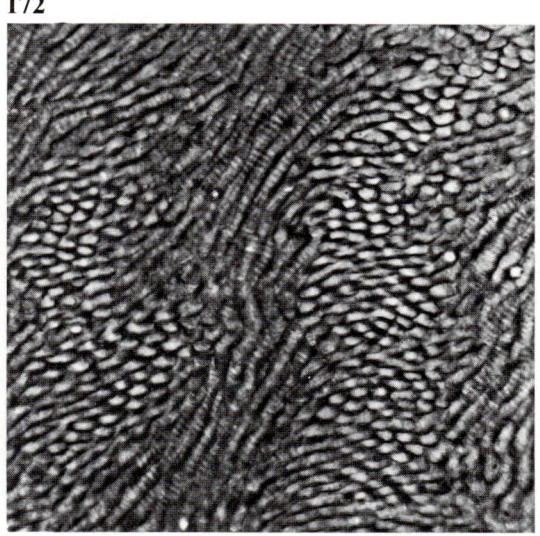

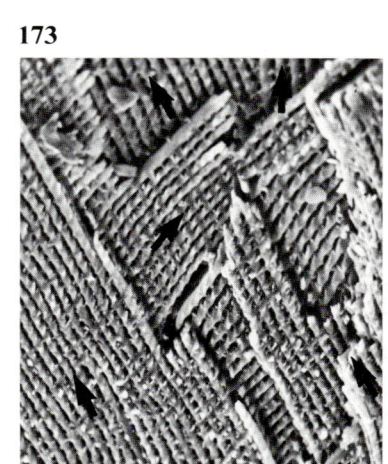

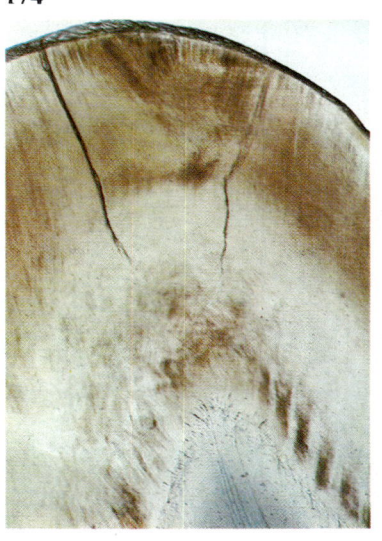

171 Hunter-Schreger bands appear as broad alternating dark and light bands of vague outline passing in the same general direction as the prisms and occupying the inner two-thirds of enamel. They are best seen in longitudinal sections of enamel in polarised or reflected lights. (*Polarised light,* × 25)

172 The optical effects which are the **Hunter-Schreger bands** can be explained with regard to variations in the course of groups of adjacent prisms. This ground, longitudinal section through enamel near the amelodentinal junction shows alternating changes in prism direction, such that some prisms being cut transversely, others longitudinally. If viewed in reflected light those prism surfaces lying more parallel to the light beam would reflect light away from the microscope and appear dark, while those prism surfaces lying less parallel to the beam would reflect light through the microscope and appear bright. In polarised light, the bands appear because of regional variations in crystallite direction within the alternating bands of prisms. The Hunter-Schreger bands are not normally visible in the outer third of enamel since here the enamel prisms become straighter and run a more similar course. (× 250)

173 Fractured enamel of rodent incisor showing changes in direction of enamel prisms in alternating planes. The tissue shown is from the inner zone of enamel near the amelodentinal junction. Single rows of prisms can be seen running in different directions. Six separate layers can be discerned, the prism direction in each layer being arrowed. (*Scanning electron micrograph,* × 500)

174 Longitudinal, ground section showing gnarled enamel. Gnarled enamel is the term used to describe the irregular twisting and decussation of prisms in enamel over the cusps. (× 30)

175 Prismless enamel. Not all regions of enamel show prisms. During the development of prismatic enamel the ameloblast is characterised by a Tomes's process at the secretory end of the cell. It is the configuration of this process which is said to be associated with the changing orientation of crystallites necessary for the appearance of prisms (see page 160). However, since during the early and late stages of amelogenesis the secretory end of the ameloblast may be flattened, all crystallites are arranged parallel to each other, producing a uniform, prismless enamel. Thus, prismless enamel may be seen adjacent to the amelodentinal junction and in the surface enamel. The electron micrograph shown is taken at a late stage in amelogenesis at the surface zone. A, ameloblast; B, prismatic enamel; C, prismless enamel. Note the absence of Tomes's processes. ($\times 2,100$)

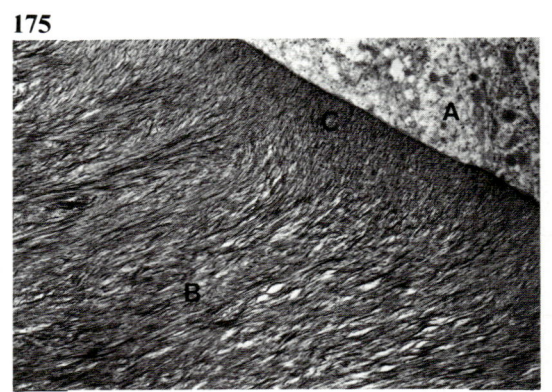

Two types of structural lines are present in enamel, the cross-striations and the striae of Retzius. Both these lines are incremental, reflecting the phasic nature of the development of the tissue.

176 Ground, longitudinal section of enamel prisms showing cross-striations. This section, viewed with a phase-contrast microscope, shows fine regular lines, the cross-striations, running transversely across each prism. The striations of adjacent prisms are in phase and are at approximately 5μm intervals. They are thought to delineate daily increments of growth. It is not known whether their appearance is due to variations in chemical and/or physical properties, though it has been suggested that they are associated with constrictions of the prisms. They have not yet been clearly identified at the electron microscope level. ($\times 350$)

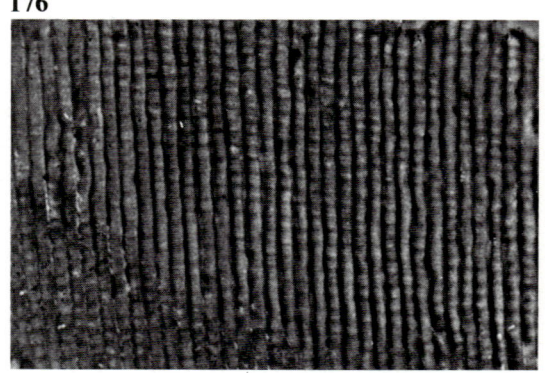

177 Decalcified section of enamel prisms showing cross-striations. (*Procyon dye*, $\times 300$)

178 The striae of Retzius are incremental lines which are spaced at varying intervals of between 20–80μm. Unlike the cross-striations, they run obliquely across the prisms from the amelodentinal junction to the surface. The figure shown is of a ground, longitudinal section of enamel. The striae are most numerous and lie closer together in the cervical region. Over the tips of the cusps and incisal margins they do not reach the surface (except following attrition, as shown in this specimen). ($\times 15$)

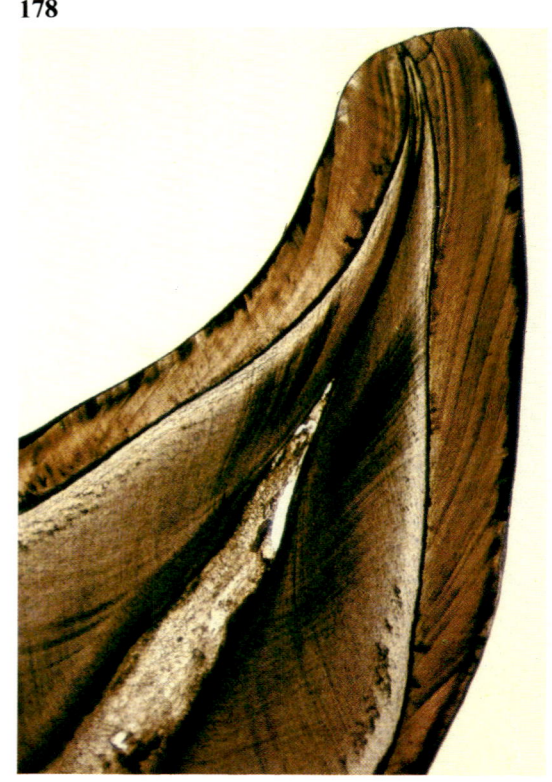

179 Ground, longitudinal section of enamel at higher power showing striae of Retzius. The striae may vary in thickness from between 4–150μm. They may be hypo- or hypermineralised and continuous or discontinuous. (× 40)

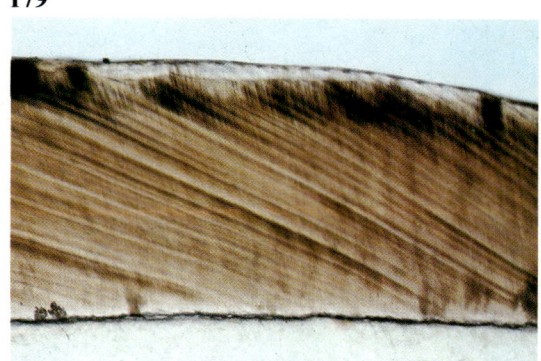

180 Decalcified, cross-section through enamel showing the concentric pattern of the striae. These resemble the annual rings of a tree. (*Light blue*, × 150)

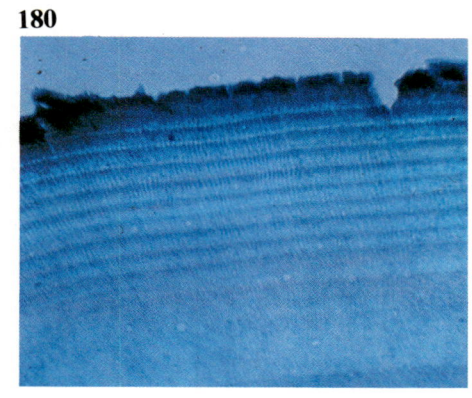

181 The nature and development of the striae of Retzius. Each stria represents a former outline of the developing front of enamel. The developing front appears as a picket-fence into which slot the Tomes's processes of the ameloblasts. In the diagram, it can be seen that each slot is related to two structural elements – a cross-striation (red) and a prism boundary (black). Periodically, where there is a disturbance in the development of enamel a stria will be formed which characteristically takes on the picket-fence appearance of the developing front (Stria 1). Striae 2 and 3 show the S-shaped appearance seen in low power microscopy. It has been suggested that this S-shaped configuration results from variations in the incremental growth rates during the early, middle and late stages of amelogenesis. The diagram shows that at the surface and amelodentinal junction where the daily increments are smallest (i.e. the intervals between the cross-striations are most narrow), the rise in the striae is shallowest. Note that the diagram shows only a 2-dimensional representation of the striae which are in reality 3-dimensional 'faults' in enamel.

At present, it is not known what events are responsible for the disturbances producing a stria, i.e. whether systemic or local, whether the organic and/or inorganic components are effected or whether the change is physical rather than chemical.

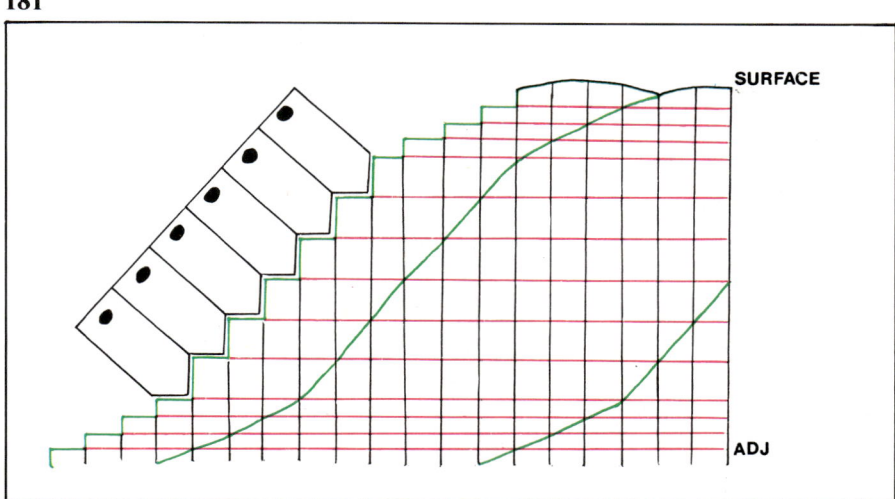

182 A ground, longitudinal section of enamel showing the picket-fence appearance of a stria. (× 1,000)

183 The appearance of striae (A) as they approach the enamel surface. Where a stria meets the enamel surface, it is associated with a furrow termed a perikyma (B). The development of perikymata may be related to cessation of enamel secretion by ameloblasts in the depth of the furrows a short time before the ameloblasts on either side. (*Electron micrograph*, × 1,000)

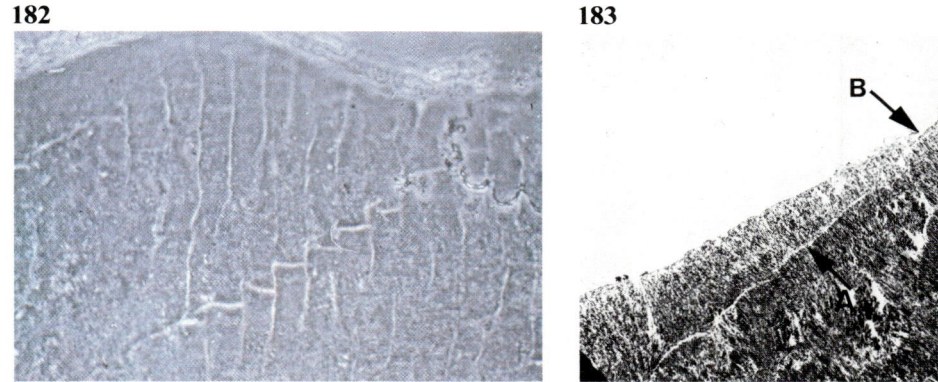

184 Surface enamel, showing perikymata. (*Scanning electron micrograph, ×200*)

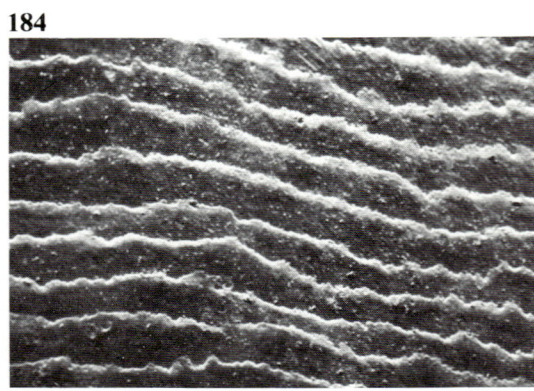

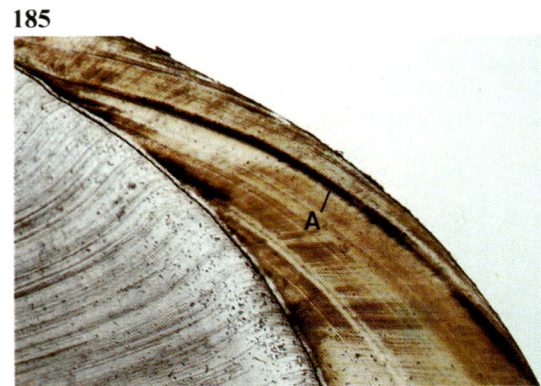

185 Neonatal line. Disturbance in the development of enamel at birth is sufficient to produce an exaggerated stria, designated the neonatal line (A). Neonatal lines are present in the enamel of all deciduous teeth and generally the first permanent molar. (*×30*)

186 A ground and acid-etched surface of enamel showing a neonatal line (A). Note the change in width and direction of the prisms at the neonatal line. (*Scanning electron micrograph, ×400*)

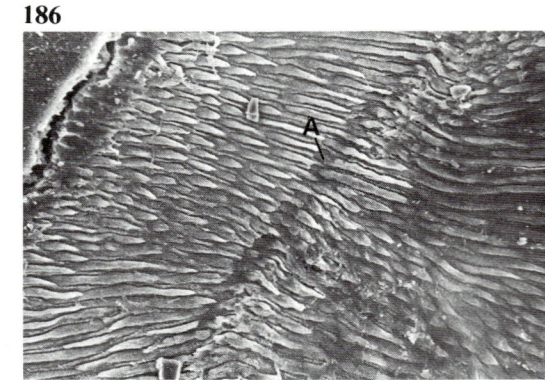

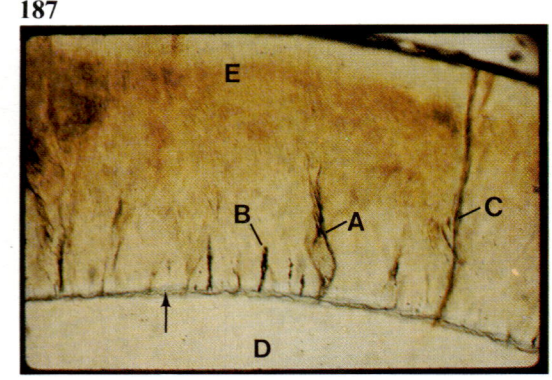

187 Ground, transverse section through enamel and dentine to show the amelodentinal junction and associated structures. Generally, the amelodentinal junction (*arrowed*) has a scalloped appearance presenting as a series of irregular elevations and depressions. The scalloping is such that the depressions or bays dip into the surface dentine (D), the elevations into the enamel (E). Certain areas of the amelodentinal junction, however, may appear smooth. It has been suggested that the scalloping has a mechanical function, helping to strengthen the union between the enamel and dentine.

Enamel tufts (A), enamel spindles (B) and enamel lamellae (C) are structural features at the amelodentinal junction. (*×60*)

188 The scalloped appearance of the surface dentine following removal of the overlying enamel by demineralisation. (*Scanning electron micrograph, ×400*)

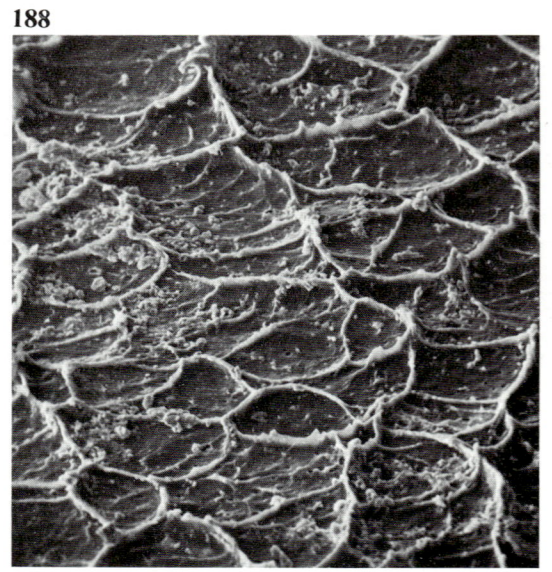

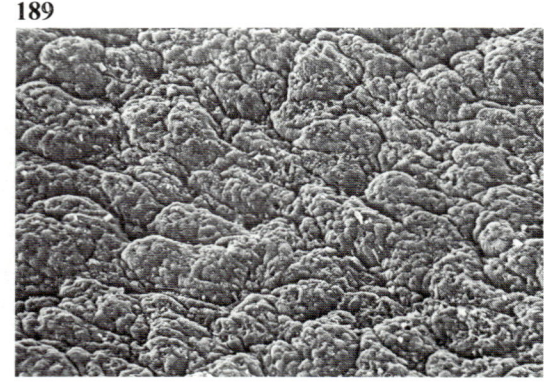

189 The enamel surface of the amelodentinal junction exposed by fracturing off the dentine following dehydration. The convexities correspond to scalloped concavities in the dentine and are complex in shape and size. Note the large number of small fissures and prism markings on this surface. (*Scanning electron micrograph, ×250*)

190 The amelodentinal junction (*arrowed*) illustrating the different sizes of the enamel (A) and dentine (B) hydroxyapatite crystallites. (*Electron micrograph,* × 18,000)

191 Ground, longitudinal section showing enamel spindles (A) at the amelodentinal junction. Enamel spindles are projections of the dentinal tubules into the enamel. They are generally seen in ground, longitudinal sections of enamel beneath the cusps. They are thin, club-shaped processes which run perpendicularly from the amelodentinal junction into the enamel for about 10μm. It is presumed that they are formed by odontoblast processes which pass between the developing ameloblasts before the onset of amelogenesis. (× 250)

192 A small opening (*arrowed*) at the dentine surface thought to be a termination of a dentinal tubule. In view of recent work suggesting that the odontoblast processes only extend for a relatively short distance into the circumpulpal dentine (see page 95), the enamel spindle is unlikely to contain the free end of an odontoblast process. (*Scanning electron micrograph,* × 1,600)

193 Replica of the amelodentinal junction showing an enamel spindle (A). (*Electron micrograph,* × 2,500)

194 Ground, transverse section of enamel at the amelodentinal junction, showing enamel tufts. Enamel tufts are ribbon-like structures extending into the inner third of enamel from the amelodentinal junction. They are so named because of their resemblance to tufts of grass. The enamel tufts are hypocalcified prismatic regions in which the prism sheaths are well marked. Because of their vertical orientation they are best seen in transverse section. (× 200)

195 Decalcified, transverse section of enamel showing an enamel lamella. Lamellae are hypomineralised structures arranged radially and vertically from the surface through enamel and are best seen in transverse section. Generally, lamellae are restricted to the outer portion of the enamel but in some instances pass through the whole thickness of enamel. In ground section, they are indistinguishable from cracks. (*Light blue,* × 150)

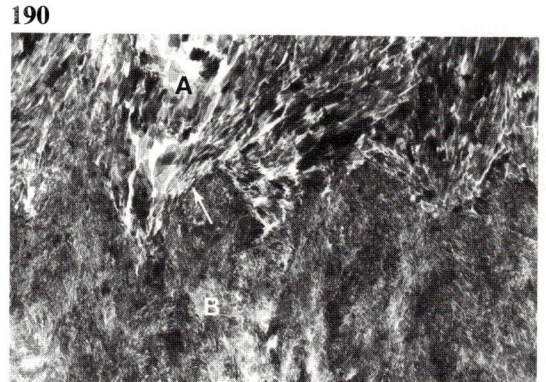
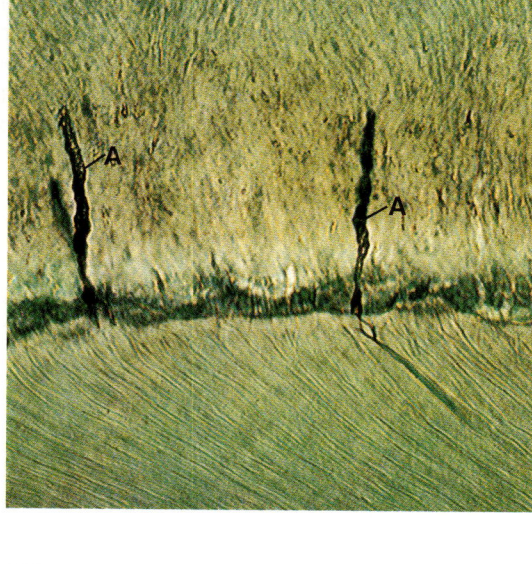
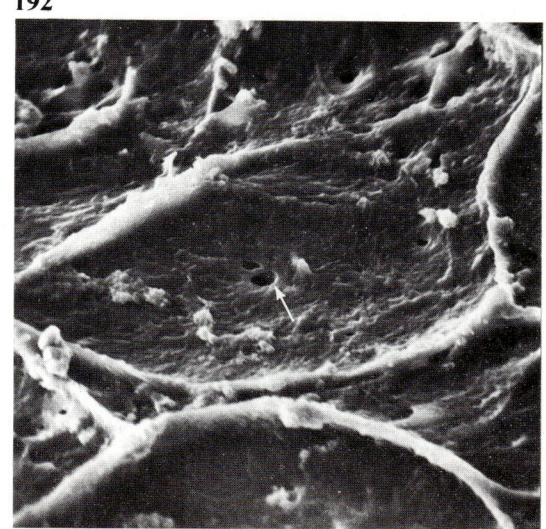
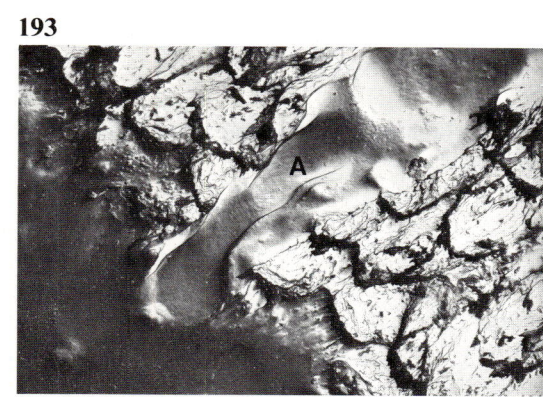
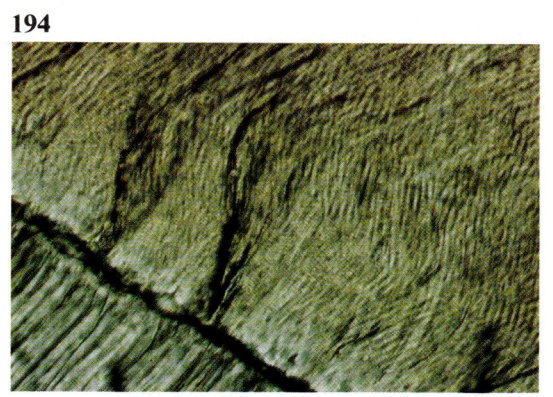
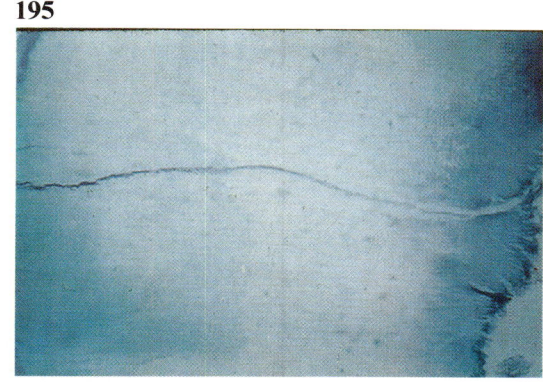

Particular attention has been paid to the surface regions of the character of the early enamel carious lesion.

Investing layers associated with the crowns of erupted teeth

205 Approximal view of an erupted premolar tooth showing its investing layers. The stained film covering the enamel surface consists of three distinguishable zones, plaque (A), primary enamel cuticle (B) and part of the junctional epithelium (C) derived from the reduced enamel epithelium. The plaque corresponds to a position above the crest of the gingival margin and around the contact point (*arrowed*). The cuticle tends to be more substantial in the gingival crevice. Where it derives additional components from oral sulcular cells, it has been termed the secondary enamel cuticle. (*Alcian blue/aldehyde fuchsin, ×4*)

206 Enamel integument. Using careful demineralising techniques it is possible to lift off the investing layers and consequently the plaque, primary enamel cuticle and junctional epithelium appear as a single continuous entity. The term 'enamel integument' has been used to describe this continuous organic layer. A thin section of this integument is shown. A, junctional epithelium; B, primary enamel cuticle; C, plaque. (*Ollett's modification of Twort, ×100*)

207 A deep surface view of enamel integument showing the three, histologically distinguishable zones, the plaque (D), primary enamel cuticle (C) and the cells of the junctional epithelium (E). In the cuticle and plaque, bands of prism end markings may be seen (**207B**) indicating the persistence of the pre-eruptively formed cuticle on the erupted enamel surface (**207A**, *Toluidine blue and erythrosin, ×20*; **207B**, *Alcian blue and erythrosin, ×20*)

208 The enamel integument at the level of the junctional epithelium. This shows the enamel surface (A) covered by the primary enamel cuticle (B) and a vestige of the junctional epithelium (C). The junctional epithelium is discussed further on pages 130–131. (*Electron micrograph, ×13,000*)

209 The enamel integument immediately above the junctional epithelium showing primary enamel cuticle lining the enamel surface. This section is taken from the enamel integument within the gingival crevice, and differs from the preceding micrograph in that the junctional epithelial cells do not overlie the cuticle. The cuticle has an electron dense outer (and often inner) border. (*Electron micrograph, ×10,000*)

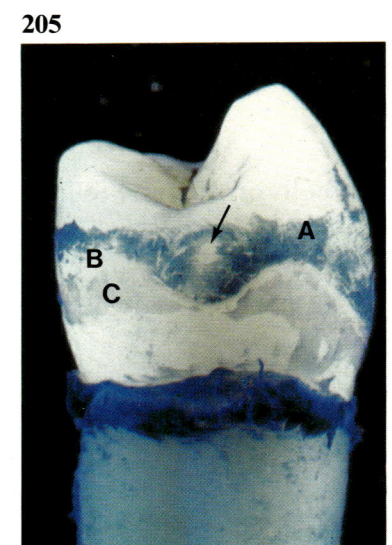

205

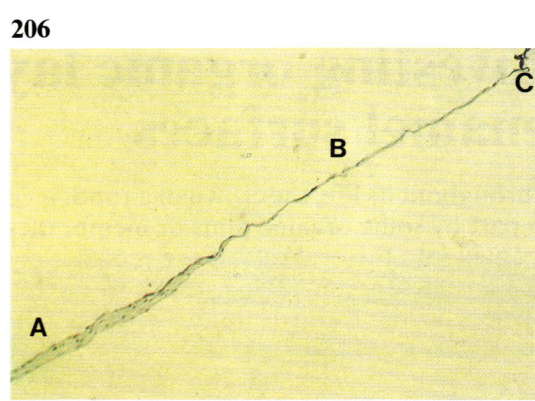

206

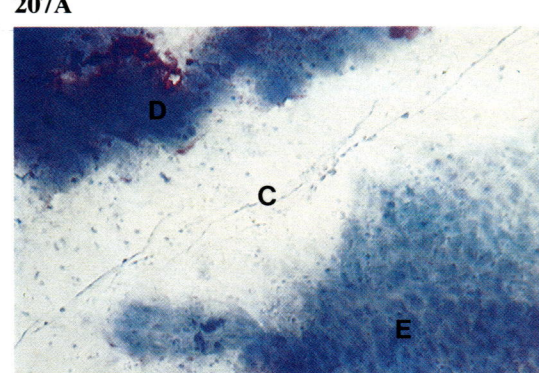

207A

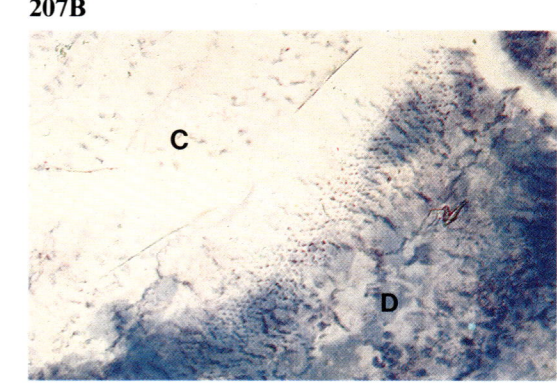

207B

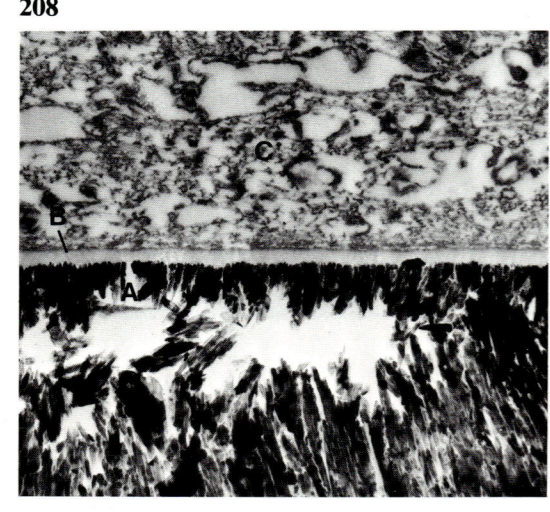

208

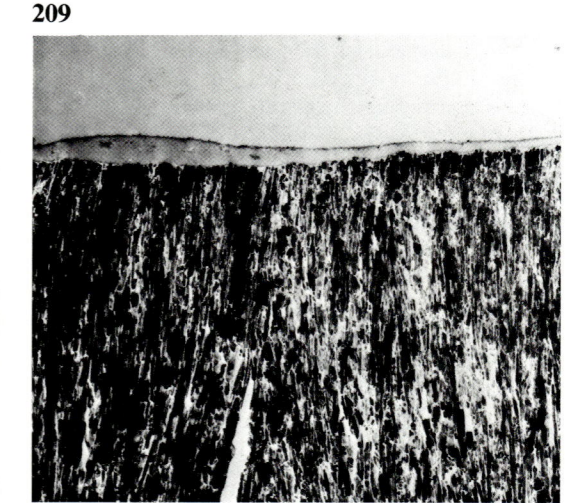

209

210 The enamel integument above the gingival crest showing bacterial colonisation forming dental plaque. Where the primary enamel cuticle is exposed to the oral environment, it may become coated with a layer of structureless material said to be derived from saliva, the acquired pellicle. In the absence of satisfactory oral hygiene, dental plaque forms rapidly as bacteria colonise the acquired pellicle. The micrograph shows a relatively clear zone of material (A) lining the enamel (B), which is probably a combined layer of primary enamel cuticle and acquired pellicle. Above this clear zone is a mass of micro-organisms (C). If allowed to accumulate, plaque may be involved in the causation of both dental caries and inflammatory periodontal disease. The deposition of mineral salts within the plaque, primarily amorphous calcium phosphate, crystalline octacalcium phosphate and hydroxyapatite, will result in the formation of a hard deposit termed dental calculus. (*Electron micrograph, ×1,500*)

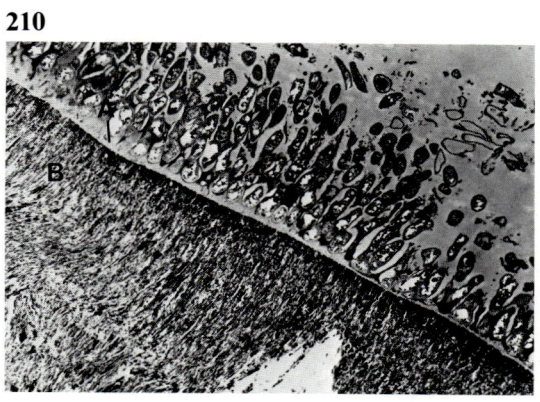

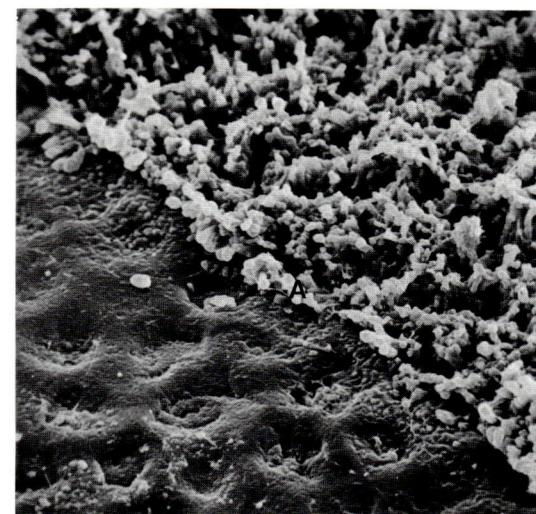

Where the enamel surfaces are exposed to abrasion and attrition (e.g. the cuspal surfaces), the integument is worn away and the only lining may be that of the acquired pellicle which reforms rapidly subsequent to abrasion. Dental plaque and calculus may also accumulate in occlusal fissures.

211 Enamel surface showing a deposit of dental plaque. The boundary of the dental plaque (A) in this micrograph corresponds to the gingival crest, the enamel surface cervical to this line being almost free from plaque. (*Scanning electron micrograph, ×1,500*)

Dentine

212 Longitudinal, ground section through a tooth showing the distribution of dentine. Dentine (A) forms the bulk of the tooth. In the crown, it is covered by enamel, from which it is demarcated by the amelodentinal junction. In the root, it is covered by cementum, the boundary between them being termed the cemento-dentinal junction. The dentine surrounds the pulp cavity. Both the dentine and pulp are derived from the dental papilla (see page 154). To indicate the close relationship between the structure, function and development of the dentine and pulp, the term pulpodentinal complex has been used to collectively describe these tissues. (×4)

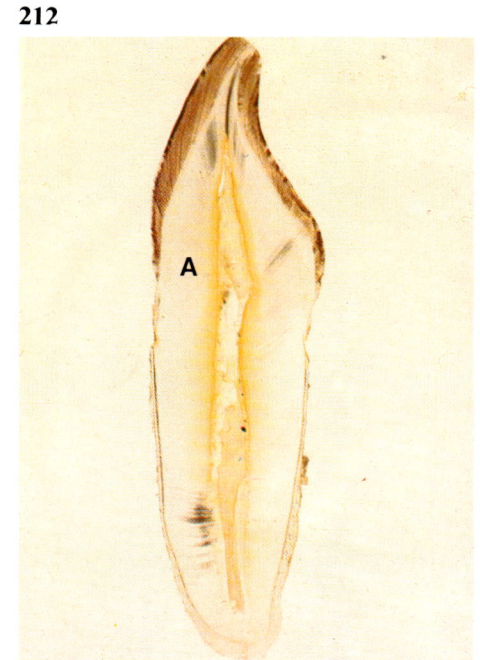

Physical properties of dentine. Dentine is pale yellow in colour, and it is this which imparts the colour to the crown of the tooth through the semi-translucent enamel. It is harder than bone and cementum but much softer than enamel. Dentine is highly elastic, though not as elastic as enamel. Unlike enamel, it is not brittle. Because it is traversed by a system of tubules, dentine is considerably more permeable than enamel. The density of dentine is approximately 2.1g/ml.

Chemical composition of dentine. On a wet weight basis, dentine is composed of approximately 70 per cent inorganic material, 18 per cent organic material and 12 per cent water. By volume, the same components comprise respectively 45 per cent, 30 per cent and 25 per cent of the dentine. Thus, dentine has a much higher content of organic material than enamel. As other hard tissues, the principal inorganic component is hydroxyapatite. The crystals of dentine are small plates and are much smaller than the crystals of enamel (figures **162** and **190**). Recent evidence suggests that, like enamel, many of the figures quoted for the length of the crystals are underestimates, because of fracturing of crystals during preparation. Small amounts of carbonate and several trace elements are also present. Most of the organic component is collagen, with small amounts of citrate, chondrotin sulphate and other protein-carbohydrate complexes, insoluble protein and lipid.

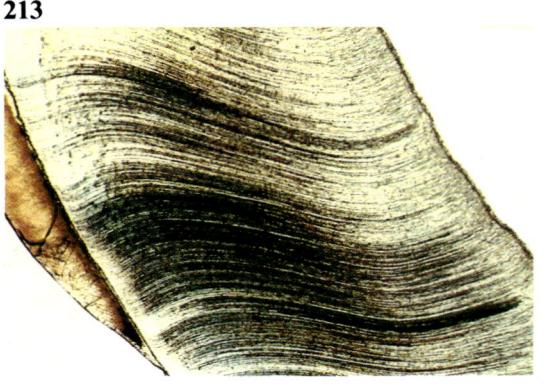

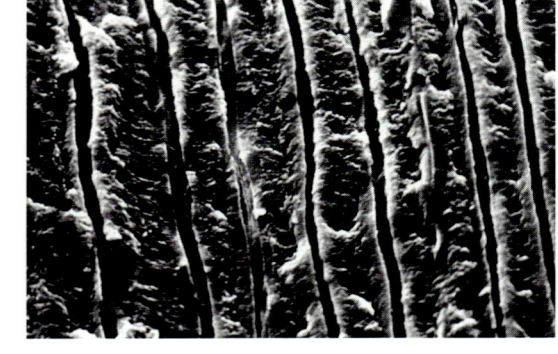

213 The dentinal tubules seen in a longitudinal ground section through dentine. Dentine is permeated by tubules which run from the pulpal surface towards the amelodentinal and cemento-dentinal junctions. *In vivo* the tubules may contain cellular processes which are derived from cells lining the pulpodentinal junction (the odontoblasts). The tubules taper from about 4μm in diameter at their pulpal ends to 1μm or less peripherally. As the surface area of the dentine is much smaller internally than externally, the tubules are more widely separated at their peripheries. Approximately 80 per cent of the total volume of the dentine near the pulp is composed of tubules, while near the amelodentinal junction they comprise only about 4 per cent of the tissue by volume. The tubules follow a curved, sigmoid course, the *primary curvatures.* The convexity of the first curve of the primary curvatures faces rootward. In the root and beneath the cusps the primary curvatures are less pronounced, the tubules running a straighter course. (× *25*)

214 Dentinal tubules in longitudinal section. (*Scanning electron micrograph,* × *1,000*)

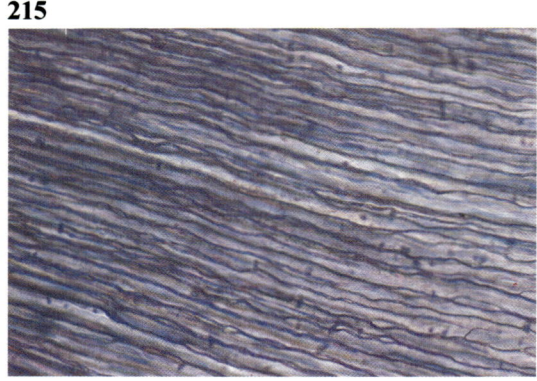

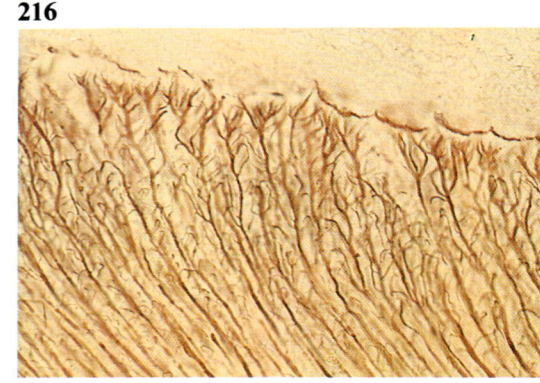

215 Longitudinal ground section of dentine showing secondary curvatures. In addition to the primary curvature, each tubule shows a series of small undulations every few microns – the secondary curvatures. The section is viewed in blue light. (× *320*)

216 Branching of the dentinal tubules. This is a longitudinal ground section near the amelodentinal junction. The dentinal tubules are not single discrete tubes running through the dentine, but give off narrow branches along their course. Branching is particularly marked at the amelodentinal junction. In the root, the dentinal tubules not only branch at their ends but also form loops which are thought to be responsible for the appearance of the granular layer (of Tomes) (see page 98). (*Picrothionin,* × *320*)

217 Transverse ground section showing dentinal tubules. In ground sections the dentinal tubules (A) appear as circular regions. The concentration of tubules varies from 15,000/mm² in outer dentine to 65,000/mm² in inner dentine. Between the tubules lies the bulk of the dentine referred to as intertubular dentine (B). Though when first formed the lumen of the tubule is approximately 4µm in diameter, it is reduced by the deposition on its wall of peritubular dentine (C). Because of its position, a more correct term for this layer might be intratubular dentine. In the section shown, the large amount of peritubular dentine deposited in the tubules has reduced the lumen to a very small diameter. The mounting medium used has not penetrated the tubules and, because of the air and debris trapped within them, the tubules appear as black dots. The section is viewed in red light. (× 1,500)

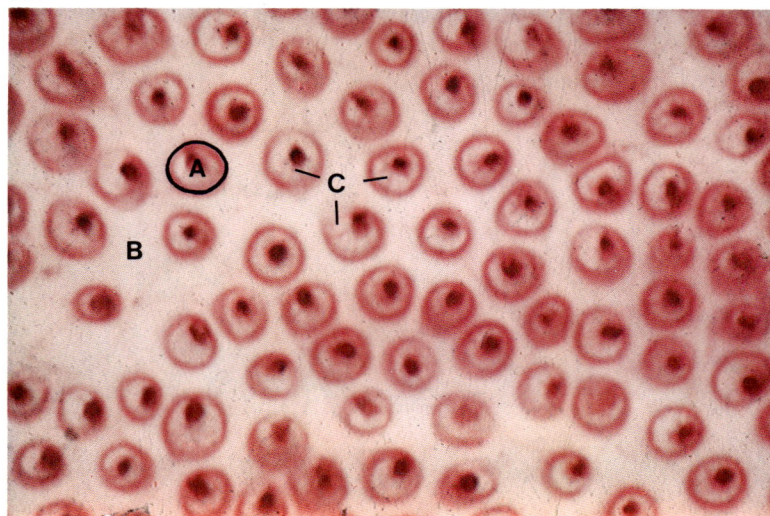

218 Transverse decalcified section of dentinal tubules. Compared with ground sections, two basic differences are seen in a decalcified, transverse section through the tubules. An odontoblast process may be seen within the lumen of the tubule and the peritubular dentine is lost so that the lumen of the tubule appears larger. (*Harris' haematoxylin, × 1,000*)

The contents of dentinal tubules

219 Peritubular dentine. (A) can be distinguished from intertubular dentine (B) as a zone of increased electron density lining the internal surface of the dentinal tubule. Peritubular dentine is more highly mineralised than intertubular dentine. Unlike intertubular dentine, the matrix of peritubular dentine is not collagenous though its precise composition has yet to be identified. In demineralised sections at the electron microscope level, the matrix appears as an amorphous material. The mineral component of peritubular dentine is calcium phosphate, but not in the form of hydroxyapatite crystallites. Although commonly considered amorphous, it has been reported as crystalline octocalcium phosphate. Although the bulk of peritubular dentine is hypercalcified relative to the intertubular dentine, hypocalcified areas bound its inner and outer surfaces. (*Electron micrograph, × 3,000*)

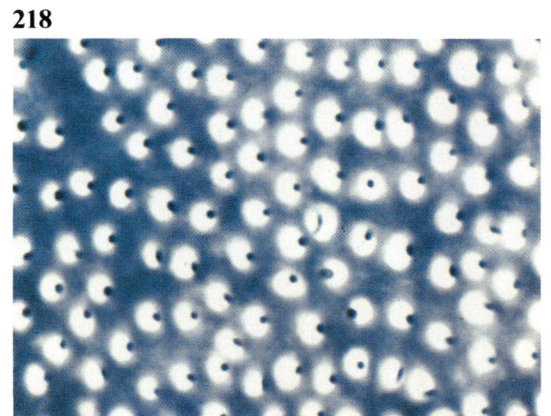

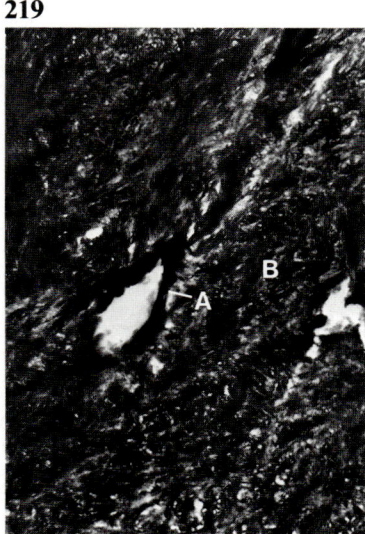

220–222 The relationship between peritubular dentine formation and tubule diameter at various levels within the dentine. (*Scanning electron micrographs*)

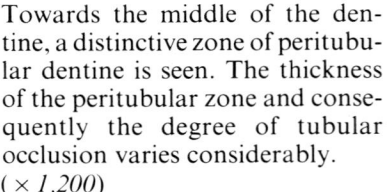

Near the amelodentinal junction, the tubule may be filled or nearly filled with peritubular dentine. ($\times 1,200$)

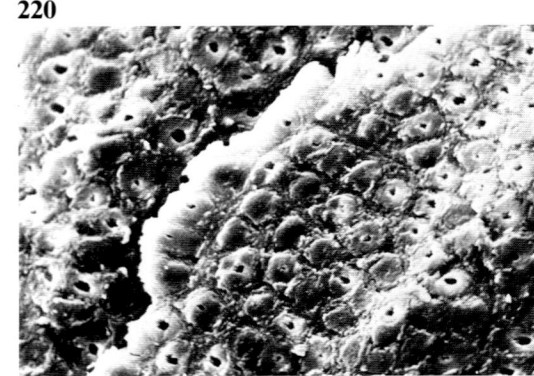

Towards the middle of the dentine, a distinctive zone of peritubular dentine is seen. The thickness of the peritubular zone and consequently the degree of tubular occlusion varies considerably. ($\times 1,200$)

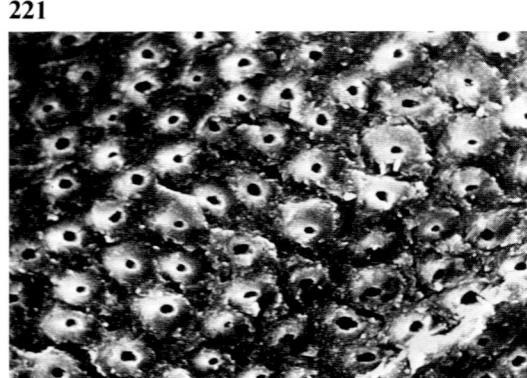

Near the pulp, where the tubule is newly formed, there may be little or no peritubular dentine. ($\times 540$)

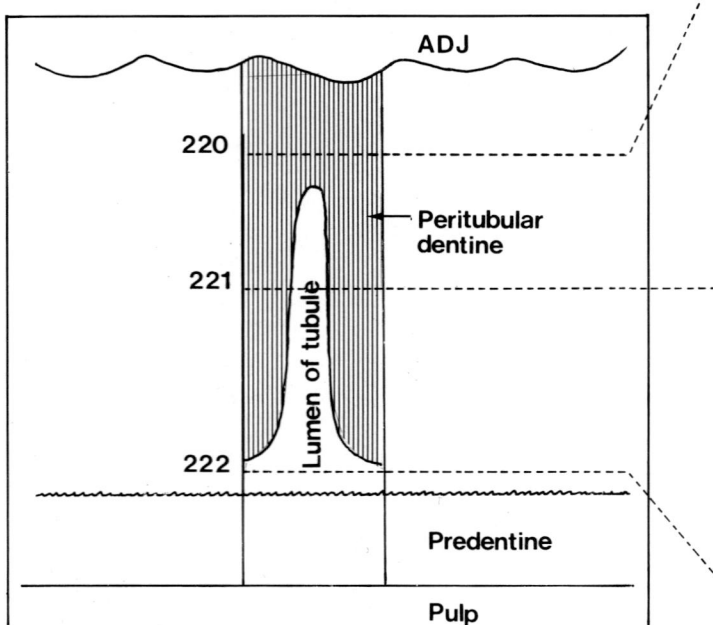

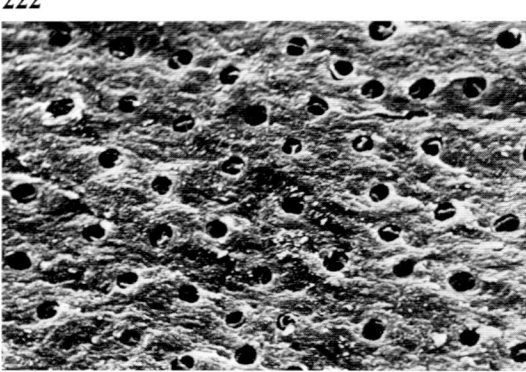

It has been suggested that variations with age in the reactions of the pulp to a noxious stimulus through the dentine may be related, at least in part, to variations in the amounts of peritubular dentine formed. Thus, in the young tooth where the tubules are relatively open, the passage of a stimulus through the dentine may be more rapid than in an older tooth where the tubules may be occluded with peritubular dentine. Peritubular dentine may also be seen in significant amounts beneath sites of attrition.

223 A ground transverse section of dentine. Peritubular dentine, being hypercalcified, is seen as a radio-opaque halo around the tubules. (In this print, radio-opaque tissues are dark.) In any one area, the degree of formation of peritubular dentine may be variable so that some tubules are completely occluded while others have little or no peritubular dentine. (*Microradiograph,* $\times 400$)

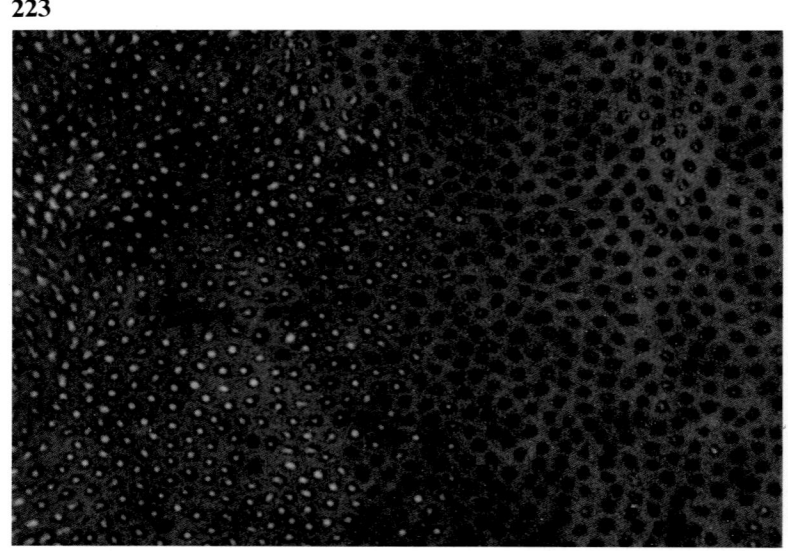

224 Classically, each dentinal tubule is said to contain a long protoplasmic extension of the odontoblast, which passes through the full thickness of the dentine. Consequently, these processes are extremely long when compared with the length of the cell body. The process is bounded by a cell membrane and in the calcified dentine contains microfilaments, vesicles and ribosomes. The vesicles may discharge their contents into the narrow space immediately surrounding the process (the periodontoblastic space). The process is considered to be in this way responsible for the production of the dentinal matrix. Near the pulp at its base, the process contains endoplasmic reticulum and an occasional mitochondrion. Near the amelodentinal junction, the cytoplasmic contents are reduced, the centre of the process being occupied by large vacuoles containing hydrolytic enzymes which compress the cytoplasm into a hyaline ring. The processes accompany the tubules as they branch. In inner dentine near the pulp, some of the tubules contain unmyelinated nerve terminals spiralling around the process.

Recent evidence suggests that, contrary to this classical view, the odontoblast process extends only a short way into the tubule.

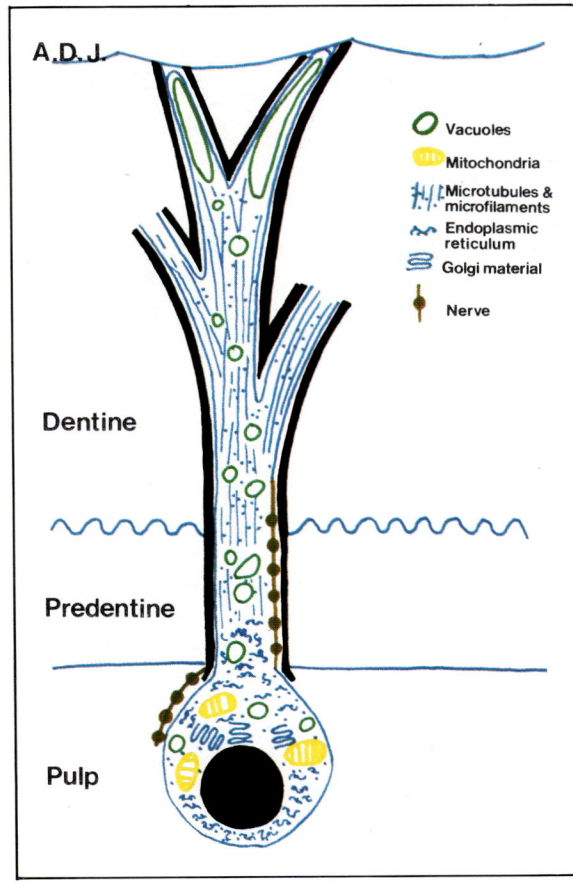

225 **Dentinal tubules cut transversely from inner dentine (225A), outer dentine (225C) and an intermediate area (225B).** These show variation in the extent of the odontoblast process. Note that all the tubules in inner dentine are occupied by processes, while in the intermediate area some are empty of cellular contents, being filled with embedding material. In outer dentine, no processes are seen in the tubules. Thus, the process appears to terminate about halfway through the width of the fully formed primary dentine. (*Electron micrographs*, A = ×4,000, B = ×5,500, C = ×4,000)

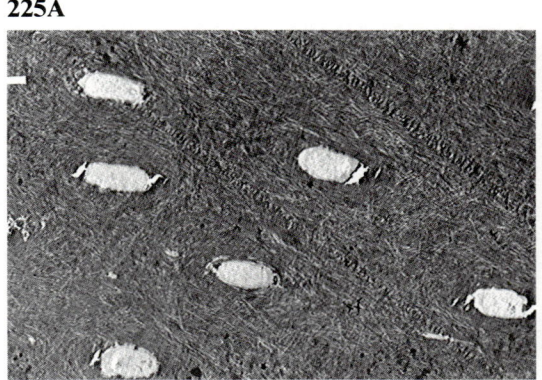

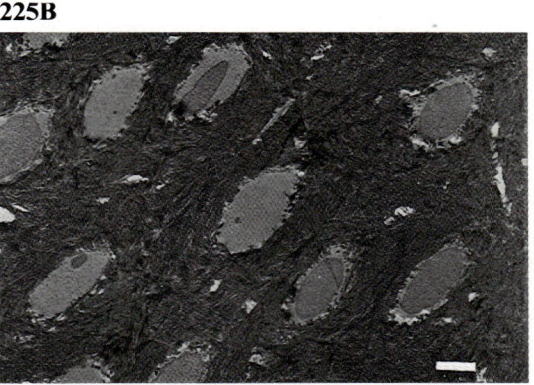

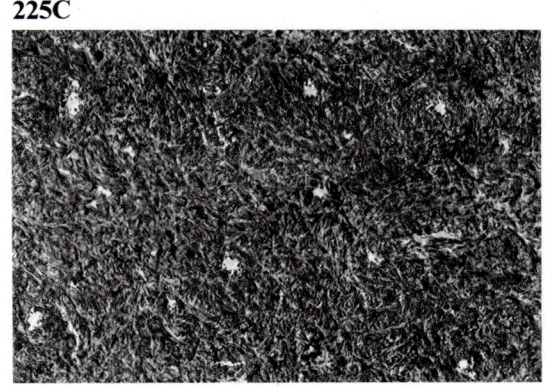

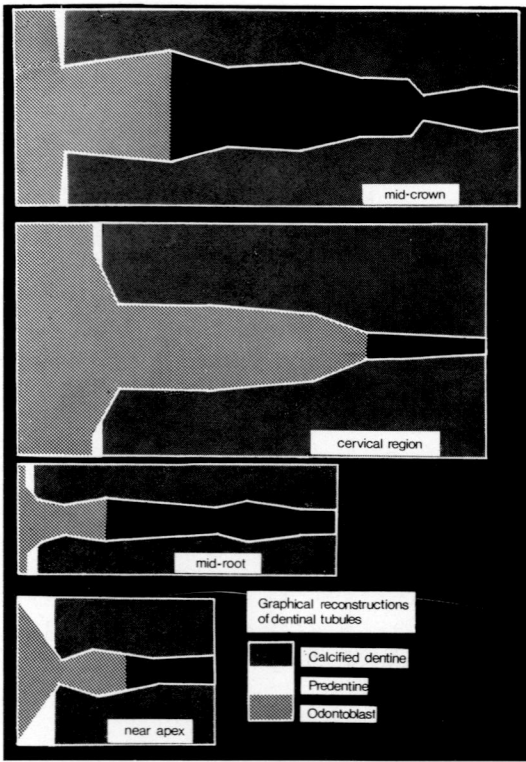

226 Graphical reconstructions of dentinal tubules at various levels in the canine of the cat showing variation in tubule size and shape and extent of the odontoblast processes.

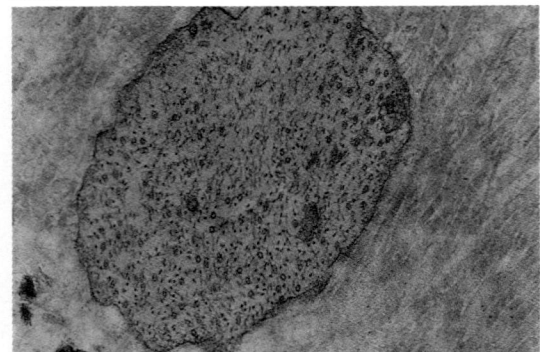

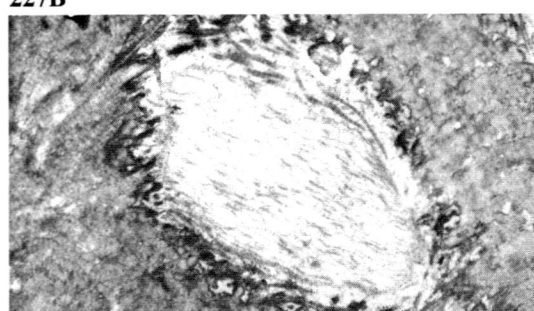

227 The electron microscopic appearance of the odontoblast process.

227A Transverse section through the base of the process in the uncalcified predentine. The odontoblast process is surrounded by the, as yet, uncalcified collagen of the predentine. The process is bounded by a cell membrane and contains many microtubules, microfilaments and vesicles. The vesicles are seen mainly at the periphery of the process. Occasional mitochondria are present at this level although none are seen in this section. (× 25,000)

227B Transverse section through the process near its termination. At this level, the odontoblast process contains few organelles, consisting mainly of microfilaments and the surrounding cell membrane. (× 16,500)

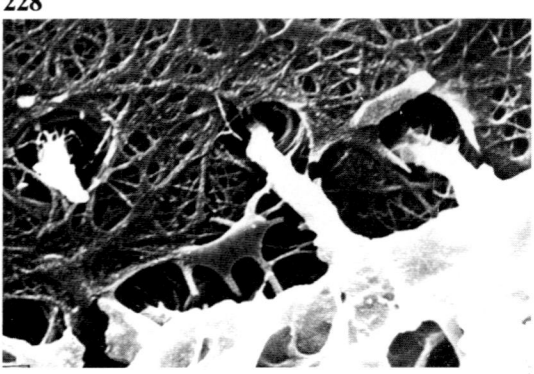

228 Odontoblast processes entering the tubules in the predentine. Note the network of uncalcified collagen fibres at the surface of the predentine. Since the odontoblasts are an integral part of the dental pulp, the structures and relationships of the cell bodies of the odontoblasts are considered on pages 102, 103. (*Scanning electron micrograph*, × 2,700)

The sensory mechanism(s) of dentine has been the object of much research. Silver staining techniques suggest that dentine is innervated by small axons which originate from the subodontoblastic nerve plexus in the pulp and which pass into the dentine up the tubules. More recent evidence for the innervation of dentine has been obtained from electron microscopic studies of the tissue.

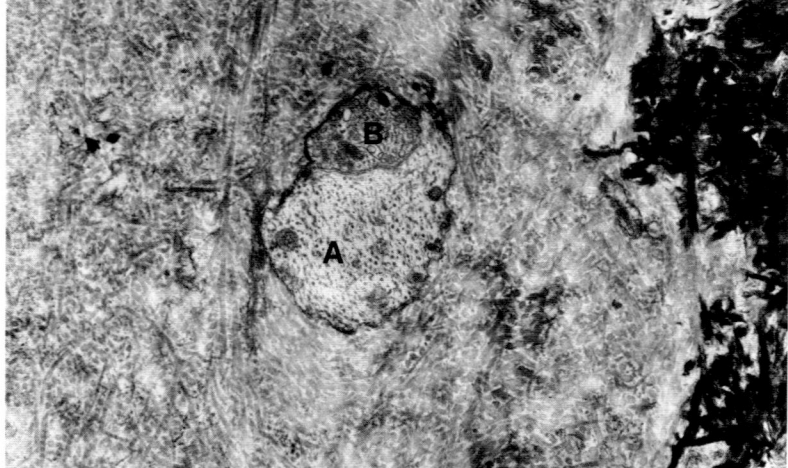

229A Odontoblast process (A) in predentine accompanied by another process (B), possibly a nerve, containing a more varied collection of organelles. The odontoblasts and nerves are said to be distinguished from each other by the appearance of 'clumps' of mitochondria in the nerves. (*Electron micrograph*, × 15,000)

The nature of the 'nerve-like processes' has now been clarified by autoradiography. In these studies, (^{3}H)-L-proline was injected into the trigeminal (Gasserian) ganglion, the label subsequently reaching nerve endings, having passed along the trigeminal nerve from the site of injection by axonal transport.

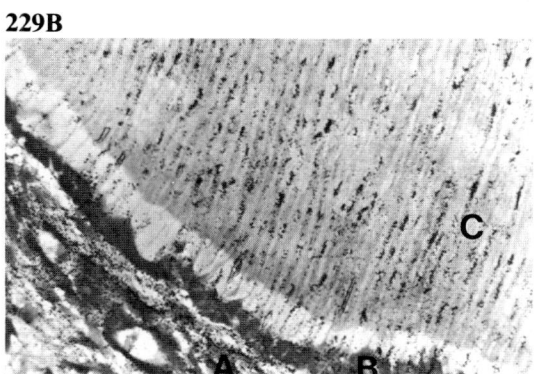

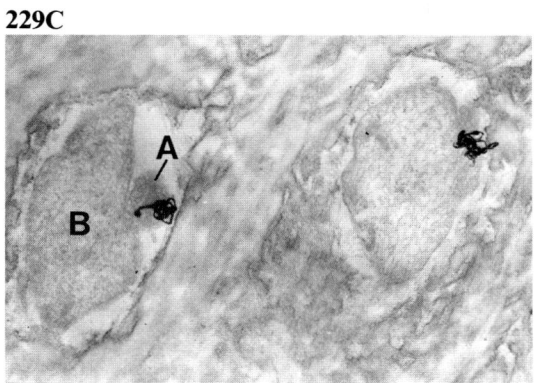

229B Light microscope autoradiograph showing the position of nerve endings in rat dentine. The presence of radioactively labelled nerve endings is demonstrated by the black silver grains developed in photographic emulsion painted over the section. Silver grains occur over the subodontoblastic plexus (of Raschkow) (A), the odontoblast layer (B) and over the dentinal tubules in the inner circumpulpal dentine (C). ($\times 600$)

229C Labelled nerve (A) adjacent to an odontoblast process (B) in the coronal dentine of a rat. Developed silver grains can be detected over the nerve-like processes which accompany odontoblastic processes in the dentinal tubules. This evidence confirms that these structures are different axons whose cell bodies lie in the trigeminal ganglion. Almost all the radioactivity remains within the nerve terminals for at least 7 days after injection and does not transfer to other cells in significant amounts. (*Electron microscopic autoradiograph, $\times 17,000$*)

Nerves in dentine appear to be limited to inner dentine and are more prevalent beneath cusps and incisal margins. Nerve frequency decreases between cusps and cervically, and nerves are absent from root dentine. At present the functional significance of the dentinal innervation is not clear. Since the evidence at present shows that the nerves may not extend into outer dentine, the most plausible current hypothesis concerning dentinal sensibility would seem to be that stimuli applied to the outer dentine cause the movement of tubule contents (either inwards or outwards) and as a result nerve terminals in the inner dentine and outer pulp are excited mechanically. Conflicting results from human and animal experiments, however, suggest that this mechanism may only be dominant in teeth in which the pulps are inflamed. In healthy teeth, stimuli cross the dentine by simple diffusion and conduction. It is possible that several mechanisms co-exist and that the dominant mechanism is determined by the condition of the pulp. The nerve-odontoblast relationship and its possible significance is described in relation to figure **261**.

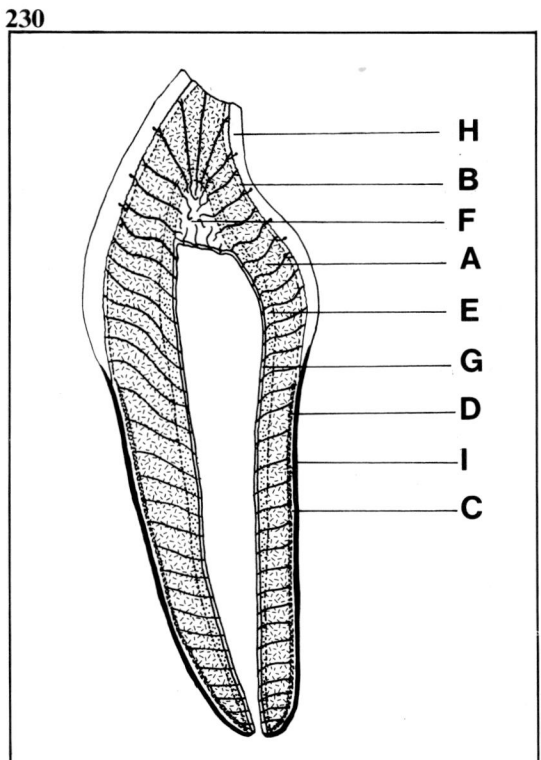

230 Regional differentiation of dentine. Dentine is not a uniform tissue but differs from region to region. The bulk of the dentine, termed circumpulpal dentine (A), differs in terms of structure and composition from the outer dentine lining the amelodentinal junction, mantle dentine (B). In the root, the mantle dentine becomes continuous with a hyaline layer (C) which lies above a granular layer (D). The term primary dentine is used to describe the first-formed dentine which produces the typical form of the tooth. Secondary dentine is deposited during the later functional life of the tooth inside the primary dentine. Secondary dentine may be subdivided into regular (E) and irregular (F) varieties, depending upon its structure (see pages 100, 101). The innermost, uncalcified layer of dentine lining the pulp is termed the predentine (G). H, enamel; I, cementum.

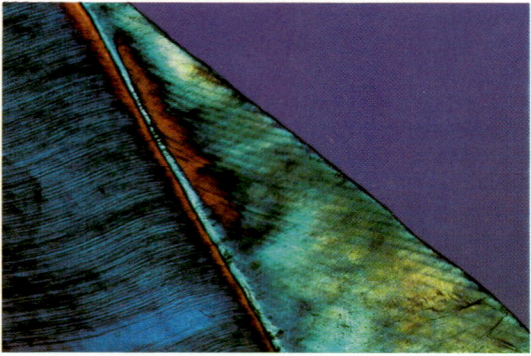

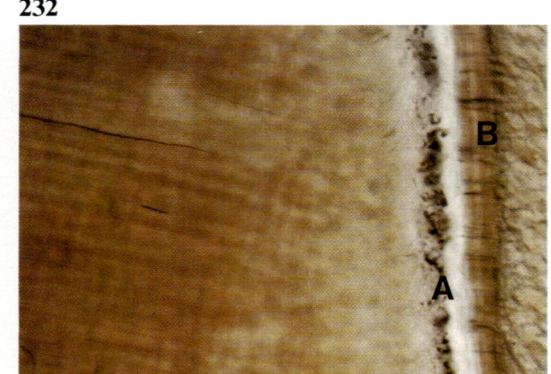

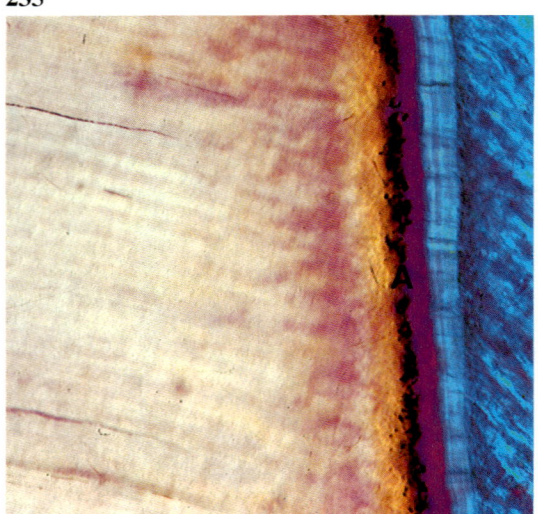

231 Longitudinal, ground section showing mantle dentine viewed in polarised light through a quartz sensitive tint. Mantle dentine appears as the orange layer immediately beneath the amelodentinal junction. The use of polarised light allows a visible distinction to be made between the mantle dentine and the circumpulpal dentine which here appears blue. The mantle dentine is a thin layer approximately 20μm wide. It is the first dentine formed. The main distinguishing feature of the mantle dentine is the orientation of a large proportion of its collagen fibres perpendicular to the amelodentinal junction. The fibres of the circumpulpal dentine are mainly parallel to the amelodentinal junction. Such differences in orientation account for the differing appearances in polarised light. Mantle dentine also differs from circumpulpal dentine in the following respects: mantle dentine is hypomineralised compared with circumpulpal dentine; many of its fibres are said to be derived from the subodontoblastic cells (see pages 164–6), the fibres of the circumpulpal dentine, on the other hand, being derived from odontoblasts; the dentinal tubules in mantle dentine branch more profusely than those in circumpulpal dentine. (×50)

232 Ground section of root dentine showing the granular and hyaline layers. The granular layer (A) is seen as a thin, dark, granular region just beneath the cementum (B), lying along the whole length of the root. It is hypomineralised compared with the circumpulpal dentine. Its appearance has been related to the presence of minute, interglobular areas produced as the result of incomplete mineralisation or, alternatively, to the scattering of light from air trapped in dilatations or loops of the terminal parts of the dentinal tubules. This layer is not seen in demineralised sections.

Immediately superficial to the granular layer is the clear and relatively structureless hyaline layer (C) which is approximately 15μm wide. The hyaline layer may be difficult to distinguish from the adjoining layer of acellular cementum. (×160)

233 The granular and hyaline layers in polarised light. The ground section illustrated in figure 232 is here viewed through polarised light with a quartz sensitive tint. The granular layer (A) appears as that seen in ordinary transmitted light. However, the hyaline layer is sharply demarcated from the overlying acellular cementum. Its purple colour indicates a lack of birefringence due to the mixed orientation of its fibres. (×160)

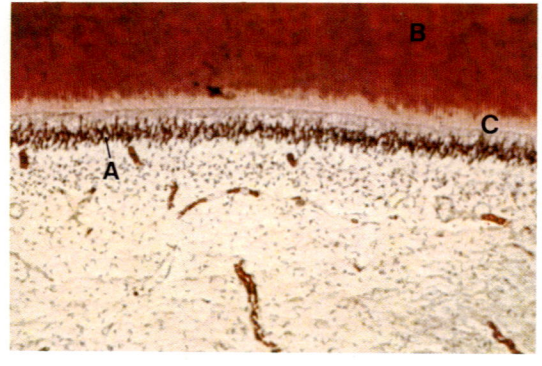

234 Decalcified section of the pulp and inner regions of the dentine showing the predentine layers. Between the odontoblast layer (A) and the darker staining circumpulpal dentine (B) lies a pale zone, the predentine (C). The border between the circumpulpal dentine and predentine is the mineralising front, predentine being unmineralised. The term intermediate dentine has been used to describe the region around the mineralising front where complex reactions involving the glycosaminoglycans of the matrix are taking place. Such histochemical changes may account for the differences in staining reactions between the organic matrix of predentine and that of circumpulpal dentine. (H&E, ×100)

Structural lines in dentine

A number of lines have been described running roughly at right angles to the dentinal tubules. However, controversy exists concerning the seemingly irreconcilable differences between the descriptions and explanations of these structures by different authorities. The following description of structural lines in dentine is essentially a compromise. Two basic types of line can be distinguished, those related to the curvatures of the dentinal tubules – Schreger and Owen's lines – and those related to disturbances in dentinogenesis or the rhythmic deposition of dentine – von Ebner and mineralising lines.

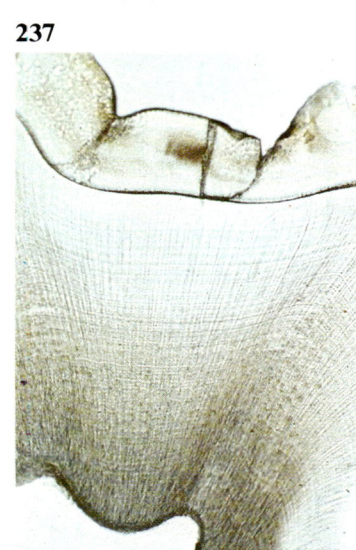

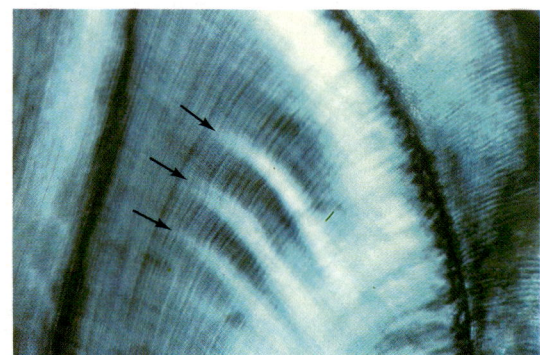

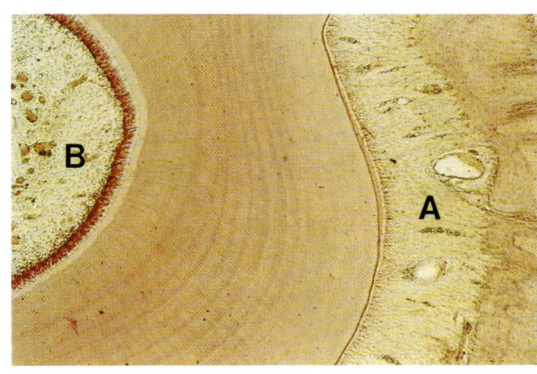

235 A Schreger line (A) seen in a longitudinal ground section through dentine. These lines result from the congruence of the primary curvatures of the dentinal tubules. In ground, transverse section two Schreger lines may be seen as concentric rings. ($\times 5$)

236 The contour lines of Owen (*arrowed*) seen in a longitudinal, ground section of dentine viewed in polarised light. Where the secondary curvatures of the dentinal tubules become coincident, the optical effect so produced gives rise to a contour line of Owen. In primary dentine Owen's lines are rare. The most distinctive and consistent Owen's line is seen at the junction of the primary and regular secondary dentine (see figures **244** and **245**). ($\times 120$)

237 Ground, longitudinal section through dentine showing von Ebner's lines. In this section, the lines of von Ebner are seen running approximately at right angles to the tubules. These lines are produced by variations in the fibre arrangement within the organic matrix of dentine. They appear as smooth lines spaced regularly at about 5μm. ($\times 12$)

238 High power view of von Ebner lines seen in polarised light. In this section, some of the dentinal tubules are highlighted (*arrowed*) and the von Ebner lines are seen running at right angles to the tubules at regular intervals. von Ebner lines are incremental lines possibly related to the phasic deposition of dentine matrix during its formation. ($\times 250$)

239 Decalcified cross-section of root dentine showing mineralising lines. Incremental lines due to variations in mineralisation may be seen microradiographically in ground sections and in demineralised sections with certain stains. Such lines are not as regularly spaced as von Ebner lines. Because the mineralising lines take on the shape of the mineralising front at different stages of dentinogenesis, they often have a more jagged appearance than the von Ebner lines. Since the mineralising front is not necessarily parallel to the inner surface of the predentine, mineralising lines often lie at an angle to the von Ebner lines. A, periodontal ligament; B, pulp. (*H&E*, $\times 80$)

240 Neonatal lines (*arrowed*) in dentine and enamel seen in a longitudinal, ground section. In the deciduous teeth and the first permanent molar an accentuated incremental line is seen separating the pre- and post-natally formed dentine. In the specimen shown, it is unusually clear and pigmented having come from the tooth of a patient who had suffered from icterus neonatorum, a disorder associated with disconjugation of bile pigment. (× 25)

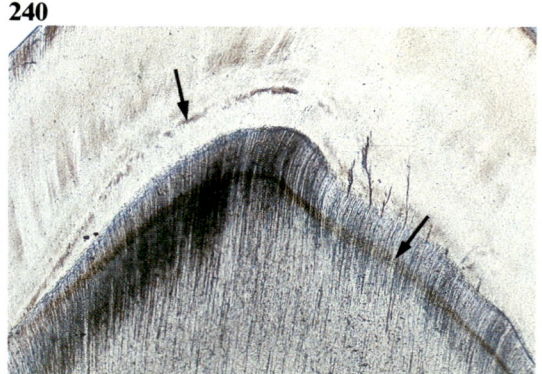

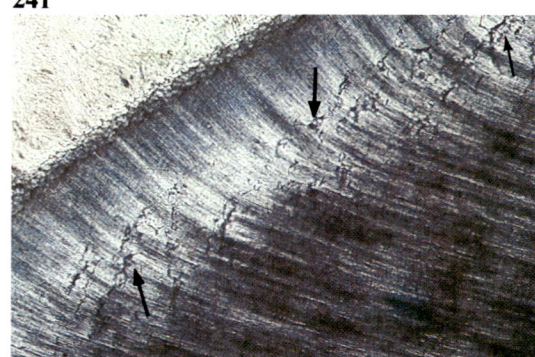

241 Longitudinal, ground section of dentine showing interglobular dentine (*arrowed*). A considerable proportion of the mineral in dentine is laid down in the form of globules, the calcospherites (see page 167). Where the calcospherites do not completely fuse, hypocalcified areas between the globules occur and these may persist in mature enamel particularly in the coronal, circumpulpal dentine close to the amelodentinal junction, as interglobular areas. (× 32)

242 The hypocalcified nature of interglobular dentine (*arrowed*). Note the tubules passing through the interglobular areas. (*Microradiograph, × 200*)

Secondary dentine and other post-eruptive features of dentine formation

Post-eruptive changes in the structure of dentine may be related to age changes or to reactions to noxious or pathological stimuli. With age, dentine formation slowly continues, and the term regular secondary dentine is used to describe this tissue. Since regular secondary dentine is laid down at the pulpal end of the primary dentine, the pulp cavity decreases in size with age. As mentioned previously, peritubular dentine generally increases with age and may completely obliterate the tubule giving rise to sclerotic dentine. In response to noxious stimuli, the odontoblasts may 'evacuate' the tubules giving rise to the so-called dead tract, and/or seal off the tubules at their pulpal ends with irregular secondary dentine.

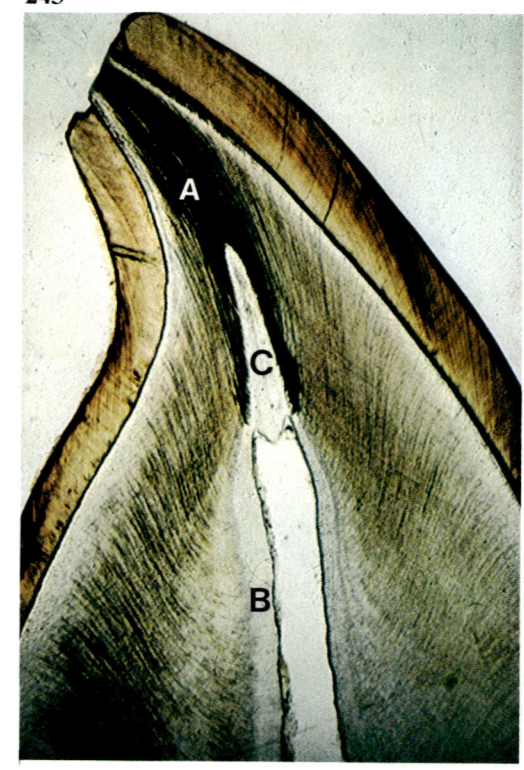

243 A dead tract (A), regular secondary dentine (B) and irregular secondary dentine (C). This is a longitudinal ground section through dentine. The dead tract shown has been produced in response to attrition. Its dark appearance is said to be related to the retention of air in the 'emptied' tubules which have not been penetrated by the mounting medium. Areas simulating dead tracts can be produced during the preparation of a ground section. A 'true' dead tract may be recognised by areas of sclerotic dentine bounding the tract laterally and pulpally. Occasionally, dead tracts are found in the dentine of unerupted teeth, possibly associated with atrophic degeneration of the odontoblast process due to excessive crowding during development. (× 15)

244A Primary (A) and regular secondary (B) dentine. This is a longitudinal ground section through dentine. Regular secondary dentine may not be easily distinguished from primary dentine. There are usually fewer tubules in secondary dentine. There is often a sudden change in tubule direction from that taken by the tubules of primary dentine, thus forming a pronounced contour line. Peritubular dentine is poorly developed in secondary dentine. (×80)

244B Longitudinal ground section viewed in polarised light with a quartz sensitive tint. This is the same specimen as figure **244A**. The colour differences illustrate the change in direction of the matrix and tubules from primary to secondary dentine. (×80)

245 The contour line of Owen separating the primary (A) and secondary (B) dentine. This is a decalcified section of dentine. (Silver, ×32)

246 Primary (A) and irregular (B) secondary dentine. This is a ground, longitudinal section of dentine in the floor of the pulp cavity. Where dentine is subjected to acute damage, e.g. dental caries, some of the underlying odontoblasts die, others lay down a form of repair tissue, irregular secondary dentine. Where there are tubules in this secondary dentine they are few in number and irregularly arranged. (×20)

247 Irregular secondary dentine filling a pulp horn. This is a decalcified, longitudinal section of dentine. (H&E, ×50)

248 Longitudinal, ground section of sclerotic root dentine viewed in polarised light with a quartz sensitive tint. With age, the tubules may become occluded with peritubular dentine. Since this peritubular dentine has the same refractive index as intertubular dentine such areas become optically homogeneous. A section of dentine mounted in a medium having a refractive index remote from dentine (e.g. water) will thus highlight tubular dentine from sclerotic or translucent 'tubular-less' dentine. In the section shown, the upper part of the dentine which is almost devoid of tubules is the sclerotic region. (×20)

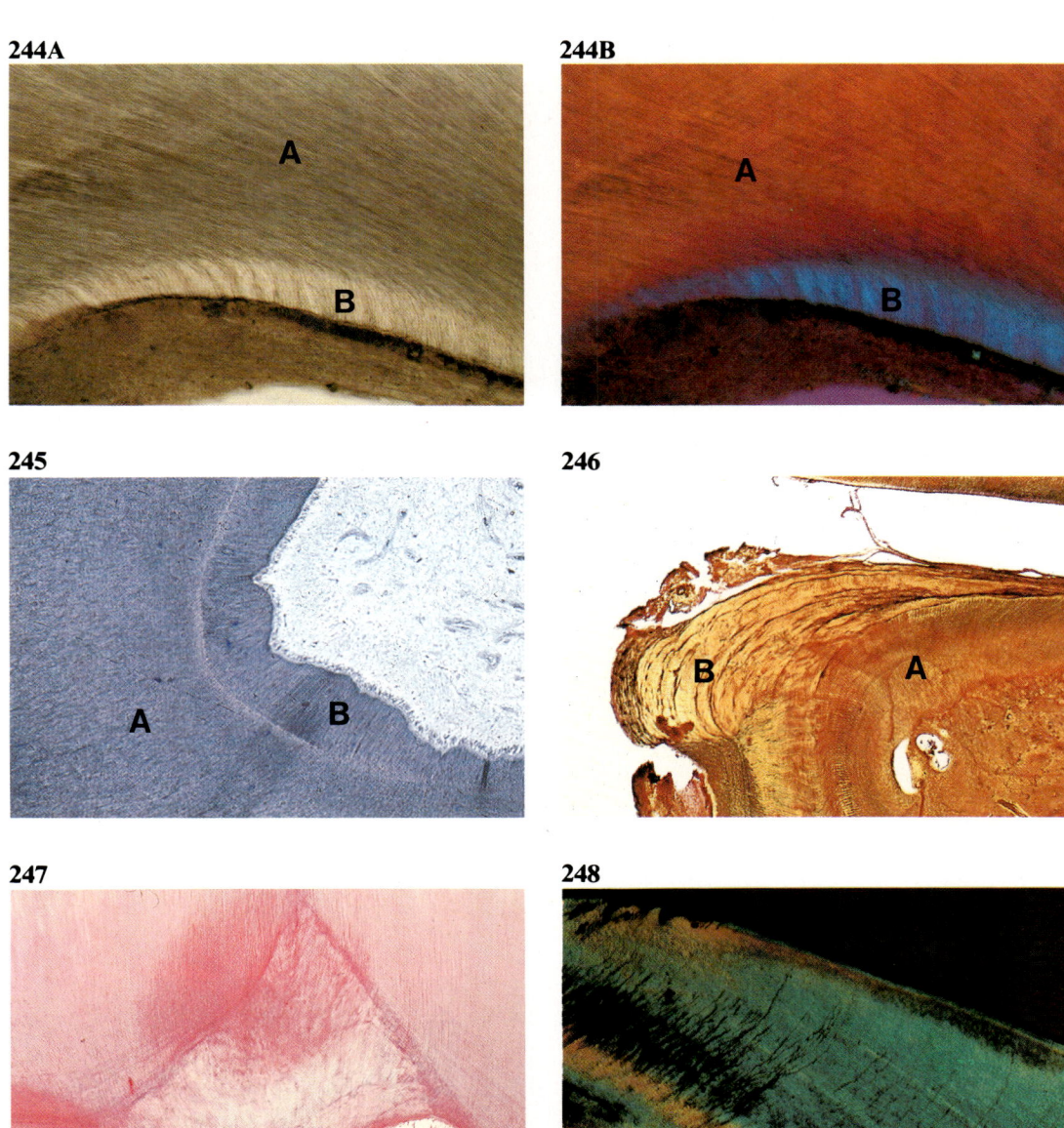

Dental pulp

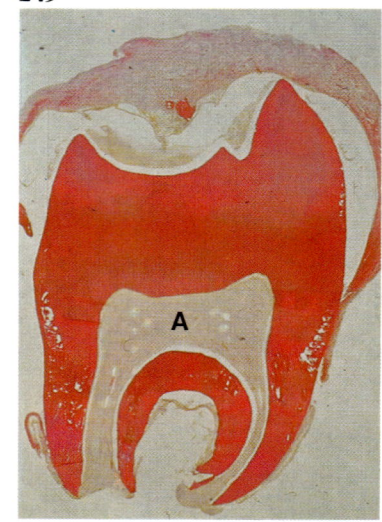

249 Longitudinal, decalcified section through a tooth showing the dental pulp (A). The dental pulp is a loose connective tissue derived from the dental papilla. It occupies a central position within the tooth. The morphology of the pulp has been described (page 34). The pulp is continuous with the connective tissue of the periodontal ligament through the apex of each root and occasionally by lateral or accessory root canals. The section shown is taken from a developing, unerupted tooth where the root apices are wide. With age, continued dentine formation narrows both the pulp cavity and the root apices. Functionally, the pulp is nutritive and sensory to the dentine. Its peripheral odontoblast layer is responsible for the development of dentine. The components of the pulp are common to all loose connective tissue, comprising cells, fibres, ground substance, blood vessels and nerves. It is composed of approximately 25 per cent organic material and 75 per cent water on a wet weight basis. The pulp differs from other loose connective tissues in having specialised dentine-forming cells, the odontoblasts, and in being contained within a rigid chamber having a high, tissue fluid pressure (approximately 20–25mm Hg above atmospheric). The pulp contains no fat cells, oxytalin fibres or mast cells. ($\times 5$)

250 Decalcified section of the outer region of the pulp. Peripherally, the predentine surface is lined by the odontoblast layer (A). Beneath the odontoblasts, at least in the crowns of older teeth, there is a zone where few if any cell bodies are located, the cell-free zone (of Weil) (B). This region would be better described as nucleus-free as cell processes, nerve fibres and blood vessels cross it in abundance. In electron microscopy, a similar zone is seen but it is usually narrower. It is possible that this layer is an artefact produced during fixation by shrinkage of the bulk of the pulp away from the odontoblasts which adhere firmly to the dentine. Beneath the cell-free zone, a cell-rich zone (C) may be distinguished. This contains not only an agglomeration of fibroblasts but also a network of nerve fibres and a capillary plexus. Central to the cell-rich zone, the pulp assumes an homogeneous pattern common to all loose connective tissues. In the middle of the pulp run the main blood vessels and nerves forming what may be called the pulpal neurovascular bundle. (*H&E*, $\times 70$)

Cells of the dental pulp

Three types of cell can be recognised in the dental pulp, the odontoblast, the fibroblast and defence cells.

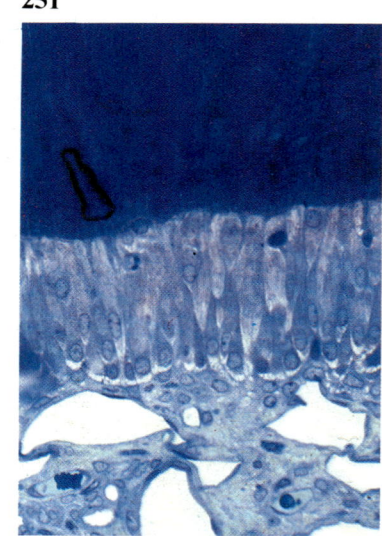

251 The odontoblast layer. The appearance of the odontoblast cell layer will vary throughout the life history of the tooth (see *dentinogenesis*, pages 164–6). In young teeth, it is only one cell thick. As dentine formation proceeds, the layer migrates pulpally and the odontoblasts become crowded producing a pseudostratified arrangement as illustrated. (*Toluidine blue*, $\times 320$)

252 The odontoblast cell layer sectioned longitudinally. The junction of the odontoblast layer with the predentine (A) is straight except where processes leave to enter the dentinal tubules. The cells are closely apposed at the dentinal surface but below this level there is an extracellular space which increases in size pulpally. The size and shape of cells and extracellular space is dependent on the fixation techniques but no matter how this is varied the close contacts at the dentinal surface are maintained. The cells are joined by junctional complexes. In the extracellular spaces around the cell, there are many cell processes some of which are probably minor odontoblastic processes. Since dentine is formed throughout life, the cells of the odontoblast layer show the full range of organelles characteristic of active protein synthesising and secreting cells. The conspicuous, oval nuclei are situated at the pulpal or basal ends of the odontoblast cell bodies; mitochondria, Golgi apparatus, rough endoplasmic reticulum and ribosomes are prominent in supra-nuclear regions. Some vesicles are present in the apical part of the cell but this feature is much more evident in the process than in the cell body. The cell body synthesises the elements which are to form the dentine but they are then transported for release by the process. Pseudostratification makes it difficult to visualise the full length and complete content of an odontoblast in any single section, the organelles appearing at different levels within the layer. The appearance of the odontoblast processes within the tubules of the dentine is described on pages 95–96. (*Electron micrograph,* × 2,000)

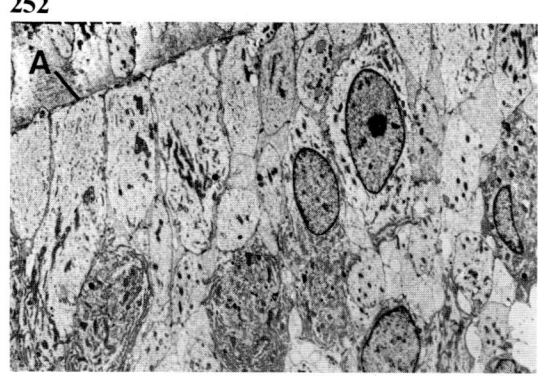

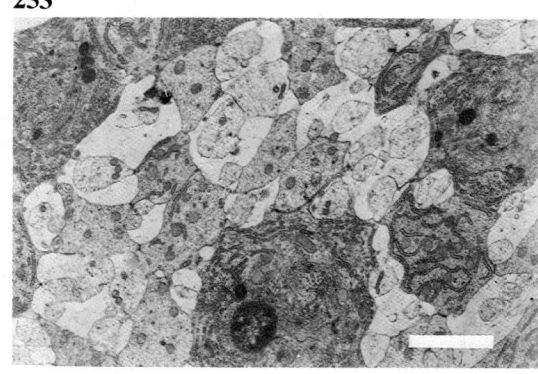

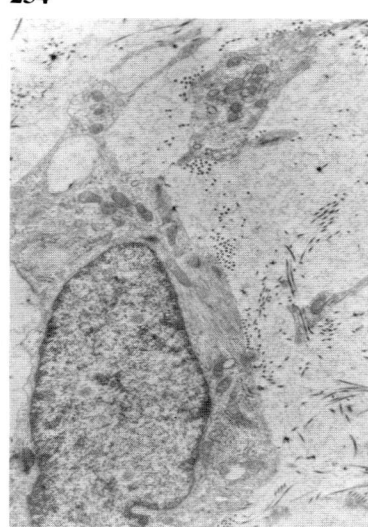

253 The odontoblast cell layer sectioned transversely. The darker staining odontoblast cell bodies show nuclei, rough endoplasmic reticulum and mitochondria. Between the cell bodies, paler staining cytoplasmic processes are seen, many of them firmly joined to the cell bodies by gap junctions (**261**). Many of these paler processes are smaller processes of the odontoblasts but some are probably terminal nerve fibres devoid of Schwann cells. (*Electron micrograph,* × 6,500)

254 A pulpal fibroblast. The fibroblast is the predominant cell type in the pulp. Pulpal fibroblasts are stellate cells, the arms of adjacent cells being joined by specialised junctions. The protein synthesising apparatus so well developed in the fibroblasts of the periodontal ligament (see figure **298**) is only poorly developed in these cells. Large areas of cytoplasm appear structureless and are crossed only by microfilaments. These cells are clearly less active than those of the periodontal ligament and this is reflected by the much lower fibre content of the extracellular space. However, when actively synthesising collagen and ground substance, the pulpal fibroblasts are markedly basophilic and in electron micrographs display an abundance of rough endoplasmic reticulum, mitochondria and Golgi apparatus. The less active cells may be called fibrocytes. (*Electron micrograph,* × 7,000)

The principal defence cell is the histiocyte or fixed macrophage. This cell appears flat or oval with a smaller nucleus than the fibroblast and a more granular cytoplasm. In inflammation, these become free macrophages. Both large and small lymphocytes are occasionally seen in the normal pulp; plasma cells are rare. Polymorphonuclear leukocytes are only found in inflamed pulps.

Defence cells are difficult to recognise in routinely prepared sections of normal pulp. Some primitive cells within the pulp retain the potentiality to differentiate into specialised cell types. These mesenchymal cells are difficult to distinguish histologically from the normal pulpal fibroblast.

Fibres and ground substance of the dental pulp

The fibres of the pulp are principally collagenous, making up 10 to 12 per cent of total pulp protein. The pulp contains no elastic fibres except in the walls of the blood vessels.

255 Collagen fibres in the pulp. The silver staining used to prepare this specimen reveals the large number of randomly arranged collagen fibres in the pulp. In the young pulp, the collagen is present in fine, single fibres or small bundles. Coarse, fibre bundles appear only at a much later stage. With increasing age, the fibrous content of the pulp increases and the cell population declines. (× 120)

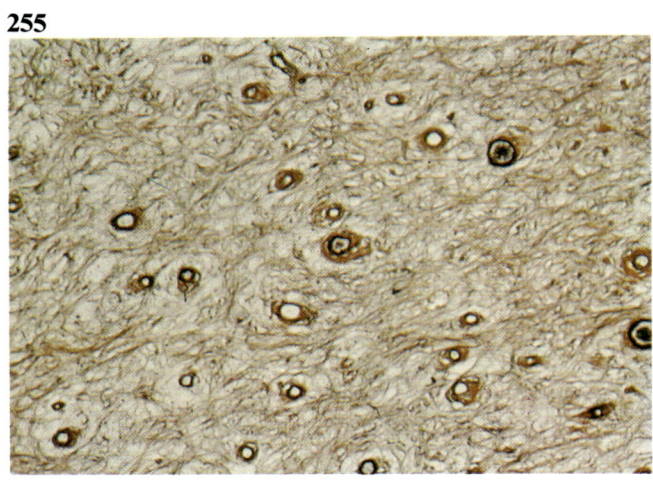

Ground substance – of the glycosaminoglycans present in the ground substance of pulp, on average 60 per cent is hyaluronic acid, 12 per cent chondroitin sulphates and 28 per cent dermatan sulphate. Some of these may be important in dentinogenesis. Glycoproteins are also present but little is known about them. The tissue fluid in the pulp appears to be a blood filtrate.

Blood supply and venous drainage of the pulp

The neurovascular bundle enters the pulp at its apical foramen which in young teeth is wide and may take the form of a delta with several canals. Lateral canals occasionally occur high up on the root. Arterioles are the largest vessels found in the pulp. The largest arterioles pass towards the occlusal surface along the long axis of the pulp but many side branches are given off en route. The arterioles terminate in a rich, subodontoblastic capillary plexus from which small capillaries pass into the odontoblast layer. Small venules drain the odontoblast layer and pass obliquely across the pulp chamber to join several small veins in the neurovascular bundle. There are numerous anastomoses between venules and arterioles. The veins are valveless and are reduced in number and diameter as the apex is reached.

256 Course of the blood vessels through the pulp. This is a decalcified, longitudinal section through a tooth. (*Iron haematoxylin,* × 6)

257 Blood vessels in the central pulp. Note the close relationship between the nerves (*arrowed*) and the blood vessels, although the larger nerves are not necessarily associated with the larger blood vessels. (*Toluidine blue,* × 380)

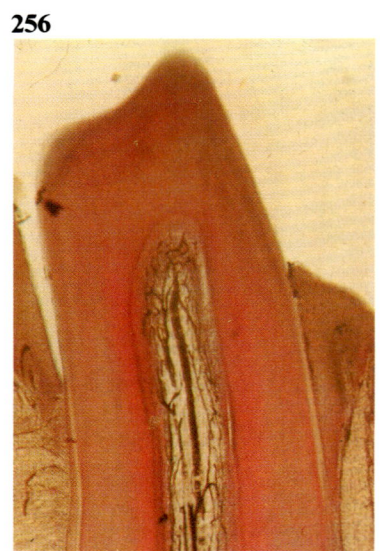
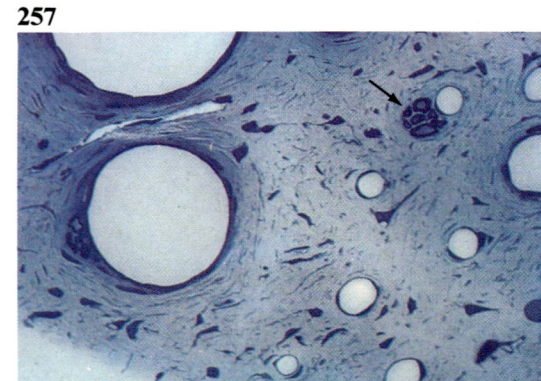

258 The subodontoblastic vascular plexus. The capillaries of this plexus have many looping branches passing between the odontoblasts towards the predentine. The capillaries of the plexus are often fenestrated, a modification which allows the rapid transfer of substrates. Occasionally, loops of capillaries are trapped in the dentine giving rise to the dentinal thorns. The subodontoblastic capillary plexus is usually absent from one wall of the root canal, and is rarely seen in areas where secondary dentine formation is in progress. Capillaries (C) of the subodontoblastic plexus are beneath the cell-rich zone (B) and odontoblasts (D). A, arteriole. (× 100)

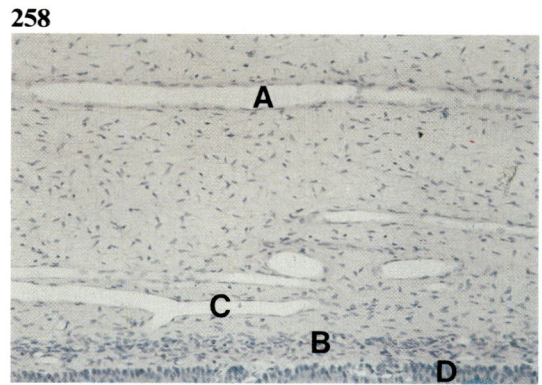

Lymphatic vessels are difficult to differentiate histologically from capillaries. Indirect evidence of their presence in the pulp has been obtained by studying the passage of dyes from pulp to local lymph nodes.

Nerve supply to the pulp

Compared to a similar volume of connective tissue elsewhere in the body, the dental pulp is richly innervated. The pulp is supplied with two groups of nerve fibres, unmyelinated fibres which are probably concerned with the control of vascular tone, and sensory, myelinated branches from the trigeminal nerve. The only sensation that can be elucidated from the pulp is pain. The course of the nerves follows closely that of the blood vessels to terminate in a dense plexus beneath the odontoblasts (Raschkow's plexus).

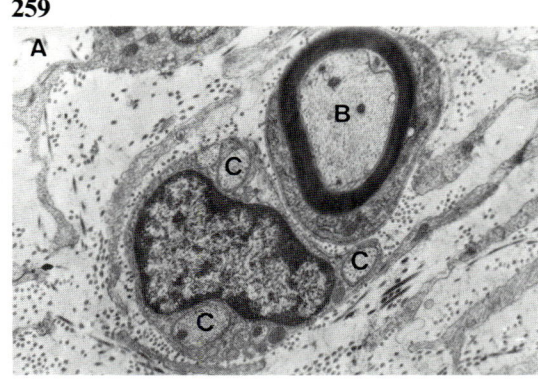

259 Central nerve bundle of the dental pulp. A, lumen of blood vessel; B, myelinated fibre; C, unmyelinated fibres. (*Electron micrograph, × 10,500*)

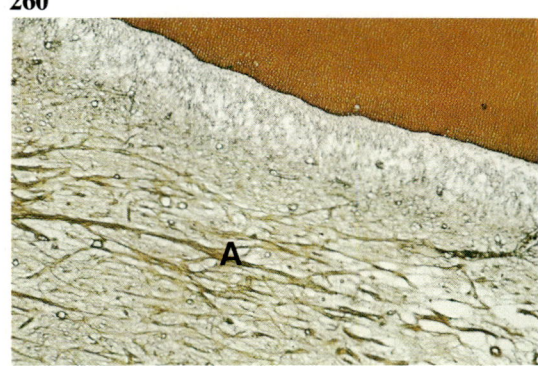

260 The subodontoblastic nerve plexus of Raschkow (A). By the time the myelinated nerves reach Raschkow's plexus, they have lost their myelin sheaths so that the axons are only surrounded by Schwann cells. Many small nerve fibres leave the plexus to cross the cell-free zone of the pulp and innervate the odontoblast layer. With age, a plexus of free nerve fibres, the marginal plexus, can be demonstrated on the predentine surface by silver staining. It is from this plexus that small, terminal, nerve fibres devoid of Schwann cells accompany the odontoblast processes up the dentinal tubules. The marginal plexus has not been seen under the electron microscope. (*Gomori's silver, × 80*)

261 A gap junction (arrow) between an odontoblast (A) and a nerve (B). Gap junctions allow ionic or 'electrical' communication between cells. They may be distinguished from occludens junctions and desmosomes (which provide a mechanical junction between the cells) by such differences as the absence of fibrils and the penetration of the substructure of the gap junction by extracellular space. Where gap junctions occur, a broad, dense intermediate line is seen between apposed cell membranes. In areas where the junction has been cut tangentially, a characteristic stippled pattern appears. The use of Lanthanam hydroxide as a marker of extracellular space shows that many of the junctions between nerve-like processes and odontoblast cell bodies are gap junctions. Since gap junctions provide a low electrical resistance pathway, they may act synaptically. This suggests, therefore, that the odontoblasts have a sensory function, though they may also be concerned with the metabolic support of nerve fibres or the transmission of mechanical disturbance. The excitability of odontoblasts has yet to be demonstrated by intracellular electrophysiological techniques. (*Electron micrograph, × 12,000*)

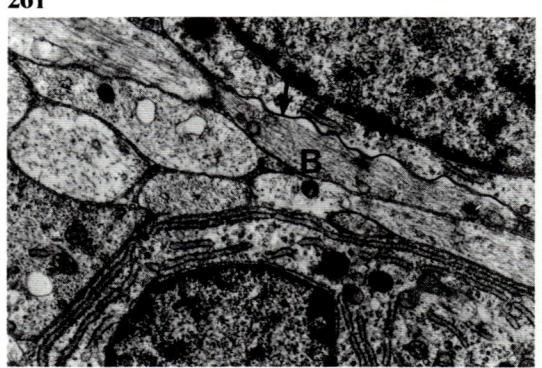

With age, the pulp decreases in size as dentine production continues, the cell density is reduced, the tissue becomes more fibrous and the blood supply declines. The pulp may become calcified either by discrete, lamellated bodies (pulp stones) or by diffuse granules of mineral throughout the entire chamber. On occasion, the pulp becomes entirely calcified.

262 Decalcified section through the pulp showing a pulp stone. Pulp stones may have a tubular structure resembling dentine (as shown here) or may be more irregular and have a laminated appearance. They may lie free in the pulp or be attached to dentine. (*Gomori's silver, × 80*)

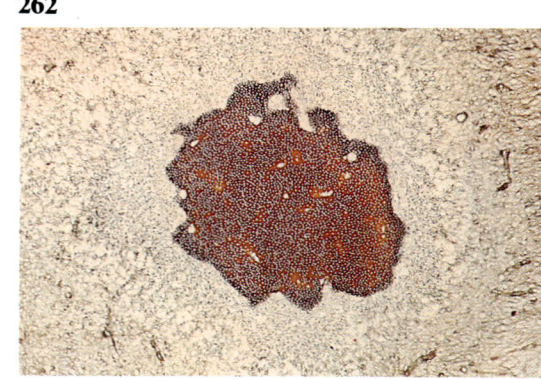

Cementum

263 Longitudinal, ground section through a tooth showing the distribution of cementum. Cementum is a thin layer of calcified tissue covering the external surfaces of the roots of the teeth. Its thickness varies according to age and site. It is usually much thicker in the apical part of the root and in the interradicular area of multirooted teeth than in the cervical region. Indeed, its thickness may exceed 600μm apically and be as little as 10μm cervically. Cementum is part of the attachment apparatus of the tooth, its outer surface being contiguous with the periodontal ligament, its inner surface being firmly bound to the underlying dentine. Cementum is derived from the inner layer of the dental follicle (see pages 170–1). It is formed throughout the life of the tooth, there being a thin layer of uncalcified matrix, the precementum, always present at its surface (see figure **270**). There are many structural and chemical similarities between compact bone and cementum. However, while bone is vascularised and innervated, cementum is avascular and has no innervation. A = cementum at root apex. (×4)

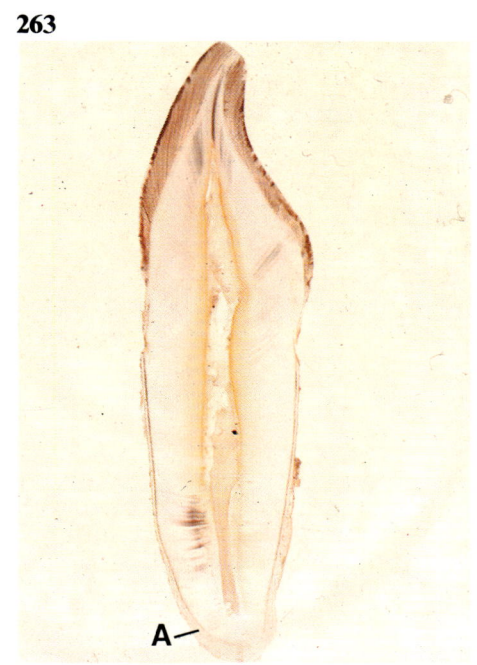

Physical properties of cementum. Cementum is light yellow in colour and lacks the lustre of enamel. It is softer and more permeable than dentine. Cementum is less readily resorbed than bone, though whether this is related to physical, chemical or biological differences between the tissues is not known. The success of physiological and orthodontic tooth movement relies upon resorption of bone without resorption of the tooth.

Chemical properties of cementum. Cementum contains approximately 65 per cent inorganic material, 23 per cent organic material and 12 per cent water on a wet weight basis. By volume, cementum is composed of 45 per cent inorganic material and 55 per cent organic material and water. The inorganic material is essentially hydroxyapatite although higher levels of trace elements are found in cementum than other dental tissues. The hydroxyapatite crystals in cementum are small, flat and plate-like, similar to those in dentine and bone. The organic matrix is composed mainly of collagen.

264 The cemento-enamel junction.
Pattern 1, where the cementum overlaps the enamel for a short distance. This occurs in 60 per cent of teeth.
Pattern 2, where the cementum and enamel meet in a butt joint. This occurs in 30 per cent of teeth.
Pattern 3, where the cementum and enamel fail to meet and the dentine between them is exposed. This occurs in 10 per cent of teeth.

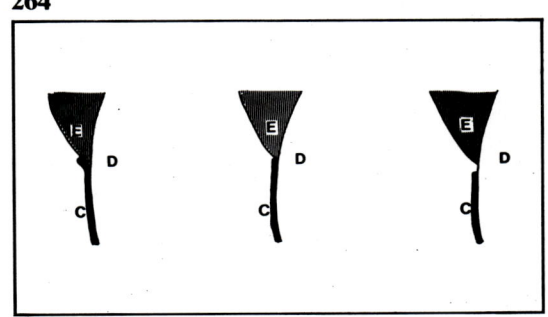

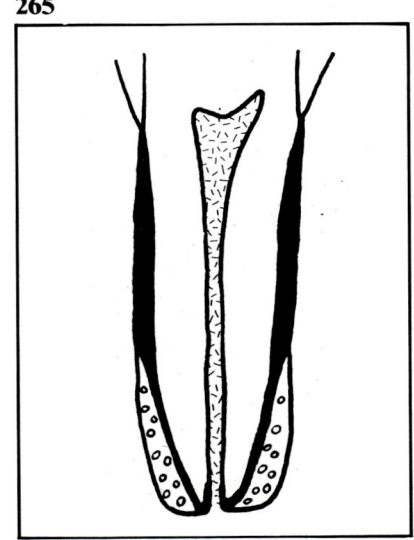

265 The types of cementum and their distribution. Two basic types of cementum have been identified, cellular and acellular cementum. As their names indicate, cellular cementum contains cells (the cementocytes), acellular cementum does not. Acellular cementum generally covers the whole surface of the root while cellular cementum is usually found in the apical third of the root covering a layer of acellular cementum. Since acellular cementum is the first-formed cementum, it has been termed primary cementum. Correspondingly, cellular cementum has been termed secondary cementum.

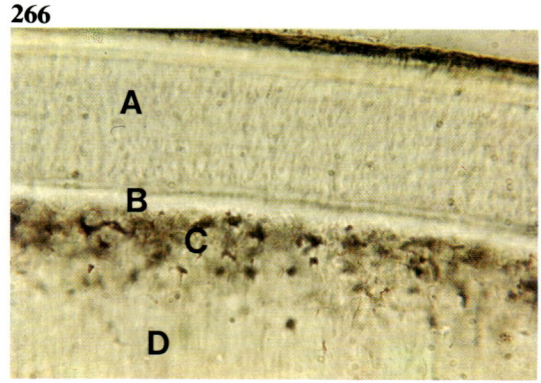 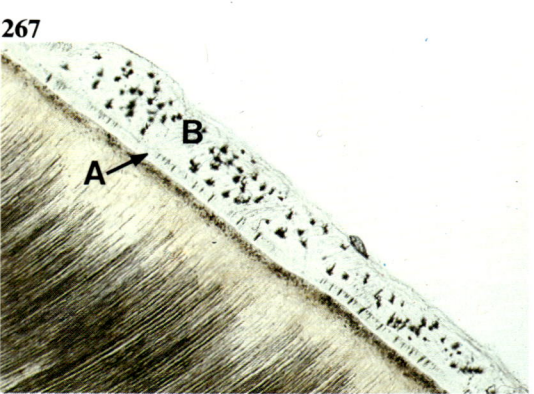 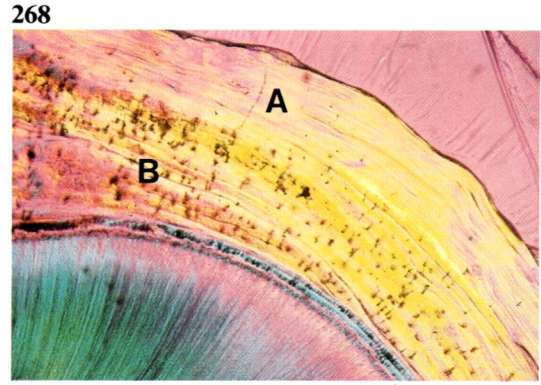

266 The relatively structureless appearance of a layer of acellular cementum. This is a ground section of a root near the cervical margin. A, acellular cementum; B, hyaline layer; C, granular layer (of Tomes); D, dentine. ($\times 200$)

267 A layer of cellular cementum (B) covering a thin layer of acellular cementum (A). This is a ground section of a root near its apex. Note the random arrangement of the cementocytes within the cellular cementum. ($\times 50$)

268 An unusual arrangement of acellular cementum (A) covering a layer of cellular cementum (B). This is a ground section of the apical part of a root. This section is viewed in polarised light with a quartz sensitive tint. ($\times 50$)

Some differences between acellular and cellular cementum	
Acellular	*Cellular*
No cells.	Lacunae and canaliculi containing cementocytes and their processes.
Border with dentine not clearly demarcated.	Border with dentine clearly demarcated.
Rate of development relatively slow.	Rate of development relatively fast.
Incremental lines relatively close together.	Incremental lines relatively wider apart.
Precementum layer narrow.	Precementum layer wide.

269A Ground section of cellular cementum showing lacunae and canaliculi. As cellular cementum is formed, many of the cement-forming cells, the cementoblasts, become embedded within the tissue. The entrapped cells are termed cementocytes. The small spaces they occupy within the cementum are termed lacunae. Small channels or canaliculi extend from the lacunae into the matrix of the cementum. The lacunae and canaliculi correspond to those found in bone though the lacunae in cementum are farther apart and more irregularly distributed than in bone and the canaliculi are not as extensive. The canaliculi of cementum are preferentially orientated towards the periodontal ligament. Canaliculi of adjacent cementocytes are connected. ($\times 60$)

269B High power view of lacunae and canaliculi seen in ground section. In the process of preparing a ground section, the cementocytes are generally lost and the lacunae and canaliculi become filled with air and/or debris thus appearing dark. ($\times 500$)

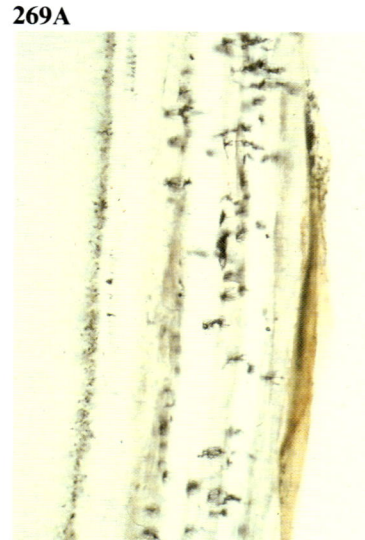 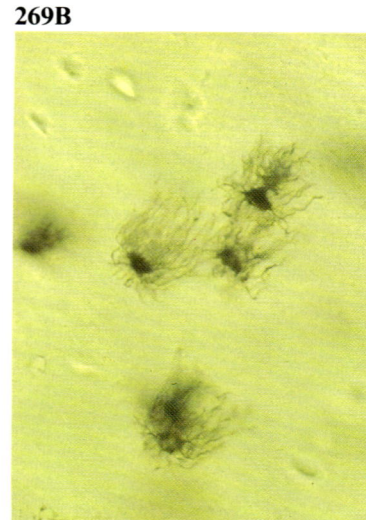

270 Lacunae with cementocytes seen in decalcified section. Also shown in this section is a layer of cementoblasts lining the periodontal surface of the cementum. This is a decalcified section through cellular cementum. Note the layer of unmineralised precementum between the layer of cementoblasts and the darker staining matrix of the mineralised cementum. The lines running parallel to the root surface are incremental lines (see also figure **275**). The collagen fibres of the periodontal ligament (A) can be followed into the cementum (Sharpey's fibres). (*H&E, ×200*)

271 A cementocyte within a lacuna. Cementocytes have relatively little cytoplasm and few organelles which is a sign of low metabolic activity. Compared with cementoblasts from which they are formed, cementocytes have relatively long processes which pass along the canaliculi. In the perilacunar space between the cell membrane and the wall of the lacuna, unmineralised collagen fibrils can be seen. (*Electron micrograph, ×4,500*)

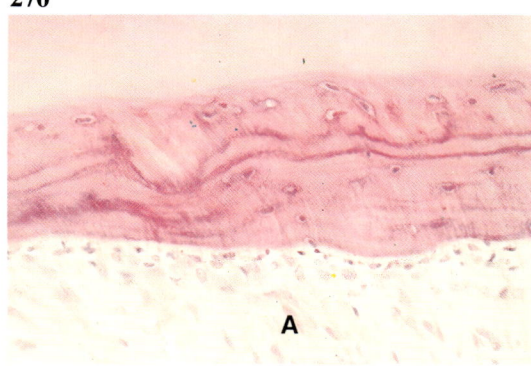

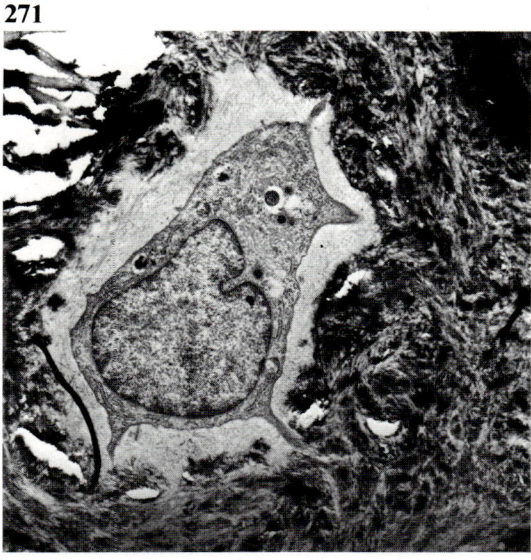

The appearance of cementoblasts, both at the light and electron microscope level, is described on page 117 in relation to the periodontal ligament.

The appearance of cementum under the electron microscope depends upon the level of sectioning.

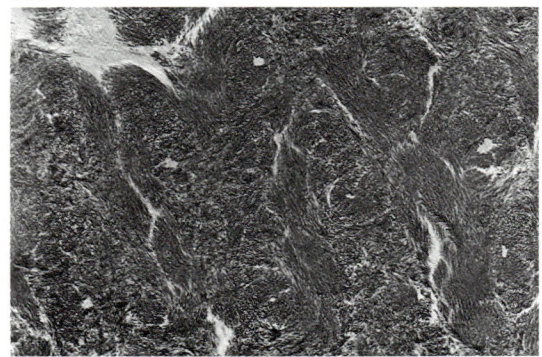

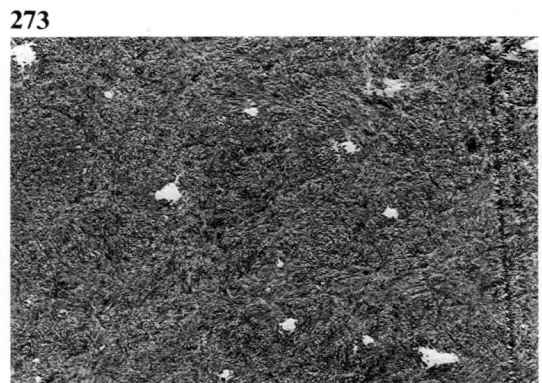

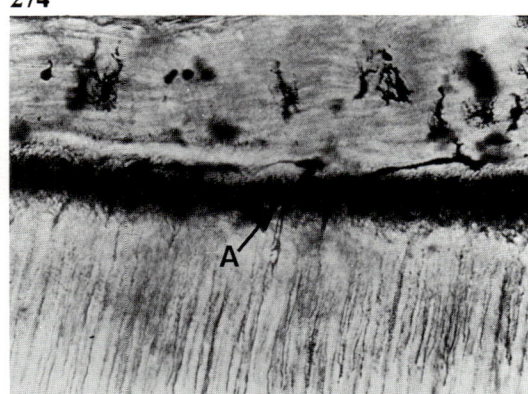

272 Cementum near its periodontal surface. Note the irregular appearance of this region where the calcification is not homogeneous. Calcification occurs on discrete bundles of fibres whose appearance is similar to that seen within the periodontal ligament. Indeed, this outer surface may simply be a calcification of the periodontal ligament. The fine channels permeating the tissue are thought to be canaliculi. (*Electron micrograph, ×1,750*)

273 Cementum near the cemento-dentinal junction. At this level, the appearance of cementum is somewhat reminiscent of that of outer dentine. Some fine channels run through the tissue. These channels may be connections between the canaliculi and dentinal tubules. (*Electron micrograph, ×1,750*)

274 Ground section of intermediate cementum near the cemento-dentinal junction. Intermediate cementum is that tissue, adjacent to the granular layer (A), which is characterised by wide, irregular branching spaces. Intermediate cementum is more commonly found in the roots of cheek teeth. The spaces in intermediate cementum may interconnect with dentinal tubules. The nature and origin of the spaces is controversial. One suggestion is that they may be related to entrapped epithelial cells. Alternatively, they may be enlarged terminals of dentinal tubules. (*×250*)

275 Decalcified section through cementum showing incremental lines. Cementum has a laminated pattern which reflects its rhythmic deposition. Such incremental lines (of Salter) are arranged parallel with the root surface. They may be hypo- or hypermineralised with respect to the remaining cementum. Since the rate of deposition of cementum is faster in cellular cementum than in acellular cementum, the incremental lines within cellular cementum are wider apart than those in acellular cementum. (*Mallory,* ×50)

Cementum, like bone, is a 'plastic tissue' allowing remodelling of the attachment as teeth move during development and growth. Changes in direction of tooth movement are often seen as pronounced reversal lines in the cementum.

The fibres within cementum are derived from two sources, namely Sharpey fibres from the periodontal ligament and intrinsic fibres from cementoblasts.

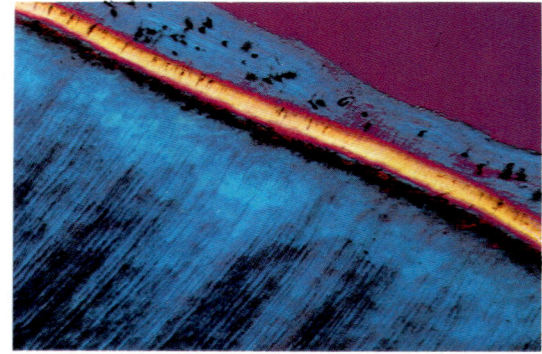

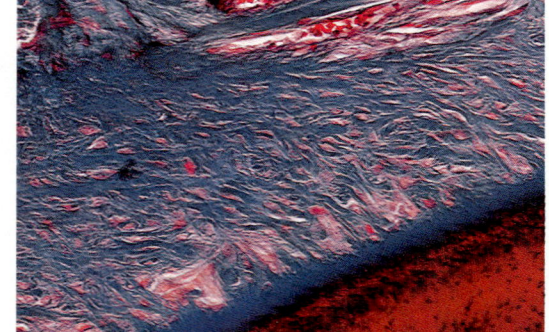

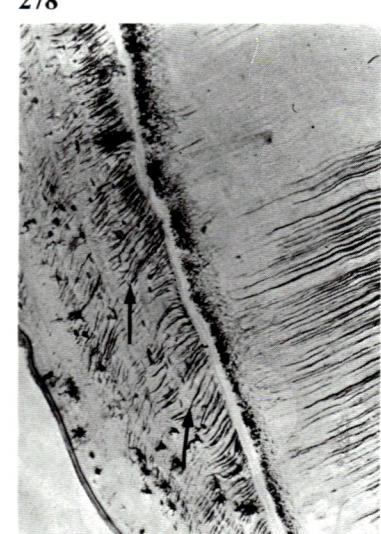

276 Fibre orientation within cementum. The tissue is shown in polarised light with a quartz sensitive tint. The different colours of acellular and cellular cementum suggest different fibre orientations within the two types of tissue. In the acellular cementum indicated by the orange zone, the fibres are chiefly orientated perpendicular to the surface. In the overlying cellular cementum most fibres are arranged parallel to the surface, though some run perpendicular to the surface (Sharpey fibres), the overall result producing a bluish colouration with some orange patches. (×50)

277 Decalcified section through cementum and periodontal ligament showing the attachment of the ligament to the cementum. The blue surface layer is uncalcified precementum, the deeper red zone, the matrix of calcified cementum. (*Masson's blue trichrome,* ×200)

278 Ground section of cellular cementum showing channels (*arrows*) for Sharpey fibres, running approximately perpendicular to the root surface. Many Sharpey fibres passing into cellular cementum have an unmineralised core only being mineralised at their periphery. During preparation of the tissue, therefore, the fibres have been removed and the resulting channels filled with air and/or debris giving the dark appearance. (×100)

279 The insertion of Sharpey fibres into cementum. A, undecalcified section; B, decalcified section. Note that the Sharpey fibres in the undecalcified section are partly mineralised. C, cementum; D, periodontal ligament. (*Electron micrograph, ×8,000, ×15,000*)

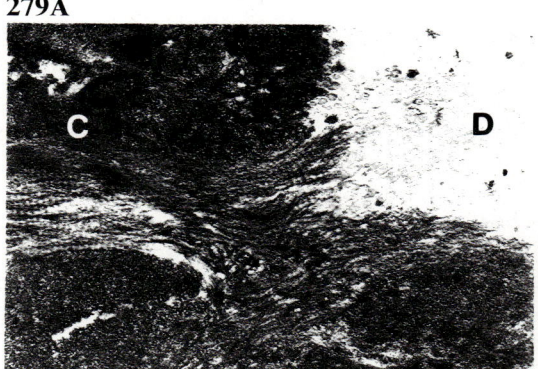
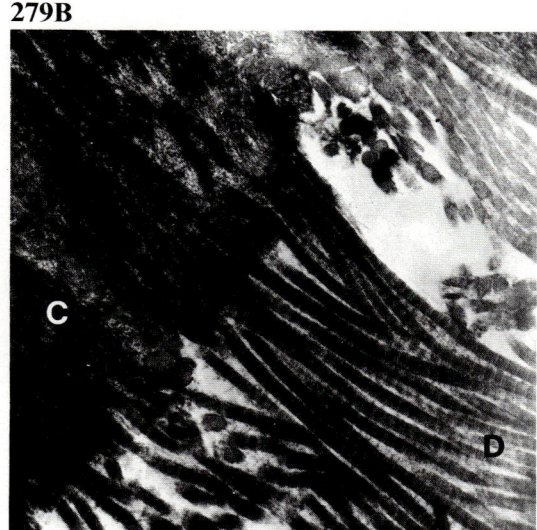

With age, there is a continued slow deposition of cementum and a decrease in permeability of the tissue. Associated with attrition of the crown of a tooth, compensatory deposition of cementum may take place at the apical region of the root. Should a root fracture, the fragments may be fused by the deposition of cementum (reparative cementum) between them. In certain situations, e.g. chronic periapical inflammation, cementum formation may be excessive giving rise to a localised hypercementosis. Hypercementosis affecting all the teeth may be associated with Paget's disease.

Periodontal ligament

280 Longitudinal, decalcified section of a tooth *in situ* showing the relationships of the periodontal ligament. The periodontal ligament is the dense, fibrous connective tissue which occupies the periodontal space between the root of the tooth and the alveolus. It is derived from the dental follicle (see pages 169–171). Above the alveolar crest, the ligament is continuous with the connective tissue of the gingiva while at the apical foramen it is continuous with that of the dental pulp. The average width of the periodontal space is 0.2mm, though there is considerable variation between and within individual teeth. The periodontal space is reduced in non-functional and unerupted teeth but is increased in teeth subjected to heavy occlusal stress. The periodontal spaces of permanent teeth are narrower than those of the deciduous teeth. The periodontal space is usually widest cervically. It is wider both cervically and apically than at its middle, and is hour-glass shaped. (*H&E, ×4*)

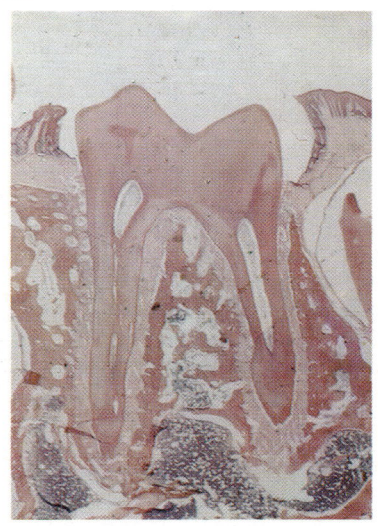

The following functions may be ascribed to the periodontal ligament:
1 It is the tissue of attachment between the tooth and alveolar bone. In this capacity it is responsible for resisting displacing forces.
2 It is responsible for the mechanisms whereby a tooth attains and then maintains its functional position. This includes the mechanisms of tooth eruption, tooth support and drift.
3 It protects the dental tissues from damage caused by excessive occlusal loads.
4 Its cells form, maintain and repair alveolar bone and cementum.
5 Its mechanoreceptors may be involved in reflex jaw activity.

The periodontal ligament has been likened to a fibrous joint (a gomphosis) and periosteum, though in both functional and anatomical terms, such comparisons, though interesting, are not strictly adequate.

Like other connective tissues, the periodontal ligament consists of a stroma of fibres in a gel of ground substance containing cells, blood vessels and nerves. The ligament is specialised in terms of its rich vascular and nerve supply, its high rate of turnover and the orientation of its fibres.

Fibres of the periodontal ligament

The principal structural element of the periodontal ligament is the connective tissue fibres which, though mainly collagenous, also consist of oxytalan, reticulin and some elastic fibres. Many of the collagen fibres are gathered together to form bundles, each bundle or principal fibre having a diameter of about 5μm, though smaller bundles may be seen.

281 Principal collagen fibres passing directly across the periodontal space from the root (A) to the alveolar bone (B). This is a transverse section through the periodontal ligament. Note the vascular nature of this fibrous tissue. (*Gomori's silver, ×250*)

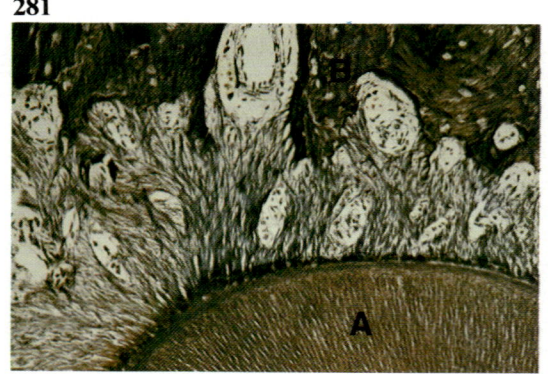

282 Periodontal ligament cut transversely to show the principal fibres and their close association with fibroblasts. Note the intimate relationship of the cells and the fibres. The fibroblasts are responsible for the synthesis and degradation of collagen. They appear as stellate cells whose processes surround or envelop the fibre bundles. Processes from adjacent cells contact and are joined by desmosomes to form a cellular network. Many of the isolated islands of cytoplasm present in this section are cell processes from fibroblasts whose cell bodies are beyond the plane of section. (*Electron micrograph, ×3,000*)

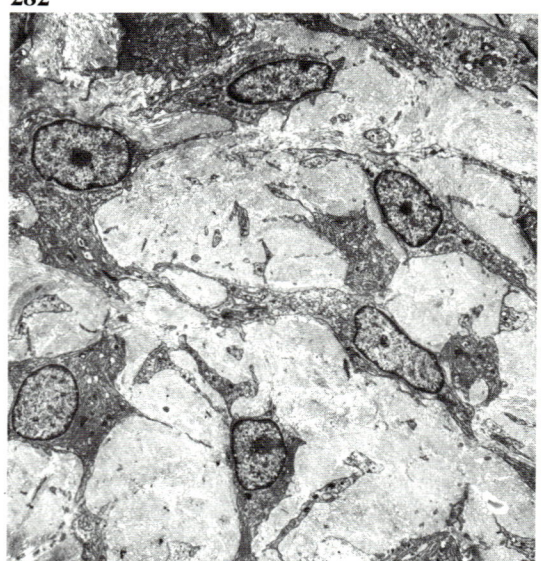

283 Fibre bundles cut in both longitudinal and transverse section. A process of fibroblast enveloping a principal fibre. Note that the individual fibrils within the principal bundle sectioned longitudinally show banding characteristic of collagen. (*Electron micrograph, ×10,000*)

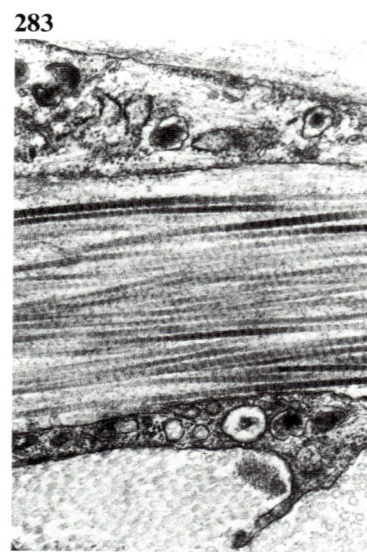

284 The orientation of the principal fibres of the periodontal ligament seen in longitudinal section. 1, dento-alveolar crest fibres; 2, horizontal fibres; 3, oblique fibres; 4, apical fibres; 5, interradicular fibres.

285 The dento-alveolar crest fibres (A) and the horizontal fibres (B). This is a longitudinal section through the periodontal ligament in the region of the alveolar crest. (*H&E, ×80*)

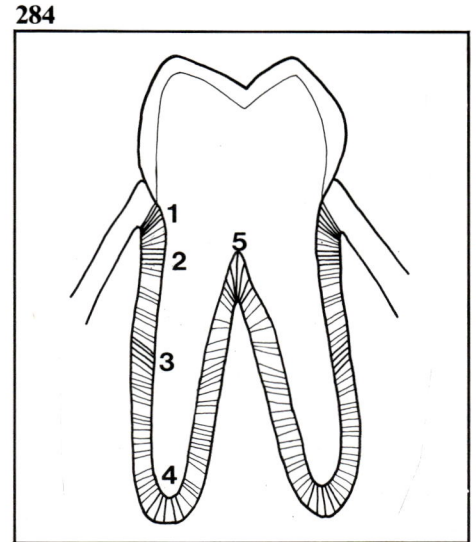

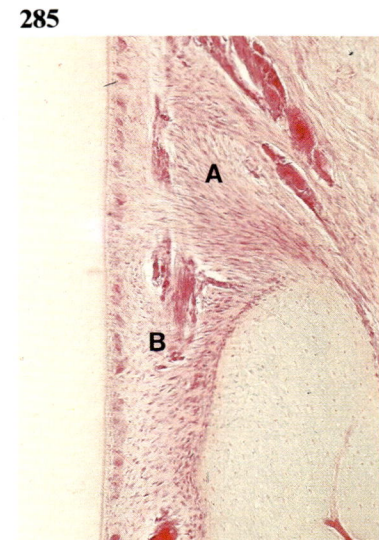

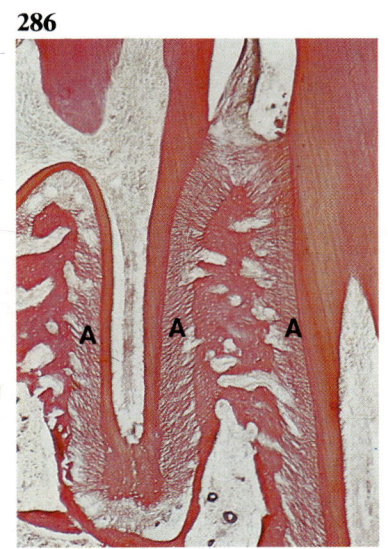

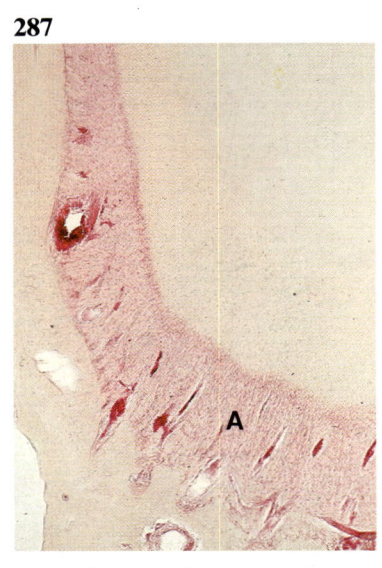

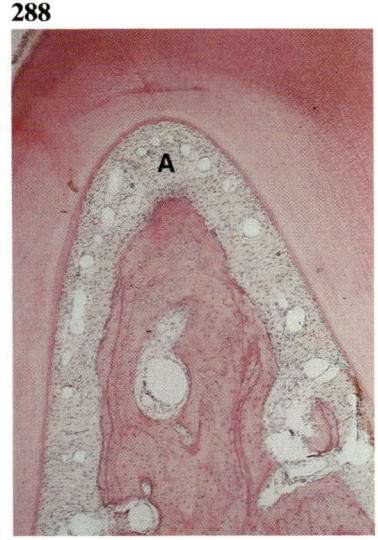

286 Longitudinal section through the ligament to show the oblique fibres (A). (*van Gieson, ×20*)

287 Longitudinal section through the ligament in the region of the root apex to show the apical fibres (A). (*H&E, ×30*)

288 Longitudinal section of the ligament in the region of a root bifurcation showing interradicular fibres (A). (*H&E, ×40*)

It has, in the past, been usual to ascribe specific functions to each of the groups of principal fibres. For example, the orientation of the oblique fibres has suggested to some that they form a suspensory ligament translating pressure on the tooth into tensional forces on the alveolar wall. No physiological evidence, however, exists to support such a concept.

Until recently, much controversy existed concerning the extent of individual principal fibres across the ligament. One view held that the fibres embedded in bone intercalated with fibres embedded in cementum via an intermediate plexus. On the other hand, recent evidence suggests that the fibres cross the entire width of the periodontal space but, en route, branch and join neighbouring fibres.

289 Longitudinal section through the periodontal ligament producing an appearance of an intermediate plexus (arrowed). (*Alcian blue, ×200*)

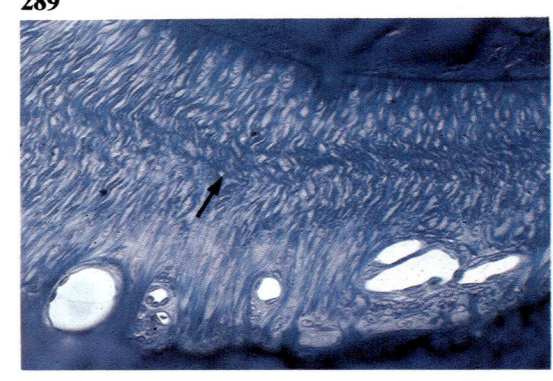

While the intermediate plexus provides a convenient model to explain axial tooth movements, the evidence suggests that it is produced artefactually by oblique sectioning. It has yet to be seen in perfectly longitudinal and transverse sections of the fibres.

290 Continuity of the principal fibres across the periodontal space. This is a periodontal ligament cut transversely. Although there is no intermediate plexus, the fibres branch and join one with another. (*Scanning electron micrograph, ×350*)

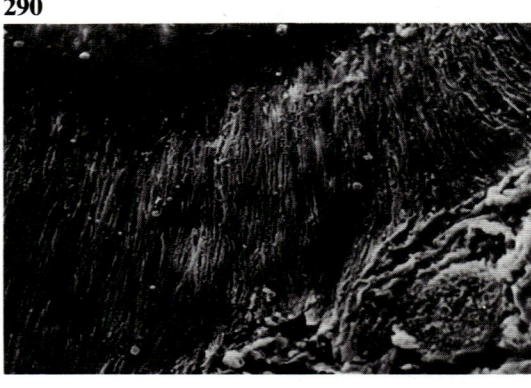

In addition to the principal fibre groups, the periodontal ligament is said to contain collagen fibres with a random orientation, forming an indifferent fibre plexus.

291 Periodontal ligament prepared with a rotating abrasive disc. Specimens prepared in this manner show the periodontal ligament to be mainly composed of a mass of fine, randomly orientated fibres, giving the appearance of an indifferent fibre plexus. (*Scanning electron micrograph, ×3,500*)

292 Periodontal ligament prepared by slicing through a demineralised tooth with a sharp razor blade. Unlike the previous illustration, the ligament consists almost entirely of branching principal fibres without an indifferent fibre plexus. Thus, the method of specimen preparation is important in determining the scanning electron micrograph appearance of the ligament. (*Scanning electron micrograph, ×3,500*)

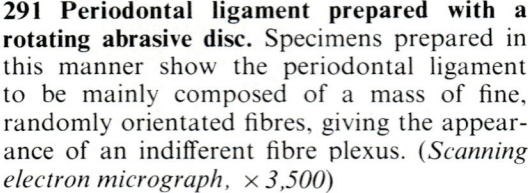 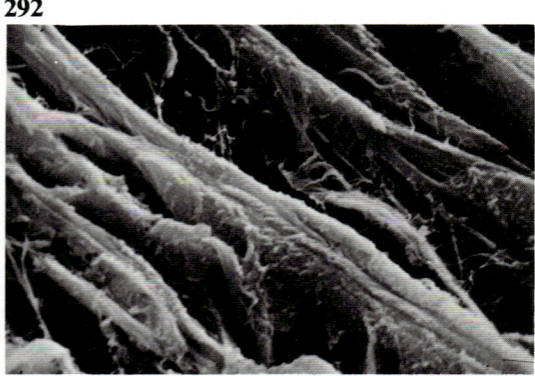

The principal fibres which are embedded in cementum and in the bone lining of the tooth socket are termed Sharpey's fibres.

293 The insertion of Sharpey's fibres into alveolar bone (A) and cementum (B). This is a decalcified section of periodontal ligament. (*H&E, ×100*) (Sharpey's fibres are dealt with further on pages 110, 111, 122 and 123.)

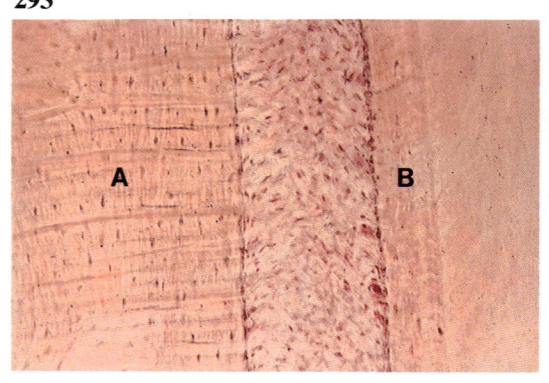

The rate of turnover of collagen fibres within the periodontal ligament is faster than in most other connective tissues. The rate varies in different parts of the same ligament and is thought to decrease with age. The high rate of turnover may relate to the changing functional demands placed upon the tooth in terms of remodelling as a reaction to occlusal stress and tooth movements. It has been suggested that collagen may contract during its maturation, thus providing a tractional force which, because of the obliquity of the principal fibres, may effect tooth eruption. However, there is, as yet, no evidence that collagen contracts under physiological conditions.

Oxytalan fibres are a recently discovered, fibrous, connective tissue component of the periodontal ligament. They appear to be more related to elastic fibres than collagen. In order to demonstrate oxytalan fibres at the light microscope level, it is necessary to oxidise tissue sections strongly prior to staining with certain elastic stains. Unlike collagen, they are not susceptible to acid hydrolysis. Little is known about their composition.

294 The course of oxytalan fibres (*arrowed*). This is a longitudinal section through periodontal ligament. The oxytalan fibres insert into the cementum and course out into the periodontal ligament in various directions, rarely being incorporated into bone. In the cervical region they follow the course of gingival and transseptal collagen fibres, but within the periodontal ligament proper they tend to be more longitudinally orientated, crossing the oblique fibre bundles more or less perpendicularly. In the outer part of the ligament they often terminate around blood and lymphatic vessels. (*Potassium monopersulphate, aldehyde fuchsin counterstained with van Gieson, × 40, × 120*)

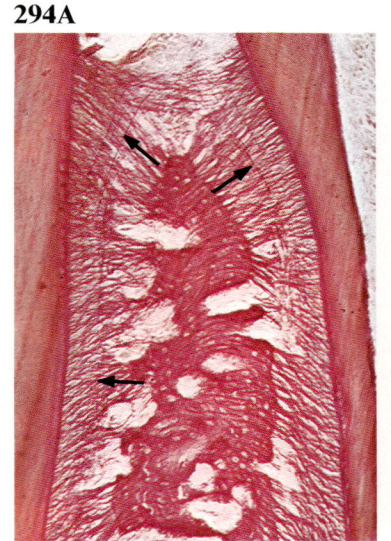
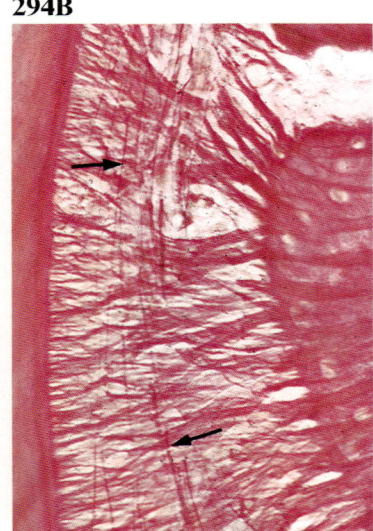

295 An oxytalan fibre. The oxytalan fibre (*arrowed*) can be recognised at the ultrastructural level as a collection of unbanded fibrils arranged parallel to the long axis of the fibre. Each fibril is approximately 15nm in diameter and an interfibrillar amorphous material is present in variable amounts. (*Electron micrograph, × 2,800*)

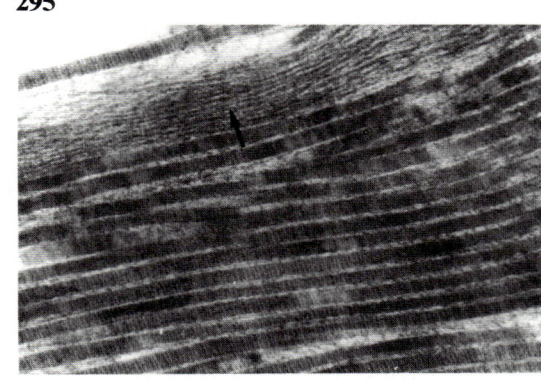

The function of oxytalan fibres remains unknown. They are thicker and more numerous in teeth which carry abnormal loads, including abutment teeth for bridges and teeth being moved for orthodontic reasons.

Elastic fibres are restricted to the walls of the blood vessels; *reticulin fibres* are related to basement membranes.

Ground substance of the periodontal ligament

Because of its relative inaccessibility, little detailed knowledge is available concerning the biochemistry of the gel. However, it is known to consist mainly of glycosaminoglycan-protein complexes and water, but also includes carbohydrates, lipids, proteins and glycoproteins. It is presumed to be secreted by fibroblasts.

As other connective tissues, the gel is associated with many important but poorly understood functions e.g. ion and water binding and exchange, control of collagen fibrogenesis and fibre orientation. Tissue fluid pressure has been found to be of the order of 10mm Hg above atmospheric. The tissue fluid has been implicated in the tooth support and eruptive mechanisms.

Cells of the periodontal ligament

The predominant connective tissue cell within the periodontal ligament is the fibroblast. Cells covering the surface of both cementum and alveolar bone are also considered part of the ligament (i.e. cementoblasts, cementoclasts, osteoblasts and osteoclasts). In addition, the periodontal ligament contains undifferentiated mesenchymal cells, defence cells and epithelial cell rests (of Malassez) as well as blood vessels and nerves.

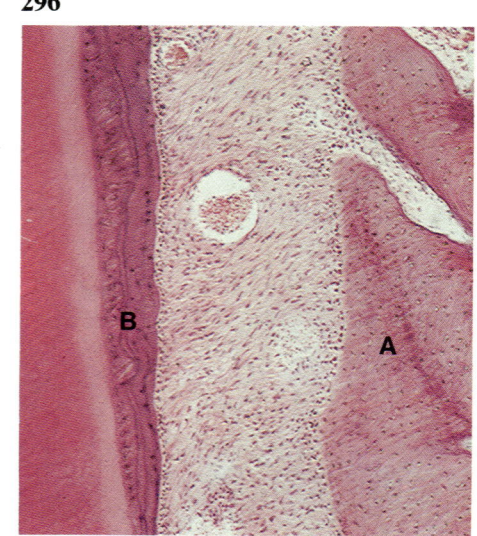

296 Decalcified, longitudinal section through the ligament, showing distribution of cells. The type and number of cells varies according to the functional state of the ligament. In addition to the numerous fibroblasts within the ligament, the surfaces of the alveolar bone (A) and cementum (B) are lined with osteoblasts and cementoblasts, indicating active deposition of bone and cementum in this specimen. (*H&E, ×60*)

The *fibroblasts* in the periodontal ligament may have a variety of shapes ranging from fusiform or tripolar cells with long, fine cytoplasmic processes to stellate cells with many short processes.

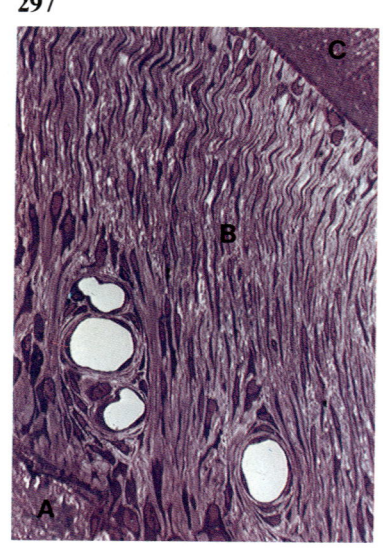

297 Decalcified, longitudinal section of a ligament (B) packed with fibroblasts. A, alveolar bone. C, cementum. (*Toluidine blue, ×300*)

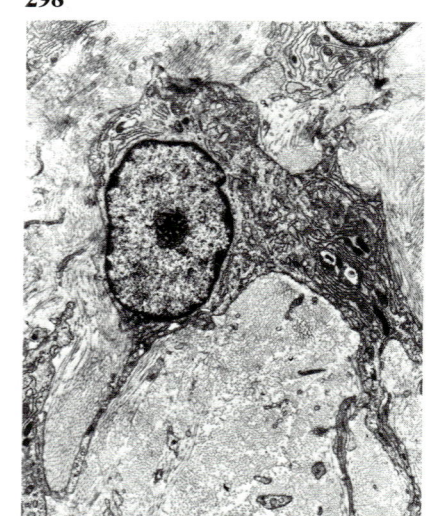

298 Periodontal fibroblast. When active, the fibroblasts have a low nuclear to cytoplasmic ratio. The nucleus is oval, contains one or more prominent nucleoli and may be folded. The typical periodontal fibroblast is rich in intracytoplasmic organelles. The cytoplasmic processes of the fibroblasts surround or envelop bundles of collagen. In the periodontal ligament where the turnover of collagen is rapid, the fibroblast shows a well-developed rough endoplasmic reticulum and Golgi apparatus and many mitochondria, these organelles being related to active synthesis and secretion of fibres and gel. Where turnover is less rapid the cells have a reduced content of intracytoplasmic organelles. (*Electron micrograph, ×6,200*)

299A Periodontal fibroblast showing intracellular collagen profiles (*arrowed*). (*Electron micrograph, ×5,000*)

299B Banded collagen fibrils (*arrows*) seen within an elongated membrane-bound vacuole. Recent evidence suggests that the intracellular collagen vacuoles are associated with the degradation of collagen which has been 'ingested' from the extracellular environment. Thus, the periodontal ligament fibroblast may be capable of both the synthesis and secretion of collagen and its degeneration, though as yet, the overall rôle of the fibroblasts in the remodelling of the periodontal ligament has not been determined. (*Electron micrograph, ×25,000*)

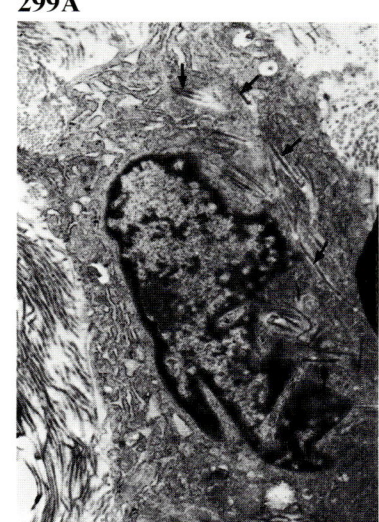
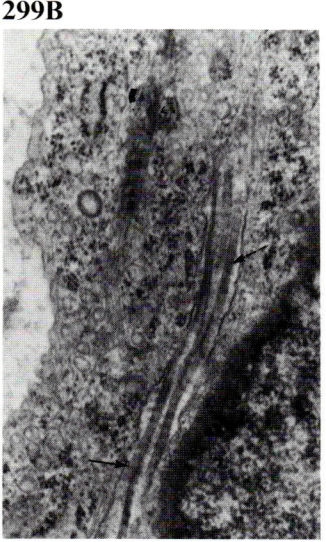

Cementoblasts are the cement-forming cells lining the surface of cementum. They are plump cells, rich in cytoplasm.

300 A layer of cementoblasts (*arrowed*) lining the cementum. This is a decalcified, longitudinal section of periodontal ligament. (*H&E, ×160*)

301 A cementoblast (A) lining cementum. Cementoblasts are not as elongated as periodontal fibroblasts being squat, cuboidal cells with large nuclei. Like fibroblasts, however, they contain all the intracytoplasmic organelles necessary for protein synthesis and secretion. The nucleus of a cementoblast is distinctly vesicular with one or more nucleoli. The appearance of a cementoblast will depend upon its degree of activity. Cells actively depositing acellular cementum do not have prominent cytoplasmic processes. However, cells depositing cellular cementum exhibit abundant basophilic cytoplasm and cytoplasmic processes, and their nuclei tend to be folded and irregularly shaped. B, precementum. (*Electron micrograph, ×3,700*)

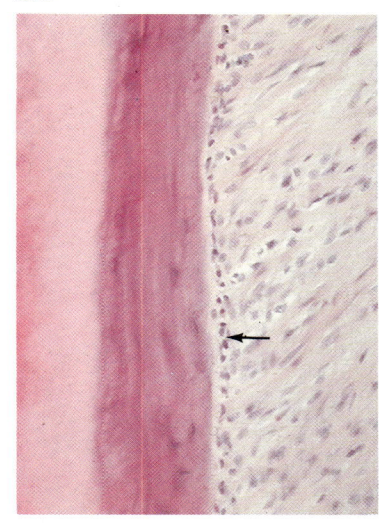
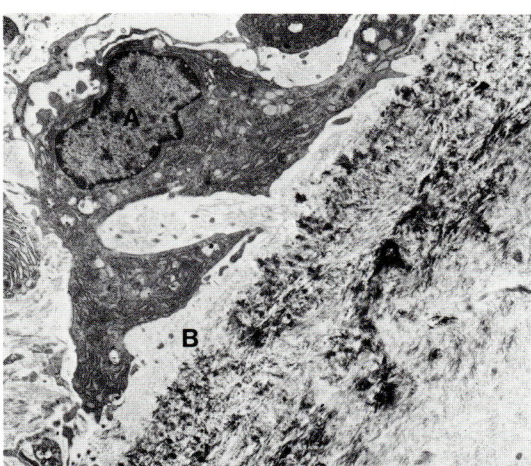

Osteoblasts are the bone-forming cells lining the tooth socket. They closely resemble cementoblasts.

Osteoclasts and *cementoclasts* are found in areas where bone and cementum is being resorbed. Recent evidence shows that these cells are actively involved in the resorption process. Osteoclasts and cementoclasts have the same cytoplasmic features.

302 A layer of osteoblasts (arrowed), shown lining the alveolar bone. This is a decalcified, longitudinal section of periodontal ligament. (*H&E, ×200*)

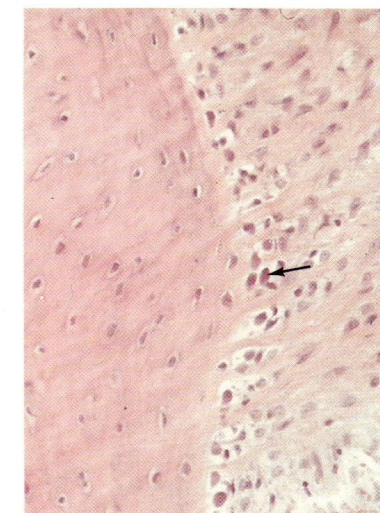

303 Decalcified, longitudinal section through periodontal ligament showing resorption of alveolar bone. The surface of the alveolar bone shows a number of resorption concavities termed Howship's lacunae in which lie the osteoclasts. Osteoclasts show considerable variation in size and shape, ranging from smaller mononuclear cells to large multinuclear cells. The cytoplasm of osteoclasts is packed with lysosomes and mitochondria. There is a paucity of endoplasmic reticulum. The part of the cell which lies adjacent to bone often has a striated appearance, the so-called brush border. (*H&E, ×120*)

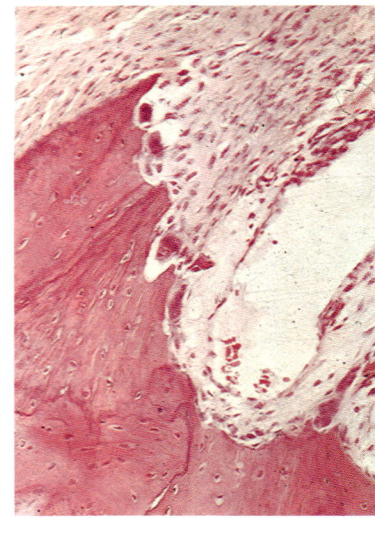

Resorption of the dental tissues is described on page 175.

Aggregations of *epithelial cell rests*, the rests of Malassez, are a normal feature of the periodontal ligament. They are the remains of the developmental epithelial root sheath of Hertwig.

304 The position of the epithelial rests (A), close to the cementum (B). This is a decalcified section through periodontal ligament. Differences have been observed in the distribution of epithelial cells according to site and age. During the first and second decades they are most prevalent in the apical zone, whereas between the third and seventh decades the majority are located cervically in the gingiva above the alveolar crest. The inset shows that in cross-section the epithelial cells appear cluster-like, though tangential or serial sections show that they form a network of interconnecting strands parallel to the long axis of the root. (*H&E, ×50, ×250*)

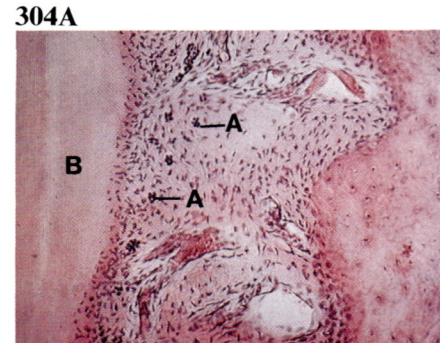
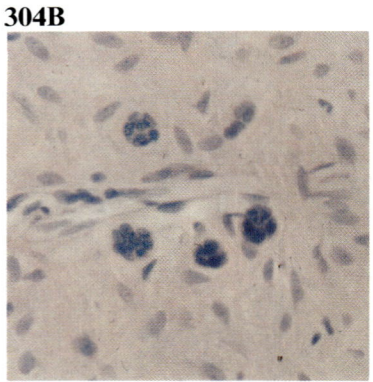

305 Tangential section through the epithelial rests. Their network appearance can be clearly seen. (*Iron haematoxylin, ×60*)

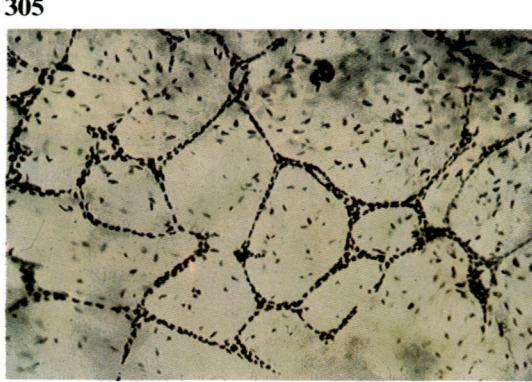

Histochemical and electron microscope studies reveal little activity in the epithelial cells. However, they may proliferate to form cysts or tumours if appropriately stimulated e.g. by chronic inflammation.

Blood vessels and nerves of the periodontal ligament

The rich blood supply to the ligament is derived from the appropriate superior and inferior dental arteries, though arteries from the gingiva, such as the lingual and palatine arteries, may also be involved. The arteries supplying the periodontal ligament are not primarily derived from those entering the pulp at the apex of the tooth, but from a series of perforating arteries passing through the alveolar bone. The dual source of the main arterial supply allows the periodontal ligament to function following removal of the root apex as a result of various endodontic treatments. The major vessels lie between the principal fibre bundles close to the wall of the alveolus. They have an average diameter of 20μm. The vessels branch and anastomose to form a capillary plexus around the teeth. Glomeruli-like structures, said to be arterio-venous shunts, have been described within the ligament.

In the region of the alveolar crest, the vessels of the periodontal ligament anastomose with those of the encircling gingiva. From this vascular circle, capillaries resembling renal glomeruli and arterio-venous shunts are given off into the attached gingiva at regular intervals.

The veins within the periodontal ligament usually accompany the arteries. Networks of veins are especially prominent beneath the junctional epithelium, at the root apex and in the bifurcation area of multi-rooted teeth. Veins also pass through the alveolar walls into intra-alveolar venous networks.

Lymph capillaries connect with lymph vessels in the periodontal ligament which then continue over the alveolar crest into the submucosa, through the alveolar bone or through the root apex.

Like the arterial supply, the periodontal ligament derives its innervation from two sources; some enter at the apex of the root and pass up through the periodontal ligament while others enter the middle and cervical portions of the ligament through openings in the alveolar walls. Fibres entering the ligament may be myelinated or unmyelinated and may be sensory fibres or autonomic fibres associated with the blood vessels. Though functionally two types of receptor are said to be present in the periodontal ligament, namely mechanoreceptors and nociceptors, numerous morphological types of nerve ending have been described in the ligament, ranging from free nerve endings to clusters of compound 'mechanoreceptors'. The functional characteristics of these morphological types have yet to be determined. The sites of the nerve endings have not been precisely determined, though the region around the apex of the tooth is richly supplied by nerves.

306A & 306B Blood vessels and nerves in the periodontal ligament. A, alveolar bone; B, dentine. Figure **306A** shows a transverse section through the periodontal ligament. Note the large number of blood vessels near the alveolar part of the ligament. Figure **306B** shows an ultrathin section of the ligament, in which the blood vessels are seen as large spaces. The nerve bundles in this section are arrowed. (**306A**, *van Gieson*, ×30) (**306B**, *Toluidine blue*, ×100)

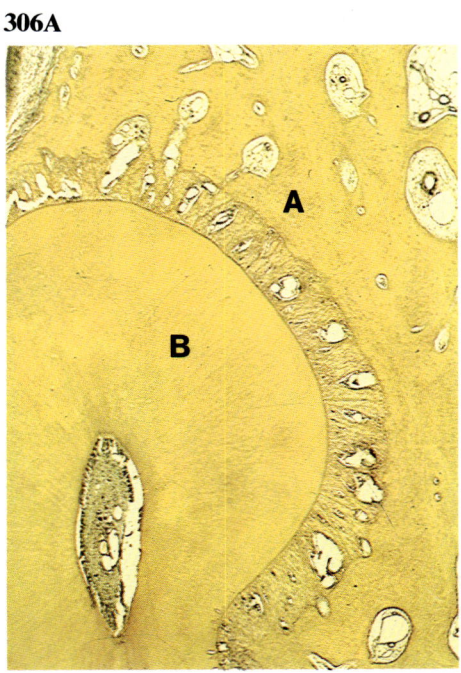

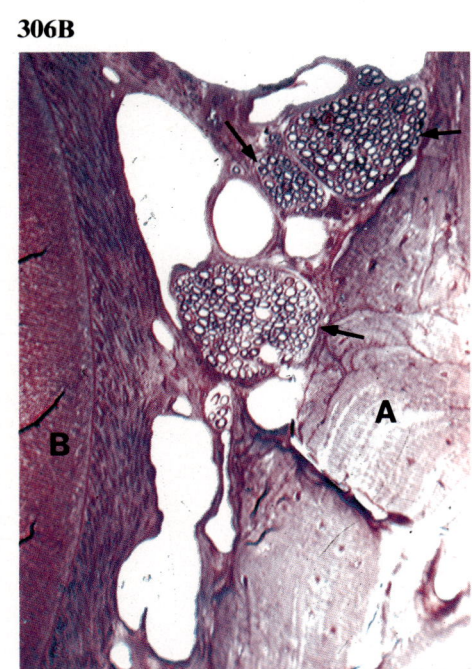

Alveolar bone

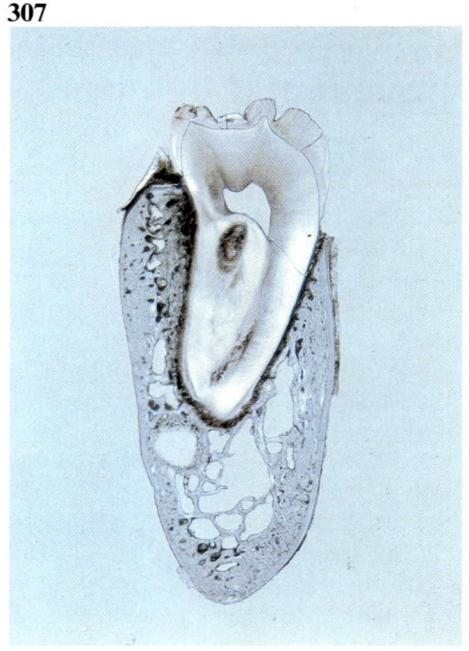

307 Longitudinal, ground section of a mandibular tooth *in situ*. Alveolar bone is that part of the mandible and maxilla in which the teeth are located. The gross morphology of the alveoli and the tooth sockets, and their radiographic appearance have been described on pages 14, 16, 73. The alveolus protects the developing teeth and, together with the periodontal ligament and cement, forms the attachment apparatus for the tooth. Alveolar bone is 'plastic' in that it can remodel according to the functional demands placed upon it. It readily adapts to the movement of a tooth during its developmental, eruptive and functional periods. Morphologically, no distinct boundary exists between the bodies of the mandible and maxilla and their alveolar processes. Two parts of the alveolar bone can be described; firstly, the thin lamina of compact bone which lines the tooth sockets and which gives attachment to the fibres of the periodontal ligament, the lamina dura; secondly, the bone which surrounds and gives support to the socket. Alveolar bone has the same physical and chemical properties as bone found elsewhere in the body. Its chemical composition is similar to that of cementum. (× 2)

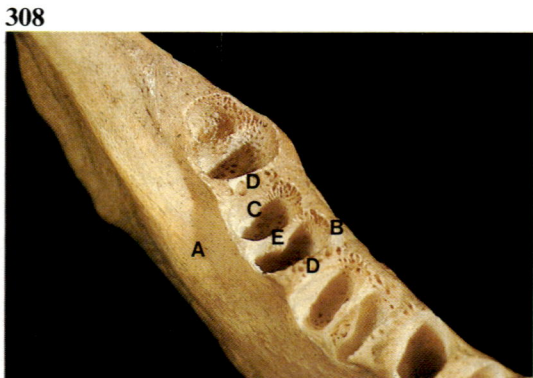

308 The morphology of tooth sockets. This macroscopic view is taken from the mandibular molar region and shows that the alveolar process is made up of outer (A) and inner (B) alveolar plates, a lamina dura (C) lining the sockets, and transverse bony septa, the interdental (D) and interradicular septa (E). The lamina dura is perforated by a large number of small, vascular openings, the Volkmann's canals. Because of this, the lamina dura has been referred to as the cribriform plate. The shape of the alveolar crest between the teeth has been described on page 73.

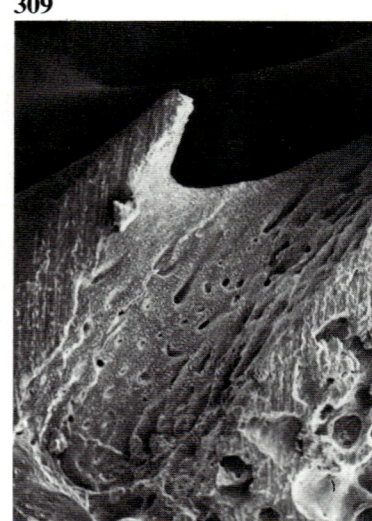

309 A fractured tooth socket showing the cribriform nature of the lamina dura. (*Scanning electron micrograph*, × 5)

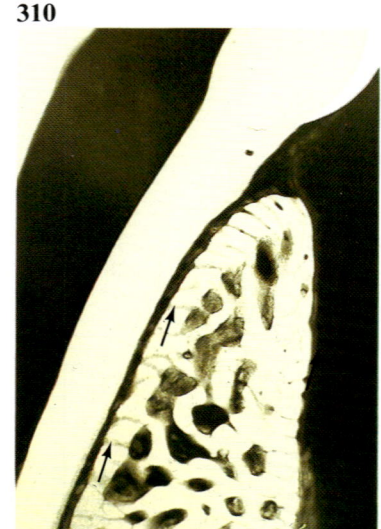

310 Part of a tooth *in situ* showing Volkmann canals (*arrowed*) passing through the alveolus into the periodontal space. (*Microradiograph*, × 7)

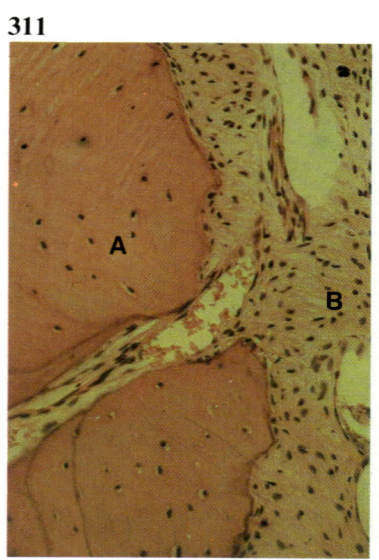

311 Decalcified section of alveolus (A) and periodontal ligament (B) showing a vascular Volkmann canal. (× 200)

The histological characteristics of alveolar bone do not differ from bone in other parts of the body. Bone is a rigid form of connective tissue. The intercellular substance appears homogeneous but is ordered according to the functional demands placed upon it. The matrix of mature bone is arranged in layers or lamellae approximately 5μm thick. The fibres within the lamellae are of even thickness, and though they take a helical course, they are approximately parallel to each other. The orientation and number of collagen fibres varies, however, from lamella to lamella. This arrangement contrasts with developing bone (woven bone) whose fibres are of varying thickness and orientation. The lamellae of mature bone contain osteocytes which lie in lacunae and are perforated by fine canals containing blood vessels and nerves. Osteoblasts, osteoclasts and osteocytes are cell types peculiar to bone.

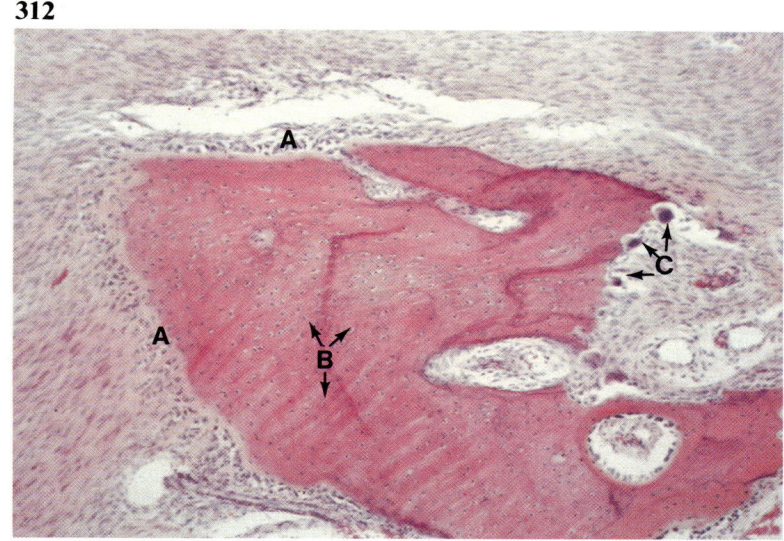

312 Decalcified section of alveolar crest region showing cell types in bone. A, osteoblasts; B, osteocytes; C, osteoclasts. *Osteoblasts* and *osteoclasts* have been described on pages 117–118. *Osteocytes* are the principal cells of fully formed bone and lie in lacunae within the calcified interstitial substance. Osteocytes are osteoblasts that have become surrounded by bone matrix during its formation. Near the surface, osteocytes have a similar intracytoplasmic organelle content to osteoblasts, but deeper within the bone these organelles undergo regression. (×75)

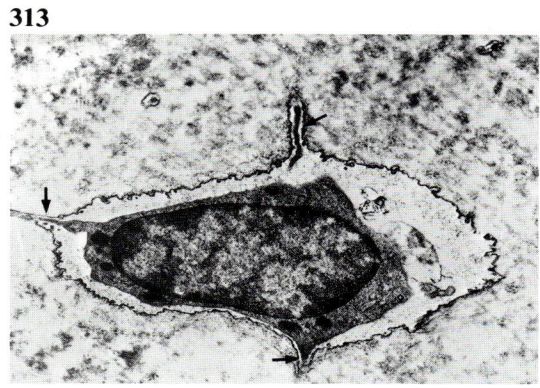

313 Decalcified alveolar bone showing an osteocyte. A number of slender processes (*arrowed*) extend from the cell body into canaliculi in the surrounding matrix. The processes of neighbouring osteocytes are in contact at their ends, forming gap junctions. Unlike the canaliculi of cementocytes, those of osteocytes are not preferentially orientated. Intracellular organelles associated with protein synthesis are visible within the cell body though they are not very numerous, suggesting that the cell has a low metabolic rate. Osteocytes are said to have an important role in calcium homeostasis and are believed to be capable of forming other cell types when released from their lacunae during bone resorption. (*Electron micrograph, ×4,000*)

Two types of bone, cancellous or spongy bone and compact bone, have been distinguished on the basis of the organisation of the bony lamellae and the size and number of vascular spaces. Cancellous bone consists of narrow, irregular, bony trabeculae which by branching and uniting form a tissue network with large spaces (marrow spaces) between the trabeculae. Compact bone, however, is dense with few marrow spaces. In the incisor and canine regions of both jaws, no cancellous bone intervenes between the outer and inner cortical plates and the lamina dura. In the molar region, some cancellous bone is usually seen (figure **19**).

In compact bone, the lamellae are often arranged circumferentially around blood vessels, thus forming longitudinal channels through the bone, the Haversian canal systems or osteones.

314 Alveolar bone viewed in ordinary transmitted light (314A) and polarised light (314B) showing compact bone with Haversian canals (*arrowed*). In polarised light, Haversian systems cut transversely show a characteristic X related to the concentric arrangement of the collagen fibres. (×80)

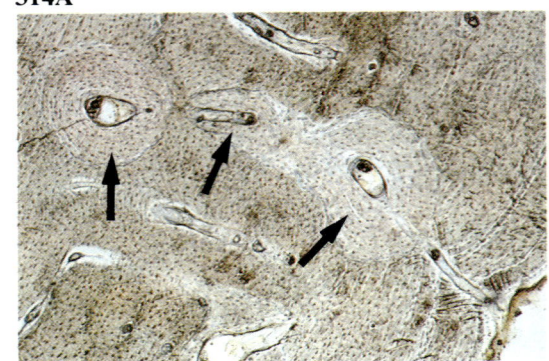
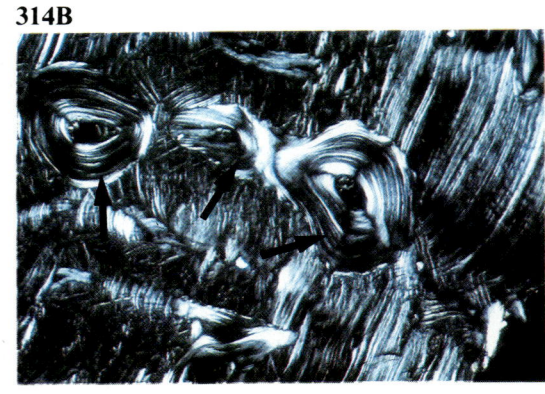

The layer of compact bone of the lamina dura lying immediately adjacent to the periodontal ligament is referred to as bundle bone, since bundles of Sharpey's fibres from the periodontal ligament pass through it.

315 Ground, longitudinal section through lamina dura, showing the appearance of bundle bone in transmitted light (315A) and in polarised light (315B). In polarised light the Sharpey's fibres are clearly seen as dark horizontal lines passing through the bone. A, periodontal ligament; B, bundle bone; C, cementum. (×70)

316 The continuation of the bundles of the principal collagen fibres from the periodontal ligament into the bundle bone as Sharpey's fibres. This is a decalcified section through the lamina dura. Osteoblasts (*arrowed*) can be seen lining the surface of the lamina dura. Between the darker staining matrix of calcified bone and the osteoblasts lies a paler zone of uncalcified osteoid. Osteocytes (A) lie within lacunae in the alveolar bone. (*H&E*, ×200)

317 The insertion of principal collagen fibres into alveolar bone. A, lamina dura; B, periodontal ligament; C, osteoblast. (*Electron micrograph*, ×5,000)

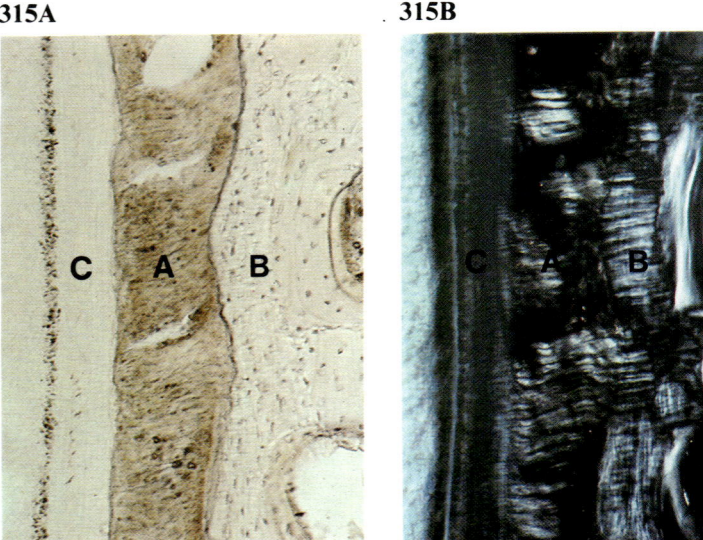
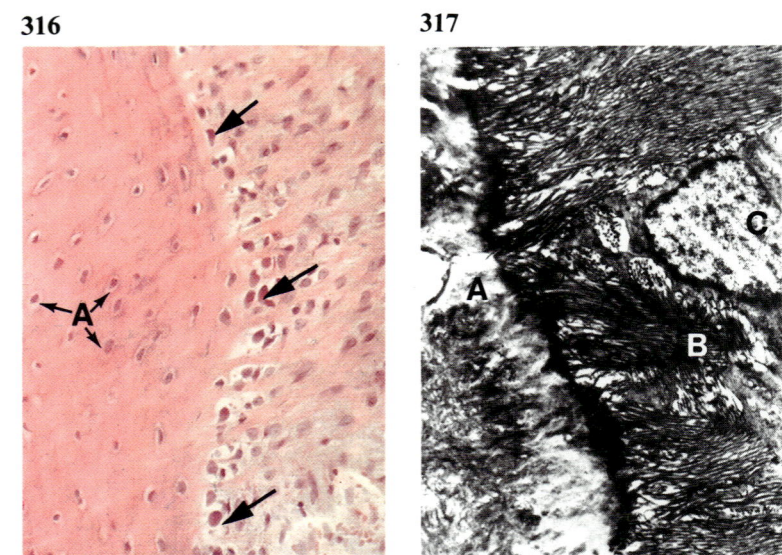

318 The periodontal surface of the lamina dura. The material shown has been treated with hypochlorite solution to remove organic material. In **318A**, the Sharpey's fibres pass into the bone for some distance without calcifying, leaving discrete channels. In **318B**, the Sharpey's fibres have calcified beyond the surface of the bone forming small, calcified prominences. (*Scanning electron micrographs, ×300*)

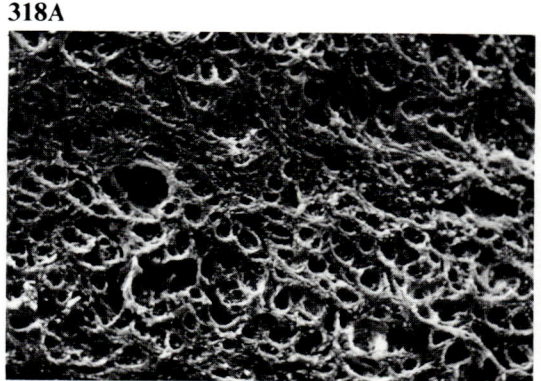
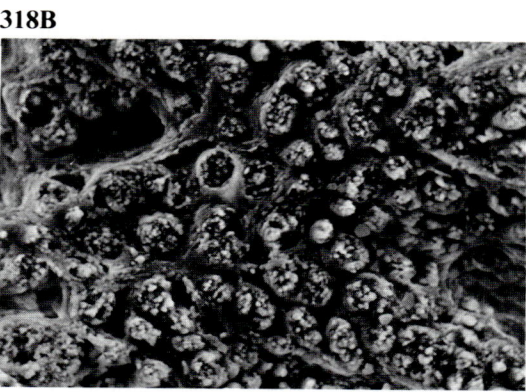

Sharpey's fibres were once thought to terminate within the lamina dura. Recent observations, however, show that in some areas the Sharpey's fibres may pass through the whole width of the alveolar bone. Such fibres have been termed transalveolar fibres.

319 Longitudinal, decalcified section through interdental bone (A) showing transalveolar fibres. B, periodontal ligament; C, root. (*Masson's trichrome, ×100*)

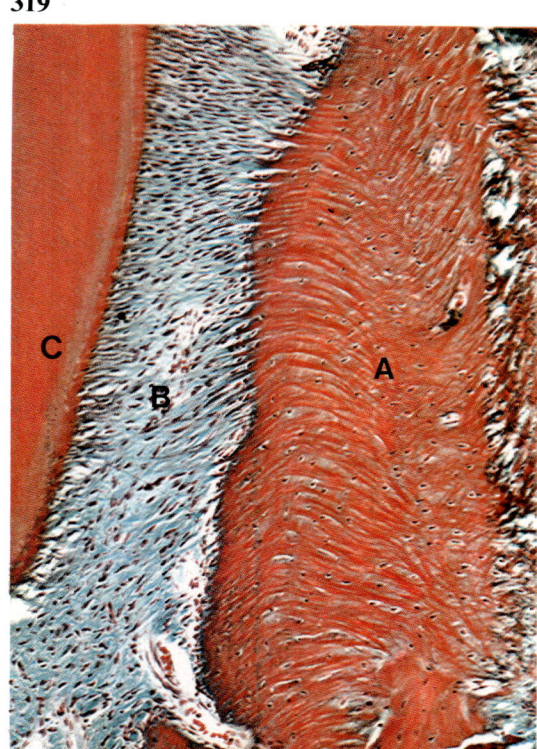

In the cervical part of the interdental septum where the bone is mainly compact, Sharpey's fibres of the periodontal ligament entering the bone in the mesiodistal plane pass straight through to become continuous with similar fibres from the root of the adjacent tooth. A similar pattern exists in interradicular bone though in this situation the fibres 'link' roots of the same tooth. Transalveolar fibres also pass through the entire thickness of the alveolar bone in the buccal and lingual planes, such fibres intermingling with the overlying periosteum or with the lamina propria of the gingiva. However, where the alveolar bone is of the cancellous type or where there are numerous Haversian systems, transalveolar fibres are not seen. In cervical regions, transalveolar and transseptal fibres form a band of connective tissue which interconnects every tooth in the arch.

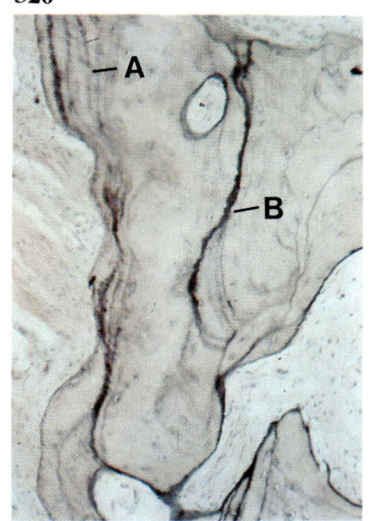

320 Longitudinal, decalcified section showing structural lines in bone. Two types of structural line may be seen within bone. One set of lines is related to the rhythmic deposition of bone during its formation (A). These lines are regular and lie parallel to each other. Because they are formed during periods of quiescence, they have been referred to as resting lines. The second type of line, reversal lines (B), mark the position where activity changed from resorption to deposition. Reversal lines are irregular lines, being composed of a series of concavities which were once sites of the resorptive Howship's lacunae. (*H&E, ×80*)

Oral mucosa

321 The morphology of the oral mucosa. This varies from region to region, being related to the varying functional demands placed upon it. As a general rule, two distinct layers of tissue can be recognised, a stratified squamous epithelium (A) and a lamina propria (B). The oral epithelium is derived from either ectoderm or endoderm and may or may not be keratinized. The connective tissue of the lamina propria is separated from the epithelium by a basement membrane. An additional layer, the submucosa, may be present attaching the mucous membrane to underlying bone or muscle. The tissue illustrated is taken from the mucosa overlying the lateral aspect of the hard palate where there is a distinct submucous layer (C). The submucosa consists of connective tissue of varying thickness and density, glands, blood vessels, nerves and adipose tissue. (*Masson's trichrome*, × 35)

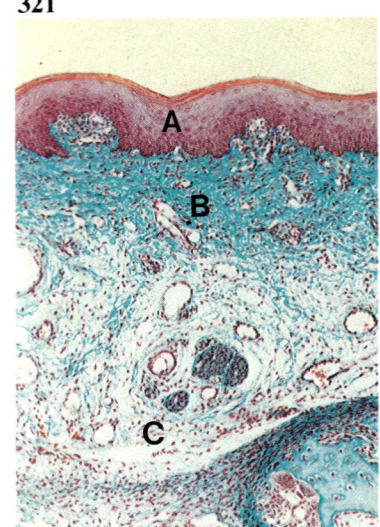

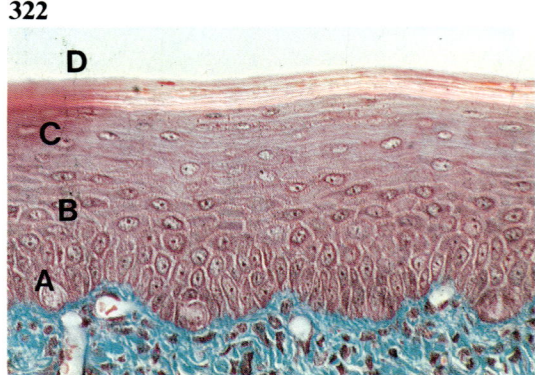

322 The constituent layers of keratinized oral epithelium. The cells of the oral epithelium are arranged in several discrete layers, each of which has a characteristic morphology. The cells in contact with the basement membrane form the basal cell layer (A). Because the cells of this layer are mitotically active, replacing cells lost at the surface, it has alternatively been termed the stratum germinativum. The basal cell layer is composed of relatively undifferentiated, low, columnar cells. Above the basal cells are several layers of larger, irregular polyhedral cells which are connected by many desmosomes. Because of their spiny appearance, this layer has been called the prickle cell layer or stratum spinosum (B). Above the prickle cell layer is the granular layer or stratum granulosum (C), the cells of which are larger and flatter than the prickle cells from which they are differentiated. The cells of the granular layer characteristically contain keratohyaline granules. Above the granular layer is the keratinized or cornified layer, the stratum corneum (D). Unlike skin, no clear layer or stratum lucidum intervenes between the granular and keratinized layers. Cells of the stratum corneum are flattened squames which lack nuclei, granules or intracytoplasmic organelles, being filled with keratin. In non-keratinized oral epithelium (e.g. the buccal mucosa), a stratum corneum and stratum granulosum are not found.

The junction between the epithelium and lamina propria is not smooth but is folded, the epithelial projections (pegs or rete) interdigitating with dermal papillae. The papillae increase the surface area between the tissues and may be important in terms of nutrition and/or bonding. The degree of interdigitation is related to wear, for in areas exposed to friction (such as the hard palate and attached gingiva) it is more pronounced. Oblique sectioning through the papillae may produce the appearance of islands of connective tissue within the epithelium, and vice-versa. (*H&E*, × 140)

323 Cells within keratinized oral epithelium.
323A Cells of stratum germinativum lining the connective tissue of the lamina propria. The cell arrowed is a lymphocyte between the basal cells. (× 2,800)
323B High power view of interface between epithelium (A) and connective tissue (B). The basal lamina consists of a lamina lucida and a lamina densa. Note the hemidesmosomes (*arrows*). (× 7,500)
323C Cells of stratum spinosum. Note the numerous bundles of tonofilaments and desmosomes. (× 3,000)
323D Cells of stratum granulosum and stratum corneum. Note the small dense keratohyaline granules within the cells of the stratum granulosum and the flattened squames lacking intracytoplasmic organelles in the stratum corneum. (× 2,800)
323E High power view of a cell from the stratum granulosum – keratohyaline granules arrowed. (× 12,000)
323F Surface cells of non-keratinized oral epithelium. Note the absence of granular and keratinized layers and the retention of nuclei and organelles within the cells. (*Electron micrographs*, × 2,000)

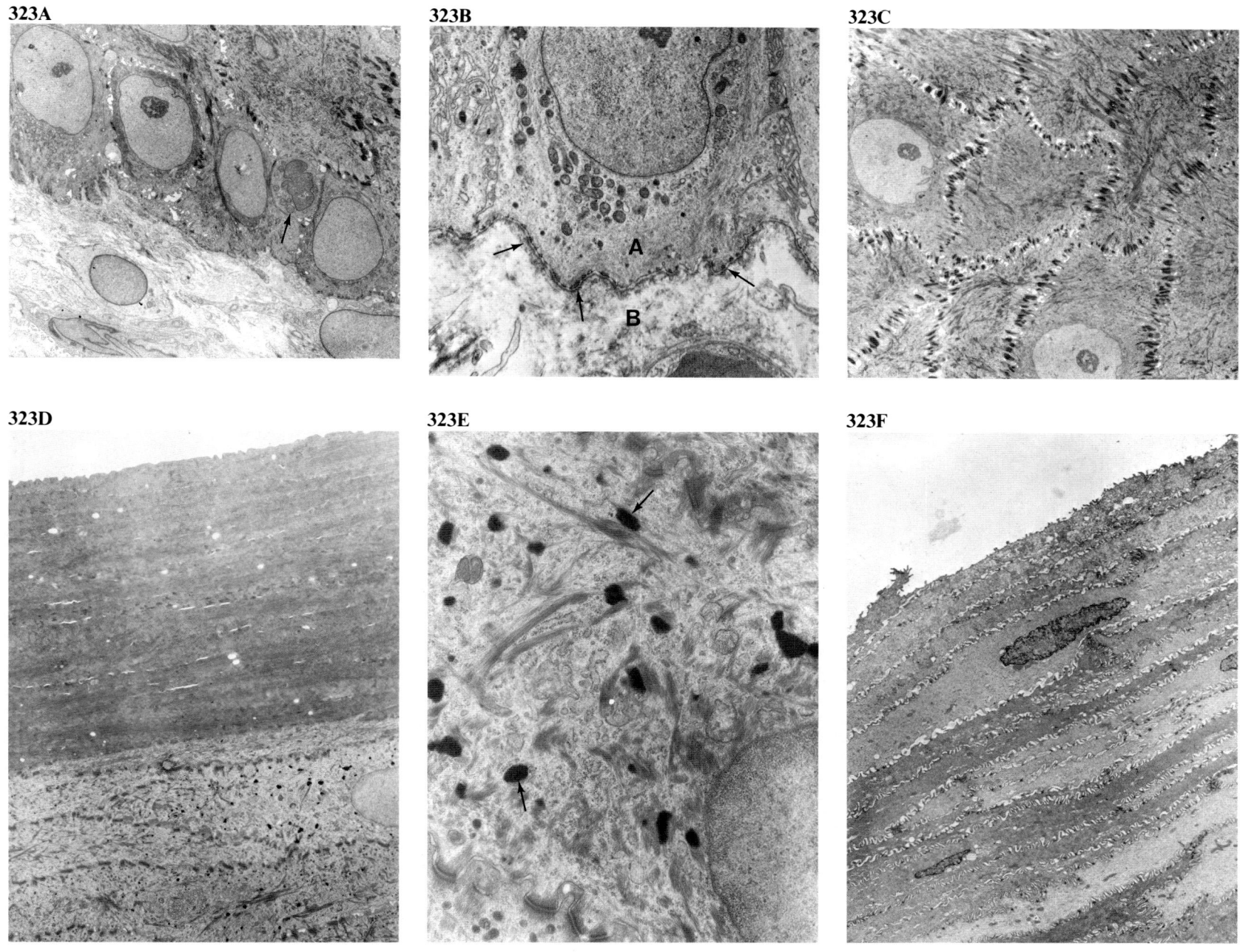

The cells comprising the stratified squamous epithelium have been termed keratinocytes to distinguish them from other cell types within the epithelium which are not involved in the differentiation of a keratin-type layer. Several types of non-keratinocytes have been described within the oral epithelium, namely melanocytes, Langerhans' cells, non-specific dentritic cells, Merkel cells and inflammatory cells. With the exception of the Merkel cell, non-keratinocytes may be distinguished from keratinocytes by the absence of desmosomes and tonofilaments.

324 Melanocytes (*arrowed*) are located in the basal layers of the epithelium and are responsible for the production of melanin pigment. The number of melanocytes varies in different regions, but differences in the degree of pigmentation between races is due to differences in the amount of pigment produced rather than to differences in the number of pigment cells. Characteristically, melanocytes have long processes which extend between neighbouring epithelial cells. The pigment is produced as small granules (melanosomes) which can be transferred to other cells in the epithelium. (*Masson's fontana, × 280*)

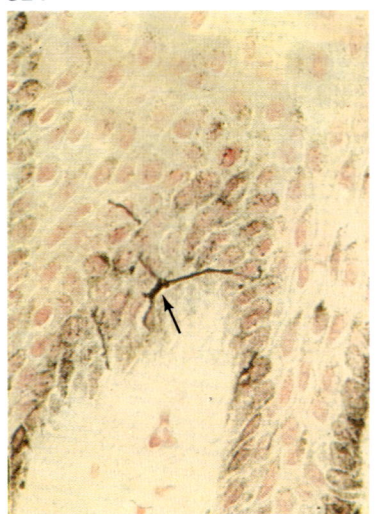

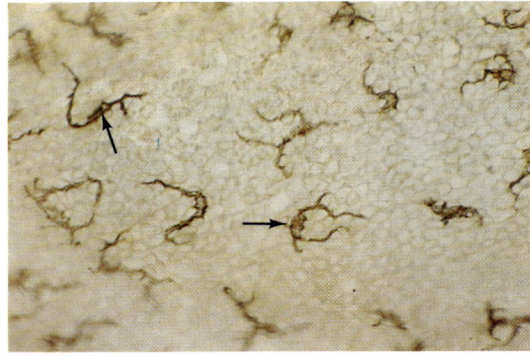

325 Langerhans' cells (*arrowed*). In sections stained with haematoxylin and eosin, Langerhans' cells appear clear. However, because of their high ATPase content, they can be distinguished from adjacent cells using a lead-capture, histochemical technique. Langerhans' cells are dendritic in form and are usually located above the basal layer. Characteristically, they contain granules which are rod-shaped but can only be seen under the electron microscope. Their origin is unknown though it has been suggested that they are effete melanocytes. The function of the Langerhans' cell is controversial. It may be a type of receptor or it may be involved in controlling the rate of cell turnover within the epithelium. (*× 200*)

Non-specific dentritic cells lack either the characteristic granules of the Langerhans' cells or the melanosomes of the melanocyte and may occasionally be seen above the basal layer of the epithelium. It has been suggested that these cells are merely portions of Langerhans' cells or melanocytes from which the characteristic granules have been inadvertently excluded during tissue preparation.

Merkel cells are non-dentritic cells lying in the basal layer of the epithelium which are closely associated with a nerve fibre. Their most characteristic feature is the small, membrane-bound granules which lie adjacent to the nerve fibre. This arrangement may be evidence in favour of the suggestion that Merkel cells are epithelial sensory receptors.

Should the oral epithelium be inflamed, then neutrophils or lymphocytes may be present within and around the basal region of the epithelium. A lymphocyte lying within the basal layer is shown in figure **323A.**

The oral mucosa shows a number of *regional* variations which include differences in the nature of the submucosa, the composition of the lamina propria, the morphology of the epithelial-connective tissue boundary, the thickness of the epithelium and the type of keratinization.

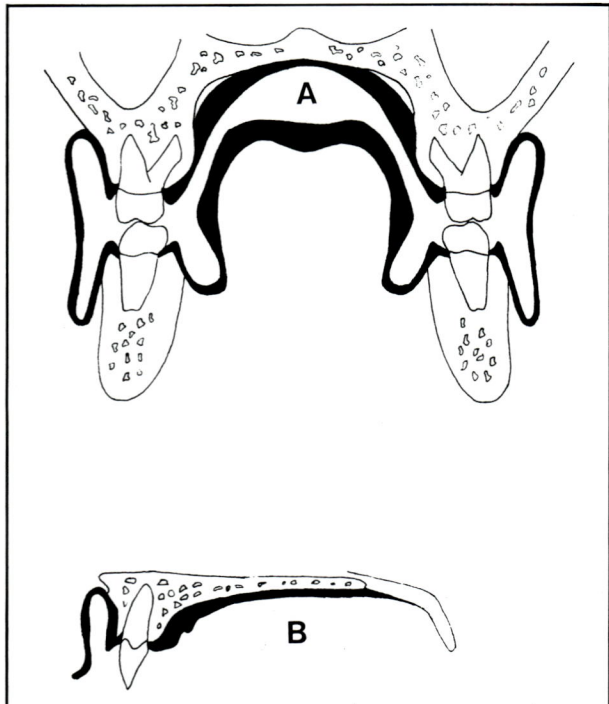

326 Regional variations in the thickness of the oral epithelium.
A Coronal section through molar region.
B Mid-sagittal section through palate.

327 Variations in the degree and type of keratinization in the oral epithelium.
A Orthokeratinization. This refers to mucosa with a keratinized layer of normal thickness.
B Hyperkeratinization. This refers to mucosa with an excessively thick keratinized layer. Hyperkeratinization is frequently associated with regions of increased irritation or trauma and with areas undergoing pathological change.
C Non-keratinized mucosa. This rarely shows a granular or a keratinized layer and the tissue has a consistent basophilic staining reaction.
D Parakeratinized epithelium. This refers to the appearance of the surface cells which, though staining like keratin, retain nuclei.

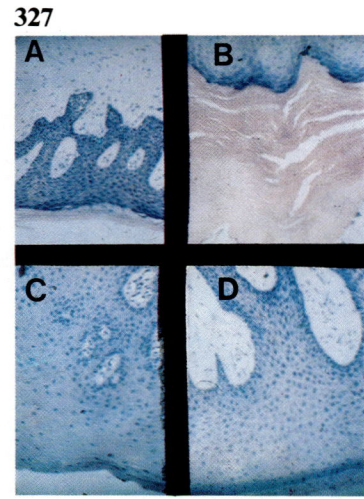

Three types of oral mucosa have been described: masticatory, lining and specialised mucosa. Masticatory mucosa is found in regions which are particularly susceptible to the stresses and strains resulting from masticatory activity. Among its characteristic features are a keratinized epithelial lining and a thick lamina propria which is tightly bound to underlying periosteum. Lining mucosa, on the other hand, is not so subjected to masticatory loads and consequently has a non-keratinized epithelium which lines a thin, elastic, lamina propria and a submucosa. The mucosa lining the gingiva and palate is masticatory mucosa, that lining the lips, cheeks, alveolus and vestibule, floor of mouth, ventral surface of the tongue and soft palate is lining mucosa. Specialised mucosa has neither the characteristics of lining mucosa nor of masticatory mucosa. The mucosa of the dorsum of the tongue is a specialised gustatory mucosa which has a well-papillated surface, some of the papillae being keratinized, others being non-keratinized. Part of the mucosa of the lip may also be regarded as specialised.

The lip

328 Low power view of lip. The skin on the outer surface of the lip (A) is keratinized and contains many hair follicles, sebaceous and sweat glands. The epithelium of the skin does not abruptly change into the non-keratinized epithelium lining the inner surface of the lip (B), a transitional zone, the red zone or vermilion border (C) interceding. The vermilion border is characteristic of man. Its red colour is caused by underlying blood vessels showing through the thin, transparent epithelium. The lips being muscular organs have, at their core, a large number of striated muscle bundles (D) associated with the circum-oral facial muscles, particularly orbicularis oris. Minor salivary glands (E) are seen in the connective tissue beneath the oral mucosa. (*Masson's trichrome*, ×5)

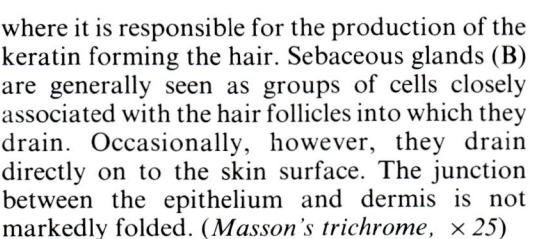

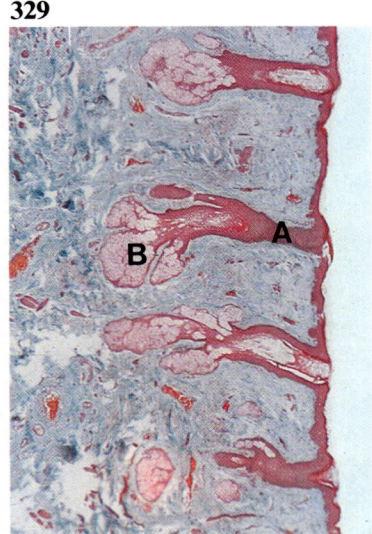

329 Skin on the outer surface of the lip is similar, histologically, to that elsewhere in the body. It consists of keratinized epithelium which rests upon a layer of connective tissue containing sweat glands, sebaceous glands and the bases of hair follicles. In this section, the hair follicles (A) are seen as channels running through the epithelium. The epithelium is continuous around the base of the hair follicles where it is responsible for the production of the keratin forming the hair. Sebaceous glands (B) are generally seen as groups of cells closely associated with the hair follicles into which they drain. Occasionally, however, they drain directly on to the skin surface. The junction between the epithelium and dermis is not markedly folded. (*Masson's trichrome*, ×25)

330 The vermilion border. At the mucocutaneous junction of the lip, the epithelium undergoes a marked change in appearance. Compared with the skin, it lacks hairs and sweat glands. Occasional sebaceous glands may be found, however, especially at the angles of the mouth. The vermilion border of the lips requires moistening with saliva by the tongue to prevent its drying. The epithelium of the vermilion border, like skin, is keratinized but is very thin and translucent. The dermal papillae are relatively long and narrow and contain capillary loops which lie close to the surface. An intermediate zone has been described between the vermilion border and the oral mucosa. In adults, the intermediate zone is covered by a thin, parakeratinized epithelium. In infants, it is thickened, possibly as an adaptation to suckling. (*Masson's trichrome, ×25*)

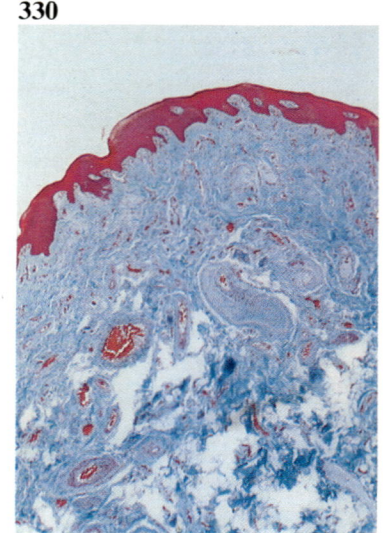

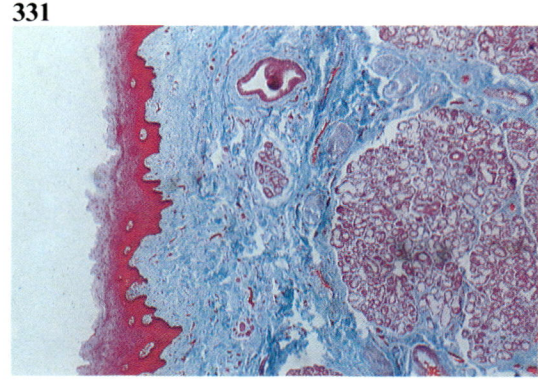

331 The oral mucosa of the lip. Unlike the vermilion border, the epithelium of the mucosa of the lip is non-keratinized. The epithelium and lamina propria are thick but the dermal papillae are short and irregular. The submucosa contains both serous and mucous minor salivary glands. Strands of dense connective tissue bind the mucosa to the underlying muscle. (*Masson's trichrome, ×25*)

The cheek

332 The buccal mucosa closely resembles the labial mucosa. The epithelium is non-keratinized and the lamina propria consists of dense connective tissue with short, irregular dermal papillae. The submucosa is firmly attached to the underlying buccinator muscle and contains minor salivary glands. After puberty in the male and menopause in the female, a series of yellowish patches, Fordyce spots, may occasionally be seen in the buccal mucosa, these being ectopic sebaceous glands. (*H&E, ×32*)

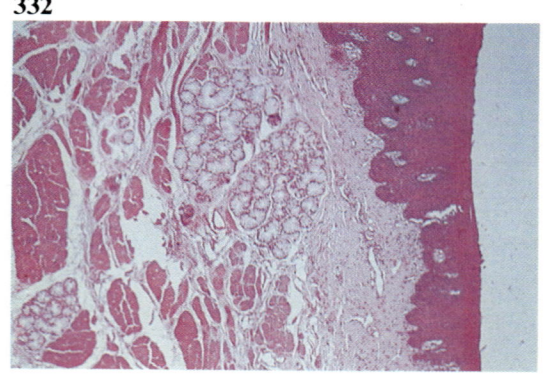

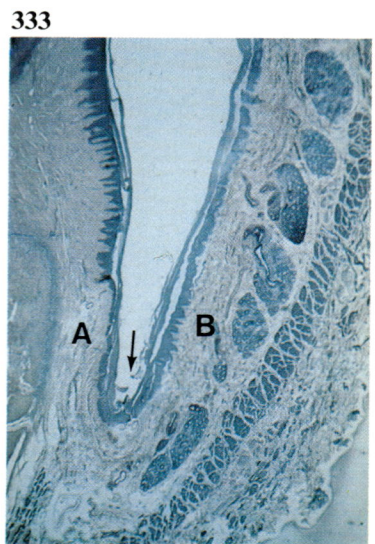

333 Transverse section through the cheek and jaw to show the vestibular fornix and buccal alveolar mucosa. In the vestibular fornix (*arrowed*), the mucosa of the lips and cheeks (B) is reflected on to the mucosa covering the lower part of the alveolus (A). The mucous membrane lining the vestibular fornix resembles that lining the cheek, though it is only loosely attached to underlying structures, thus allowing for movement of the cheeks and lips. (*H&E, ×8*)

The gingiva and alveolar mucosa

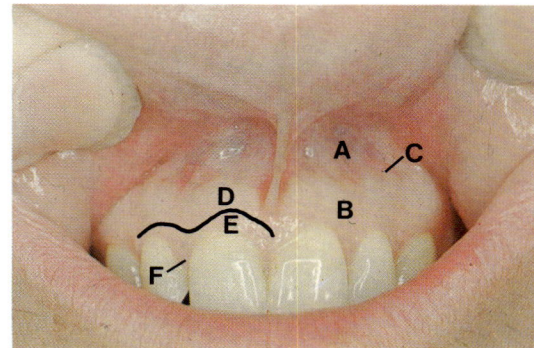 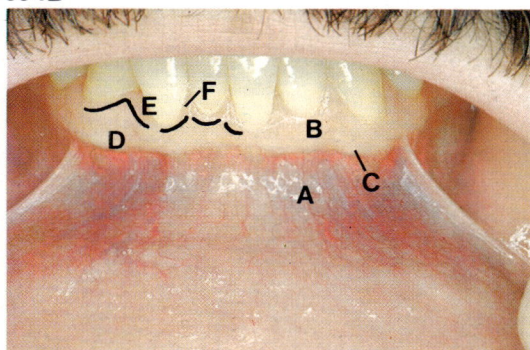

334 The gingiva *in vivo*. The mucosa lining the lower part of the alveolar process is loosely attached to the periosteum via a diffuse submucosa and is termed the alveolar mucosa (A). It is delineated from the gingiva (B) by the mucogingival junction (C). The alveolar mucosa appears dark red, the gingiva pale pink. These colour differences result from differences in the type of keratinization and the proximity to the surface of underlying blood vessels. Indeed, small blood vessels may readily be seen coursing beneath the alveolar mucosa. The gingiva may be subdivided into the attached gingiva (D) and the free gingiva (E). The attached gingiva is firmly bound to the periosteum of the alveolus and to the teeth, the free gingiva lies unattached around the cervical margin of the tooth. Between the free and attached gingiva a groove may be seen, the free gingival groove. The interdental papilla (F) is that part of the gingiva which fills the space between teeth. A feature of the attached gingiva is its surface stippling. However, the degree of stippling varies from individual to individual and also according to age and sex and the health of the gingiva. The free gingiva is not stippled. On the lingual surface of the lower jaw, the attached gingiva is sharply differentiated from the lining, non-keratinized mucosa of the floor of the mouth. On the palate, there is no obvious division between the attached gingiva and palatal mucosa.

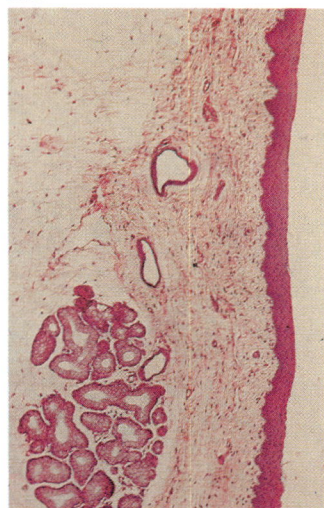 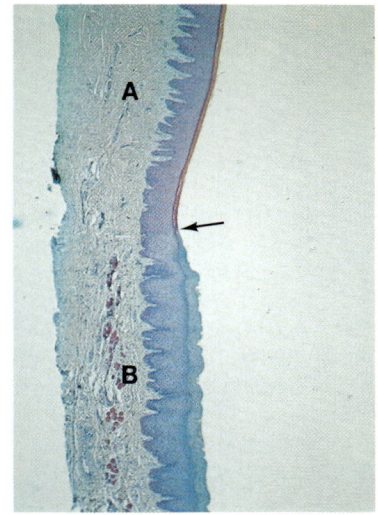

335 The alveolar mucosa. The epithelium is relatively thin and non-keratinized. Its red coloration is related to the blood vessels lying close to the surface within the lamina propria. The dermal papillae are short or may even be absent. Differences between the papillae of the alveolar mucosa and attached gingiva are best seen in figure 333. The alveolar mucosa is loosely attached to the underlying periosteum through a submucosa which may contain minor mixed salivary glands. (×15)

336 The oral mucosa in the region of the mucogingival junction (*arrowed*). The attached gingiva (A) and the alveolar mucosa (B) have been removed from the underlying alveolar bone. Note the differences in surface keratinization between the attached gingiva and alveolar mucosa. (*Papanicolou*, ×20)

337 The attached gingiva is a masticatory mucosa, its stratified squamous epithelium being keratinized. However, as much as 75 per cent of the cornified surface cells may retain their nuclei (parakeratosis) and as much as 10 per cent may be non-keratinized. In dark-skinned races, melanin granules in the gingiva (especially beneath the interdental papillae) may be sufficient to produce patches of pigmentation. The lamina propria of the attached gingiva is a dense collagenous tissue which is not particularly vascular. The numerous dermal papillae are long and narrow. There is no submucosa, the lamina propria being bound to the periosteum of the alveolar bone forming a mucoperiosteum. Note the stippled appearance of the epithelium (*arrowed*). (*H&E*, ×75)

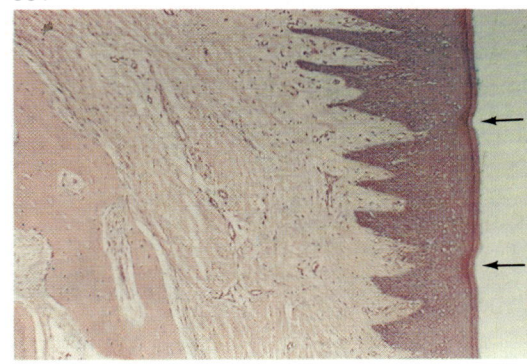

338 Appearance of the attached (A) and free (B) gingiva and the gingival cuff. This is a decalcified, longitudinal section of a tooth *in situ*. The outline of the enamel prior to decalcification has been drawn in. The epithelium of the external surface of the free gingiva is similar to that of the attached gingiva. However, it is not firmly bound to the periosteum of the adjacent alveolar bone and does not appear stippled. The junction between the tooth and the gingiva has been termed the gingival cuff. The cuff consists of two different zones. Coronally lies the sulcular epithelium (C) which is separated by a small space, the gingival sulcus, from the enamel. In health, the gingival sulcus may only be about 0.1mm deep. The sulcular epithelium differs significantly from the epithelium on the external surface, being non-keratinized and having shallow epithelial rete. At the base of the gingival sulcus, the sulcular epithelium merges with the junctional epithelium (D). The base of the gingival sulcus lies approximately at the level of the free gingival groove. The junctional epithelium forms a thin, epithelial lining directly attached to the tooth. It is derived from the reduced enamel epithelium (see page 173).

Note the infiltration of inflammatory cells in the connective tissue beneath the junctional epithelium. The degree of infiltration appears to be independent of the volume of inflamed connective tissue. Evidence of some inflammation may be apparent in clinically normal gingiva. (*H&E, ×30*)

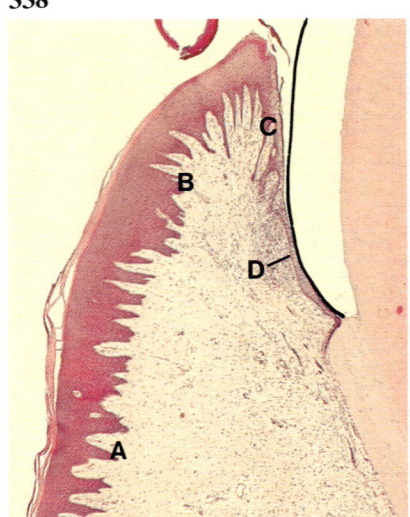

338

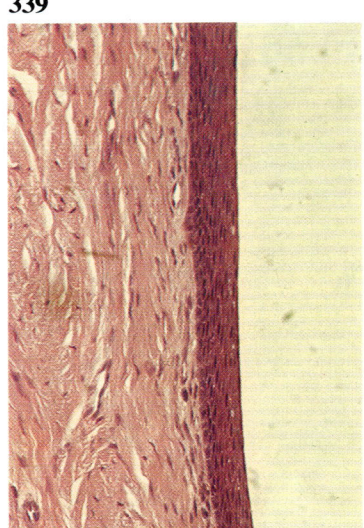

339

339 The junctional epithelium is a specialised layer of non-keratinized, stratified squamous epithelium. It consists of a stratum germinativum of cuboidal cells above which are several layers of flattened cells orientated parallel to the enamel surface. These cells may be considered equivalent to a stratum spinosum. There is no equivalent of a stratum granulosum or stratum corneum. The epithelial-connective tissue interface is smooth. The underlying connective tissue contains numerous capillaries and is relatively more cellular than that in the central part of the gingiva. (*H&E, ×150*)

340 Part of a junctional epithelial cell facing the enamel surface. A, enamel space. The attachment of the cell to the enamel surface is mediated by hemidesmosomes (*arrowed*) and a basement lamina-like structure (B). The cytoplasm contains numerous free ribosomes, cisternae of rough endoplasmic reticulum and a prominent Golgi apparatus (C) which are probably related to the synthesis and transport of materials needed to maintain the basement lamina. A few small bundles of tonofilaments (D) are also present but these are less well-developed than those in cells of the gingival, palatal or vestibular epithelium. (*Electron micrograph, ×12,000*)

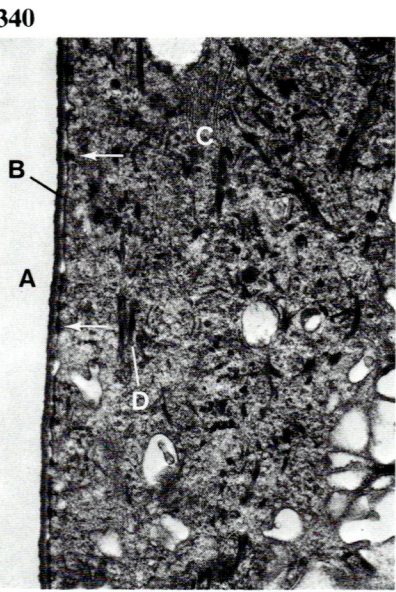

340

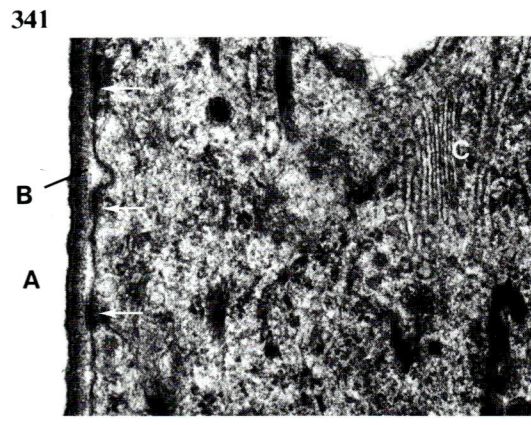

341

341 *At higher magnification*, the basement lamina (B) is seen to be composed of an electron-lucent zone adjacent to the plasma membrane of a junctional epithelial cell and a finely granular, electron-dense zone adjacent to the enamel space (A). Unlike the basement lamina between stratum germinativum and connective tissue in most regions of the oral mucosa (see figure **323**), the lamina adjacent to the enamel cannot as readily be divided into a lamina lucida and a lamina densa. However, its width (approximately 100–140nm) is comparable to the combined width of the lamina lucida and lamina densa usually found in oral mucosa.

The hemidesmosomes of the cells adjacent to the enamel are of varying length. Nevertheless, they are comparable in structure to those seen along the basal plasma membrane at most epithelial-connective tissue junctions (see figure **323**). The hemidesmosomes (*arrows*) are comprised of thickenings of the inner leaflet of the plasma membrane (the attachment plaque) with relatively few tonofilaments. Opposite the attachment plaque at the enamel surface there is a peripheral dense line comparable to that seen in the lamina lucida of the basement lamina between epithelium and connective tissue. Note the prominent Golgi apparatus (C). (*Electron micrograph, ×36,000*)

The length of junctional epithelium attached to the enamel surface varies according to the stage of eruption (see page 173). When the tooth first erupts into the oral cavity, most of the enamel will be covered by junctional epithelium. By the time the tooth reaches the occlusal plane about one-fourth of the enamel surface is still covered by junctional epithelium. With time, the junctional epithelium proliferates apically and, as a consequence, may establish a firm union with the cement surface.

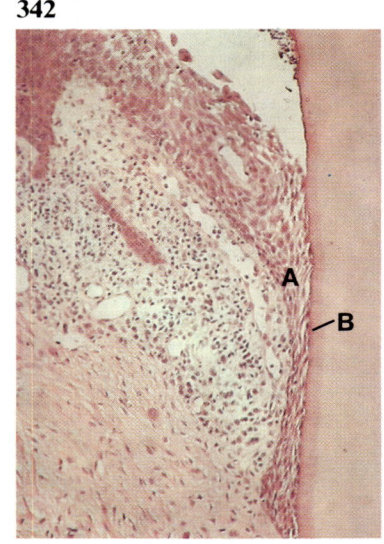

342 Junctional epithelium (A) on cementum (B). The apical migration of the junctional epithelium may be a response to inflammatory change within the periodontium though alternatively it may be considered a physiological process (passive eruption) related to ageing. Either way, this migration will involve the removal of gingival fibres and alveolar bone and the exposure of cervical root tissue into the oral cavity. (*H&E*, ×60)

The dento-gingival junction seals the underlying connective tissue of the periodontium from the oral environment. The strength of this seal is thought not only to be dependent upon the attachment of the junctional epithelium to the tooth but also upon the pressure exerted by the fibres and tissue fluid of the underlying connective tissue. The weakness of the dento-gingival junction lies in its situation, the gingival crevice being a stagnation site. The epithelium provides little resistance against the toxic products resulting from the consequent bacterial accumulation. The epithelium of the gingival sulcus is permeable. Indeed, tissue fluid and cells, as well as experimental substances such as dyes, carbon particles and horseradish peroxidase, pass readily through the epithelium from the connective tissue to the sulcus. The permeability of the junctional epithelium may be related to the presence of particularly wide intercellular spaces. A fluid containing molecules of low molecular weight, gingival or cervicular fluid, is said to pass continuously from the subepithelial tissues into the gingival crevice. Other oral epithelial surfaces do not show such exudation of tissue fluid. Since gingival fluid contains γ-globulins and polymorphonuclearcytes, it has been suggested that the immunological and phagocytic properties of the fluid are important in the defence mechanism of the dento-gingival junction. It is thought by some, however, that gingival fluid only passes into the gingival crevice as a response to pathological stimuli.

The turnover of the junctional epithelial is rapid. The epithelial cells migrate in a coronal direction to be shed into the oral cavity via the gingival crevice. The continual breakdown and reformation of lamina densa, hemidesmosomes and desmosomes allows cells to alter their relationships as they migrate through the junctional epithelium. The rate of turnover is dependent upon the demands placed upon the tissue and appears to be directly related to the degree of inflammation. Following the surgical removal of gingiva, a new junctional epithelium rapidly forms which has all the original characteristics.

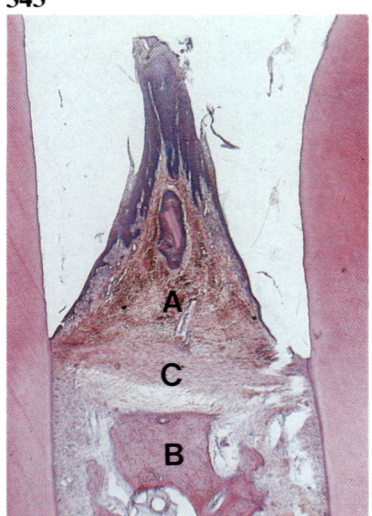

343 The interdental papilla (A) viewed buccally or lingually appears wedge-shaped. Deep to the epithelium, above the alveolar crest (B) can be seen transseptal fibres (C). (*H&E*, ×20)

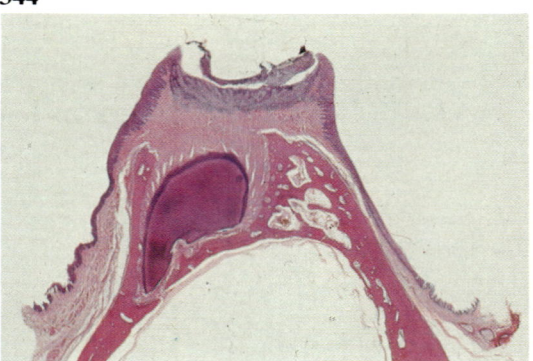

344 A buccolingual section through an interdental papilla shows that only the buccal and lingual corners are raised, the central region being concave to form an interdental col beneath the contact point of a tooth. The interdental col is lined by an extremely thin, non-keratinized, stratified squamous epithelium which is said to be derived from the reduced enamel epithelium. In teeth which are spaced, however, the interdental papilla does not appear as a col but is dome-shaped having a relatively thick, keratinized epithelium. (*H&E*, ×4)

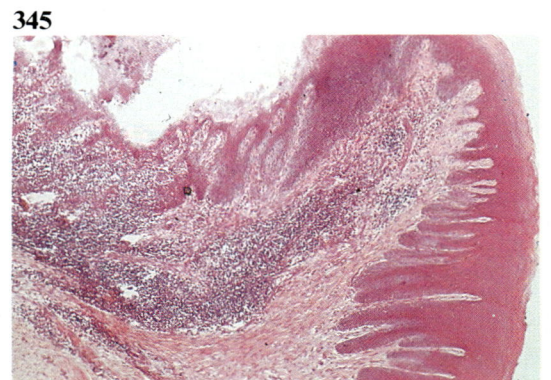

345 Interdental col. Note the thin, lining epithelium. The susceptibility of this region to inflammatory disease is said to be related to this thinness. Note the mass of inflammatory cells beneath the epithelium. (*H&E*, ×40)

Support of the free gingiva and the gingival cuff depends mainly upon turgor mediated by the vascular system and upon the interlacing of gingival collagen fibre bundles.

346 The arrangement of the principal collagen fibre groups of the gingiva.
346A Buccolingual section.
346B Mesiodistal section.
346C Horizontal section.
346D Buccolingual section through the interdental col.

a *Dentogingival* group arising from the root surface above the alveolar crest. Its fibres radiate out to be inserted into the lamina propria of the gingiva. The uppermost fibres lie beneath the sulcular epithelium, the middle group lie almost horizontal while the lowermost fibres course between gingiva and alveolar bone.

b *Longitudinal* group extending throughout the whole length of the dental arch.

c *Circular* group encircling each tooth. Some fibres are attached to cementum, others to alveolar bone.

d *Alveologingival* group passing from the alveolar crest into the overlying lamina propria.

e *Dentoperiosteal* group arising from the root and passing over the alveolar crest to be inserted into the periosteum.

f *Transseptal* fibre group passing horizontally from the root of one tooth above the alveolar crest to be inserted into the root of the adjacent tooth.

g *Semicircular* group arising from cementum near the cemento-enamel junction and crossing the free marginal gingiva to be inserted into a comparable position on the opposite side of the tooth.

h *Transgingival* group arising from the cementum of one tooth and crossing the free marginal gingiva of an adjacent tooth.

i *Interdental* group.

j *Vertical* group arising in the alveolar mucosa or attached gingiva and passing coronally towards the marginal gingiva and interdental papilla.

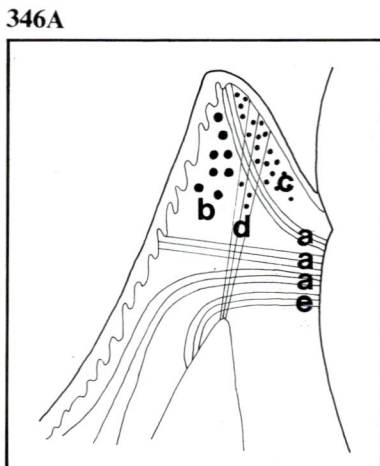

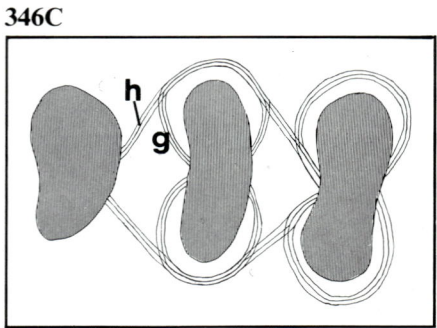

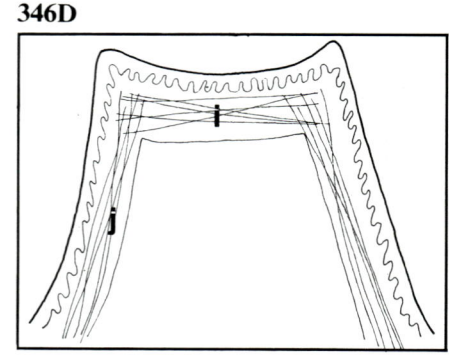

347 Decalcified, longitudinal section in the mesiodistal plane showing transseptal fibres. (*Silver, ×10*)

348 Decalcified, longitudinal section in the buccolingual plane showing dentogingival fibres (*arrowed*) passing over the alveolar crest. (*Masson's trichrome, ×80*)

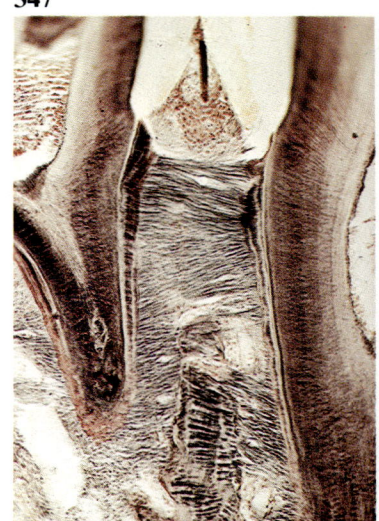 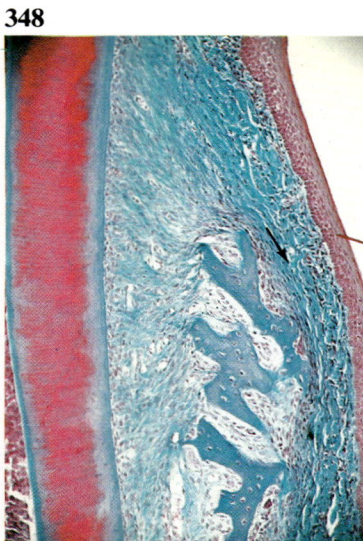

The palate

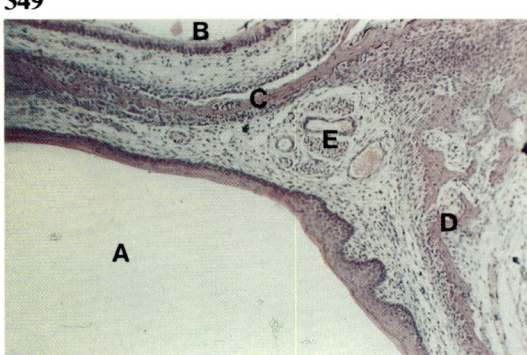

349 A coronal section of developing hard palate.
A oral cavity.
B nasal cavity.
C developing palatal process of maxilla.
D developing alveolar process of maxilla.
E neurovascular bundle.

Although this section is taken from a foetus, it nevertheless shows the basic appearance of the oral mucosa of the hard palate and demonstrates regional variations in its submucosa. In all regions, the oral surface is lined by keratinized, stratified squamous epithelium. In the midline of the hard palate, there is no submucosa, the consequent mucoperiosteum being called the palatine raphe. A distinct submucosa, however, is found between the palatine raphe and gingiva in the premolar regions though the lamina propria is firmly attached to the underlying periosteum by vertically orientated fibres. In this submucosa is found the neurovascular bundle associated with the anterior palatine nerves and vessels, mucous glands and fat. Note the lack of submucosa in the gingiva on the palatal side of the alveolus, its lamina propria being firmly attached to the periosteum. The nasal surface of the hard palate is lined by a respiratory mucosa of ciliated columnar epithelial cells. (*H&E, ×15*)

350 The mucosa of the hard palate near the midline. The keratinized stratified squamous epithelium exhibits deep epithelial pegs. The lamina propria is composed of thick, dense, collagenous tissue. (*H&E, ×20*)

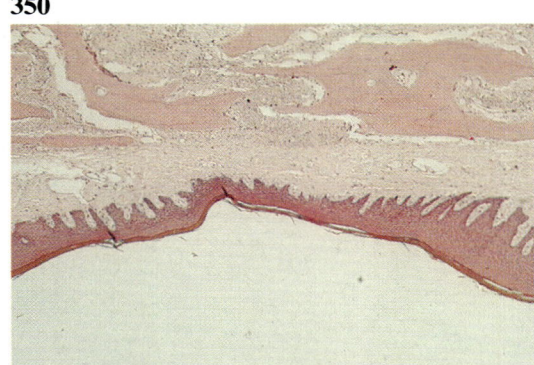

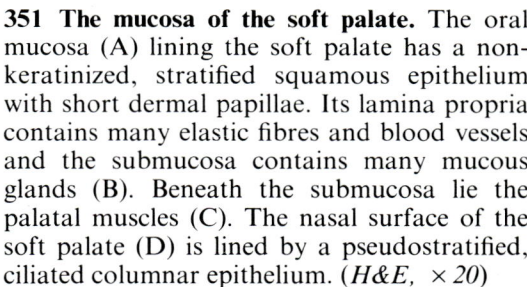

351 The mucosa of the soft palate. The oral mucosa (A) lining the soft palate has a non-keratinized, stratified squamous epithelium with short dermal papillae. Its lamina propria contains many elastic fibres and blood vessels and the submucosa contains many mucous glands (B). Beneath the submucosa lie the palatal muscles (C). The nasal surface of the soft palate (D) is lined by a pseudostratified, ciliated columnar epithelium. (*H&E, ×20*)

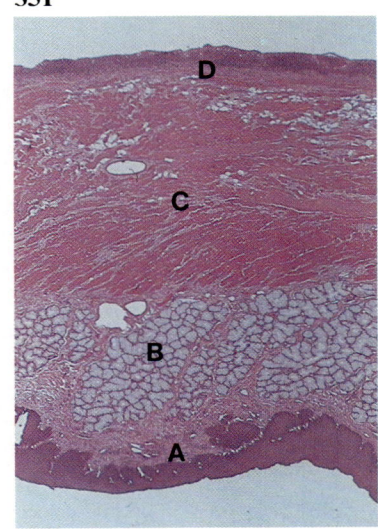

The tongue and floor of mouth

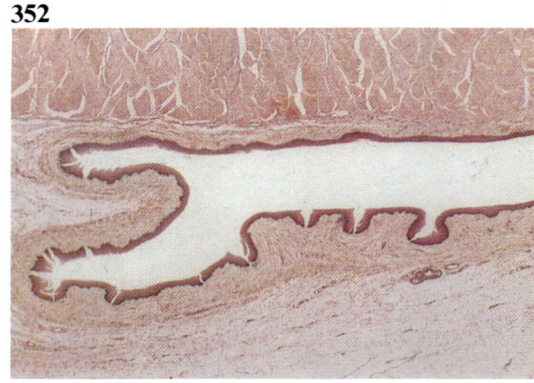

352 The appearance of the mucosa on the ventral surface of the tongue and its reflection over the floor of the mouth. The epithelium in this region is thin and non-keratinized and the dermal papillae are short. The submucosa of the floor of the mouth is only loosely attached to the underlying structures thus allowing free mobility of the tongue. The submucosa of the ventral surface of the tongue is indistinct, though what connective tissue there is binds the mucosa to the tongue muscles. ($\times 20$)

The dorsum of the tongue can be subdivided into an anterior two-thirds (the palatal surface) and a posterior one-third (the pharyngeal surface). The palatal surface of the tongue has numerous papillae which, according to their morphology, are of three types, filiform, fungiform and circumvallate papillae. The pharyngeal surface of the tongue is studded with lymphatic nodules.

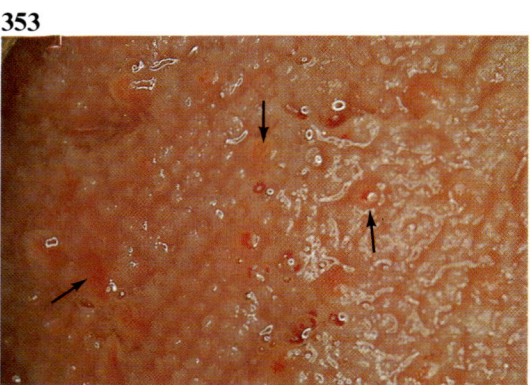

353 Dorsal surface of tongue showing filiform and fungiform papillae. The surface is covered with numerous, whitish, conical elevations, the filiform papillae. Interspersed between the filiform papillae are isolated, reddish prominences, the fungiform papillae (*arrowed*). The fungiform papillae are most numerous at the tip of the tongue.

354 Section through the palatal surface of the tongue to show the histological appearance of filiform papillae. Each filiform papilla consists of a central core of lamina propria carrying secondary papillae. The overlying stratified squamous epithelium is keratinized and forms hair-like tufts at the apex of the papillae. (*H&E, ×40*)

355 Section through a fungiform papillae. These mushroom-shaped elevations have a vascular, connective tissue core covered by a relatively thin, non-keratinized stratified squamous epithelium. They may contain taste buds. (*Masson's trichrome, ×40*)

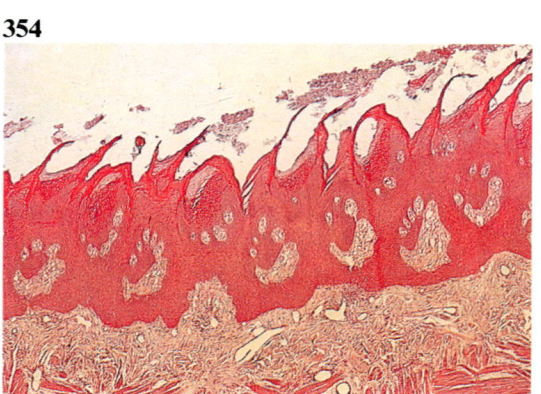

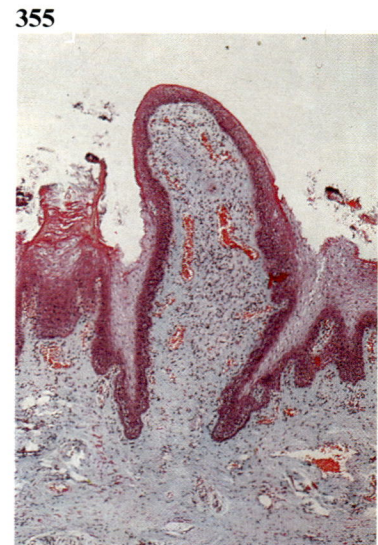

356 The circumvallate papillae (*arrowed*) are considerably larger than either the filiform or fungiform papillae. They lie immediately in front of the sulcus terminalis. They do not project beyond the surface of the tongue. They are surrounded by a circular 'trench'. The surface of the posterior third of the tongue, lying behind the sulcus terminalis, is covered by a number of smooth elevations produced by underlying lymphoid tissue.

357 Section through a circumvallate papilla. The papilla narrows at its base where ducts from serous glands (A) open. The papilla is covered by a non-keratinized, stratified squamous epithelium. Within the epithelium are small, pale, barrel-shaped structures, the taste buds (*arrowed*). (*Masson's trichrome, × 40*)

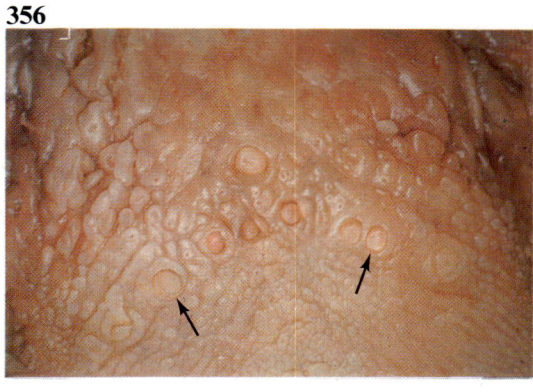

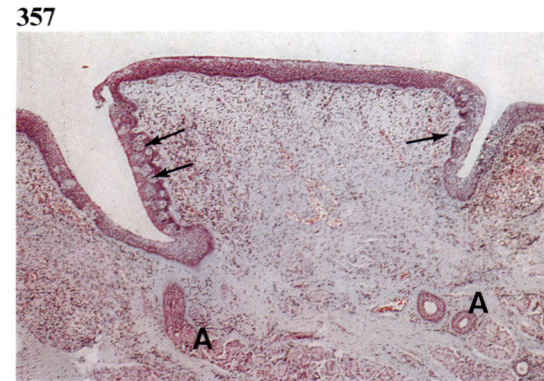

358 The taste bud appears as a pale staining structure which is composed of two different types of cells, the taste cells centrally and the surrounding supporting or sustentacular cells. (*Masson's trichrome, × 300*)

359 Section through the pharyngeal surface of the tongue showing a lingual follicle (*arrowed*). The overlying epithelium of the follicle is thin and non-keratinized. Lingual follicles are deep epithelial-lined crypts containing a mass of lymphoid material. The follicles usually open on to the surface of the tongue. (*H&E, × 40*)

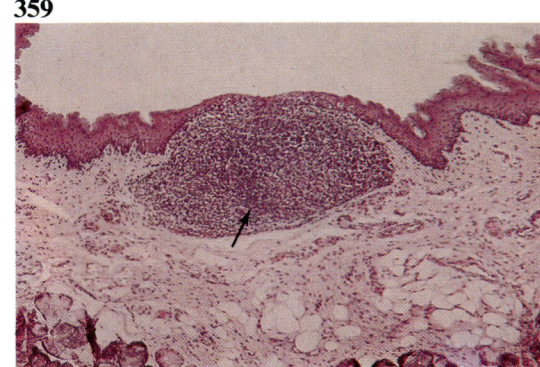

Principal features and regional variations of the oral mucosa

Region	Epithelium		Lamina propria		Submucosa		Type of mucosa
	Thickness	*Keratinization*	*Papillae*	*Fibre types*	*Density*	*Attachment*	
Labial and buccal mucosa	Thick	Non-keratinized	Short and irregular	Collagen and some elastic	Dense	Firmly to underlying muscle	Lining
Transitional (red) zone of lip	Thin	Keratinized	Long and narrow	Collagen and some elastic	Dense	Firmly to underlying muscle	Specialised
Alveolar mucosa	Thin	Non-keratinized	Short or absent	Many elastic fibres	Loose	Loose attachment to periosteum	Lining
Attached gingiva	Thick	Keratinized and parakeratinized	Long and narrow	Dense collagen firmly attached to underlying periosteum	No distinct submucosa		Masticatory
Floor of mouth	Thin	Non-keratinized	Short and broad	Collagen and some elastic	Loose	Loose attachment to underlying muscle	Lining
Ventral surface of tongue	Thin	Non-keratinized	Short and numerous	Collagen and some elastic	Not very distinct layer; attached to underlying muscle		Lining
Dorsum of tongue (anterior two-thirds)	Thick	Primarily keratinized	Long	Collagen and some elastic	Not very distinct layer; attached to underlying muscle		Specialised gustatory
Dorsum of tongue (posterior one-third)	Variable	Generally non-keratinized	Short or absent	Collagen and some elastic	Not very distinct layer; attached to underlying muscle		Lining gustatory
Hard palate	Thick	Keratinized	Long	Dense collagen in submucosa laterally, but lamina propria firmly bound to periosteum without submucosa in midline			Masticatory
Soft palate	Thick	Non-keratinized	Short	Many elastic fibres	Loose	Loose attachment to underlying tissues	Lining

Temporomandibular joint

The gross morphology, relationships and functional characteristics of this joint are described on pages 43–46.

360 Longitudinal, decalcified section through the temporomandibular joint.
A Articular disc within joint cavity.
B Glenoid fossa of temporal bone.
C Condyle of mandible.
D Ramus of mandible.
E Capsule of joint.
F Lateral pterygoid muscle.
(*Masson's blue trichrome, × 5*)

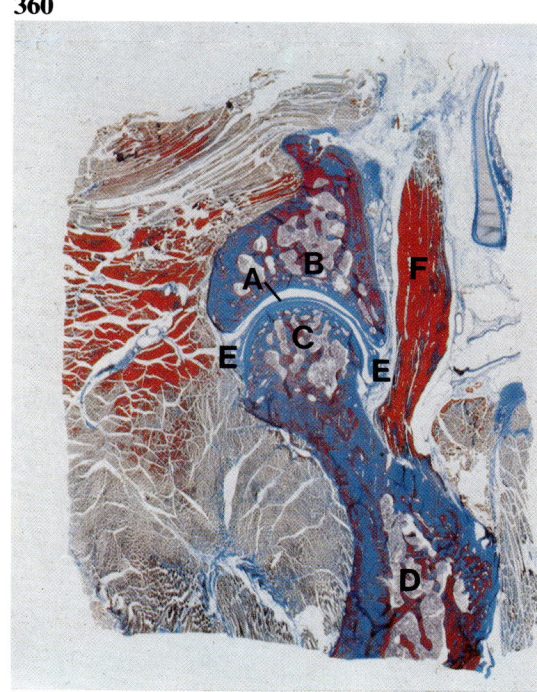

361 Longitudinal, decalcified section through the joint showing the arrangement of tissues on the articulating surfaces. The glenoid fossa (B) and the articular surface of the condyle (C) are lined by dense, fibrous, connective tissue. This joint, therefore, differs from most other synovial joints in that the articular surfaces are not lined by hyaline cartilage. This reflects the fact that the bones associated with the temporomandibular joint develop in membrane (page 150). The articular disc (A) which subdivides the joint cavity into upper and lower joint spaces, is also composed of compact fibrous tissue. (*Masson's blue trichrome, × 32*)

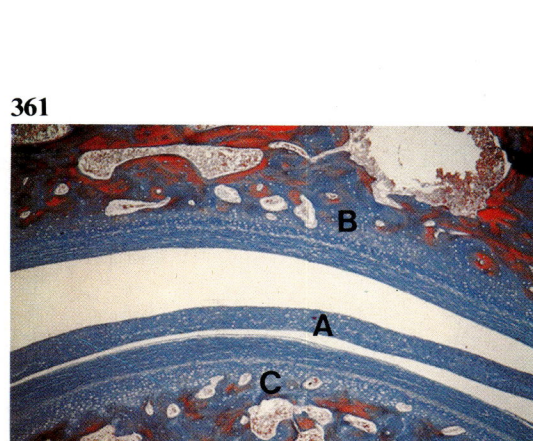

362 The articular disc. 362A anterior part; **362B** posterior part. Anteriorly, the collagen fibres are arranged as transverse and anteroposterior bundles; the disc, while clearly cellular, is relatively avascular. The posterior part of the disc is a loose-textured, fibrous, connective tissue which is vascular and richly supplied with sensory nerve endings. In this region, the disc may be covered by a thin synovial membrane. (*Masson's blue trichrome, × 320*)

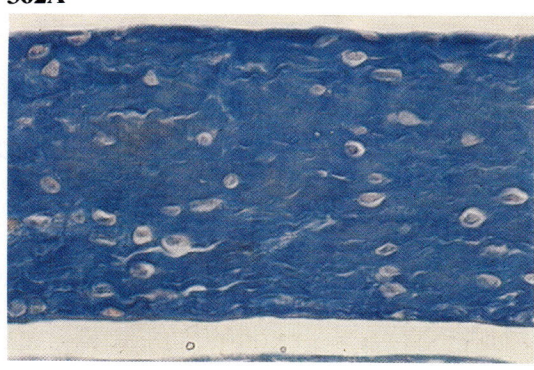

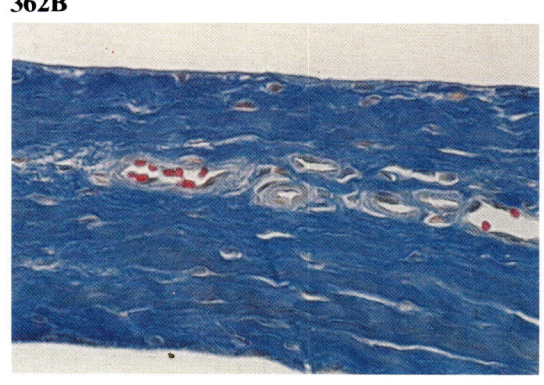

363 The articular part of the mandibular condyle. The condyle of the mandible is composed of a core of cancellous bone covered by a thin layer of compact bone. During the period of growth, a layer of hyaline cartilage (A) lies immediately beneath the fibrous, articulating surface of the condyle (B). This articulating surface is of even thickness and contains many elastic fibres. (*Masson's blue trichrome, × 200*)

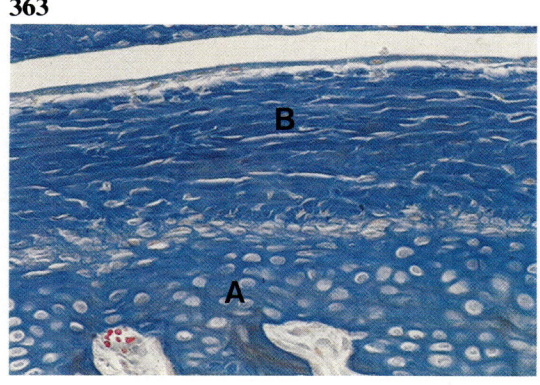

Salivary glands

Salivary glands are compound, tubular, acinous, merocrine glands whose ducts open into the oral cavity. They secrete a fluid, the saliva, which, among its many functions aids in the mastication, digestion and deglutition of food. The supporting connective tissue framework of salivary glands is termed the stroma. From a capsule of connective tissue which surrounds the gland run septa which divide the glandular tissue or parenchyma into lobes and smaller lobules. The parenchymal cells are of two kinds, mucous and serous. Mucous cells synthesise and secrete a viscous fluid which consists almost exclusively of mucin. Serous cells elaborate a watery secretion that lacks mucin but contains salts, proteins and the enzyme ptyalin or salivary amylase. Both the mucous and serous cells are arranged in secretory units, the acini or alveoli, which lie at expanded terminal parts of the ducts. All the salivary glands have extensive branching duct systems which consist of several differently structured segments:

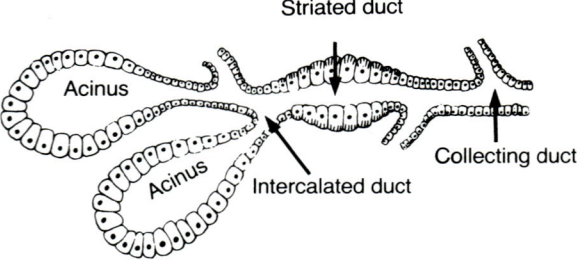

The intercalated and striated ducts are intralobular, the collecting ducts are interlobular lying within the connective tissue septa. The ducts not only transport the salivary secretions towards the oral cavity but also affect their composition.

There are three major salivary glands, the parotid, submandibular and sublingual glands, and numerous minor salivary glands scattered throughout the oral mucosa.

Parotid gland

This, the largest of the salivary glands, is enclosed within a well-defined capsule which is continuous with the deep cervical fascia. The glandular tissue is composed almost entirely of serous elements, though up to 5 per cent of the secretory cells may be of the mucous type. In the adult, the main parotid duct opens into the oral cavity opposite the upper second permanent molar.

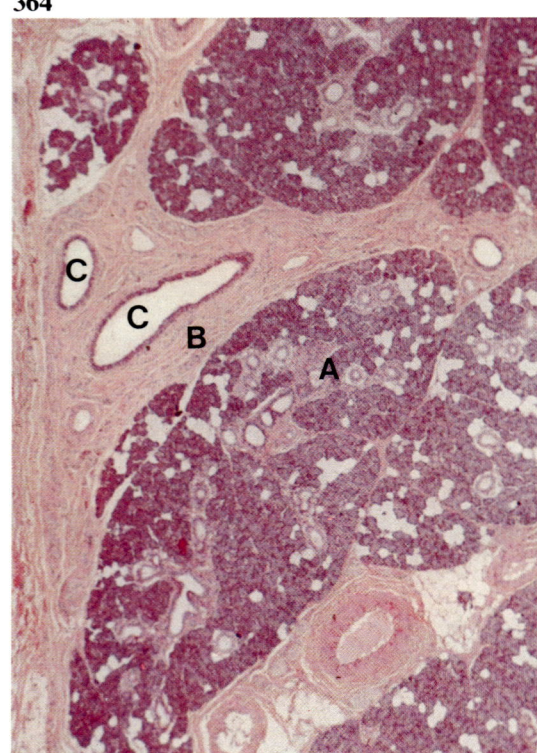

364 The lobular nature of the serous parenchyma (A) of the parotid gland. The connective tissue stroma (B) contains a number of main collecting ducts (C). (H&E, ×36)

365 The appearance of serous acini in the parotid gland. Each acinus consists of a number of serous cells which border a lumen whose size is dependent upon the secretory activity of the surrounding cells. Although not distinctly seen in light microscopy, the serous cells tend to be pyramidal in shape. The nucleus is prominent, rounded and located in the basal third of the cell, away from its serosal surface. Note the granular appearance of the cytoplasm produced by numerous refractile granules in the distal portion of the cell near its serosal surface. These granules, which contain enzymes, are termed zymogen granules.

Also shown in this section are a number of intercalated ducts (A) opening into a striated duct (B). There are also fat cells (C). With age, there is an increase in the number of fat cells, particularly within the connective tissue stroma. (*H&E*, × *360*)

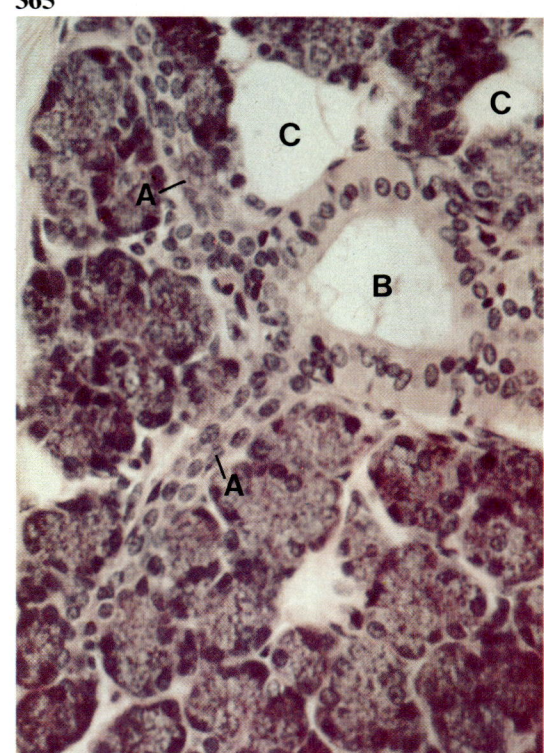

366 A serous acinus. The basal parts of the serous cells comprising the acinus contain the nuclei (A) and roughened endoplasmic reticulum (B). The distal parts of the cells contain zymogen granules (C). A basement lamina defines the acinus basally. The distal surface that borders the lumen (D) of the acinus may show a number of microvilli. The appearance of the serous cell varies according to its functional state. The appearance shown here is that of resting cells. When the cell is stimulated to secrete, there is a decrease in the number of granules, the contents of which are secreted into the lumen of the acinus by the process of exocytosis. Associated with active secretion, invaginations of the lumen into the cells may be seen, such invaginations being termed intercellular secretory canaliculi. It has been suggested that canaliculi which are involved in the transport of some secretory material from the cell into the lumen may also lie between adjacent serous cells. However, there is some controversy as to whether these canaliculi are preparatory artefacts. E, red blood cell. (*Electron micrograph*, × *2,000*)

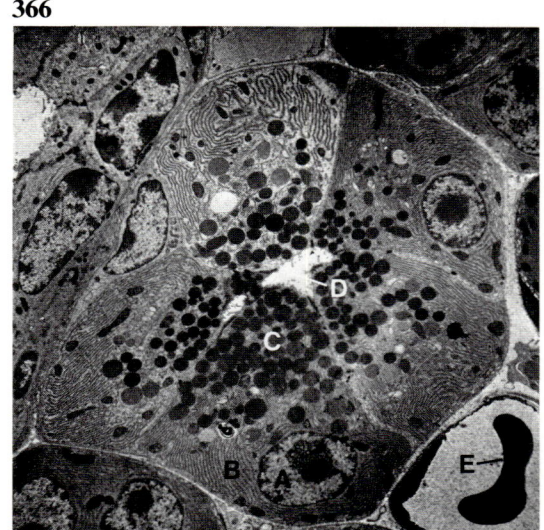

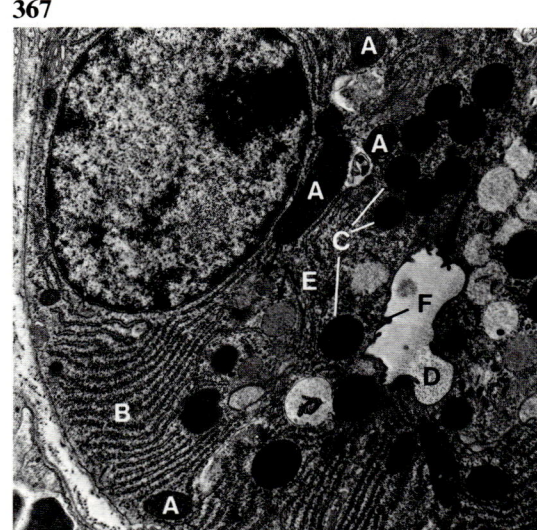

367 Part of a serous cell.
A Mitochondria.
B Roughened endoplasmic reticulum.
C Secretory granules.
D Exocytotic profile.
E Golgi material.
The granules about to be 'budded' from the Golgi material (*arrowed*) are of pale electron density. F, microvillus. Note the characteristic position of the intracytoplasmic organelles. (*Electron micrograph*, × *6,700*)

The duct system of the parotid gland consists of intercalated, striated and collecting ducts. The appearance under the light microscope of intercalated and striated ducts in parotid gland tissue is seen in figure **365**, the appearance of main collecting ducts in figure **364**.

mucous cells. Occasionally, however, the demilunes abut directly on to the lumen. Also seen in this section is a myoepithelial or basket cell (D) with one of its branching processes (E). These cells lie between the glandular or ductal epithelium and the basement membrane. They characteristically have numerous, long, branching processes. They are contractile and are thought to be involved in the flow of secretions into and along the ducts. (*Electron micrograph*, × *3,200*)

The duct system in the submandibular gland is similar to that in the parotid gland. However, the intercalated ducts of the submandibular gland are shorter and the striated ducts longer than those of the parotid gland.

368 An intercalated duct sectioned transversely. Each intercalated duct drains several acini. The ducts (A) are lined by a single layer of low cuboidal cells. Each cell has a relatively small amount of cytoplasm and the nucleus is centrally positioned. Little endoplasmic reticulum is present and there are few granules. In the parotid gland, intercalating ducts are long, narrow and branching. (*Electron micrograph*, ×5,700)

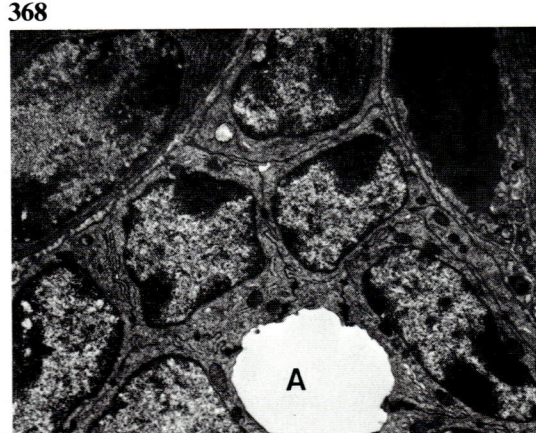

Sublingual gland

As with the submandibular gland, the sublingual gland is mixed. However, the mucous elements predominate over the serous in the ratio of approximately 3:1. Serous acini are rare, most of the serous cells occurring as demilunes. There is no conspicuous, connective tissue capsule surrounding the gland, though the septa separating the lobes and lobules are more pronounced than those in the submandibular or parotid glands. Usually, a number of main collecting ducts open independently into the floor of the mouth on the sublingual fold.

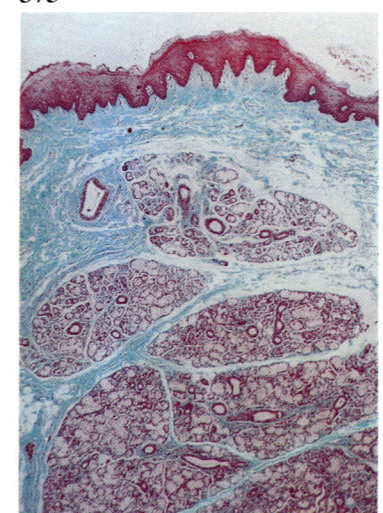

375 Section through the sublingual gland. Note the predominance of the pale staining mucous cells. (*Masson's trichrome*, ×25)

376 Section through the parenchyma of sublingual gland. The mucous acini appear pale, the demilunes (*arrowed*) are darker staining. A, striated duct. (*Masson's trichrome*, ×240)

The duct system of the sublingual gland differs from that of the submandibular and parotid glands in that there are no intercalated ducts and few striated ducts.

Minor salivary glands

The minor salivary glands include the labial, buccal, palatoglossal, palatal and lingual glands. The labial (see figure **328**) and buccal glands are mixed, containing both mucous and serous elements. The palatoglossal glands are located in the region of the pharyngeal isthmus and are mucous glands. The palatal glands lie in both the soft palate (see figure **351**) and the hard palate and are mucous glands. The anterior and posterior lingual glands are mainly mucous. The anterior glands are embedded within muscle near the ventral surface of the tongue and open by means of four or five ducts near the lingual frenum. The posterior glands are located in the root of the tongue. Around the circumvallate papillae are serous glands (of Von Ebner) (see figure **357**).

Development of oro-dental tissues

Development of the face

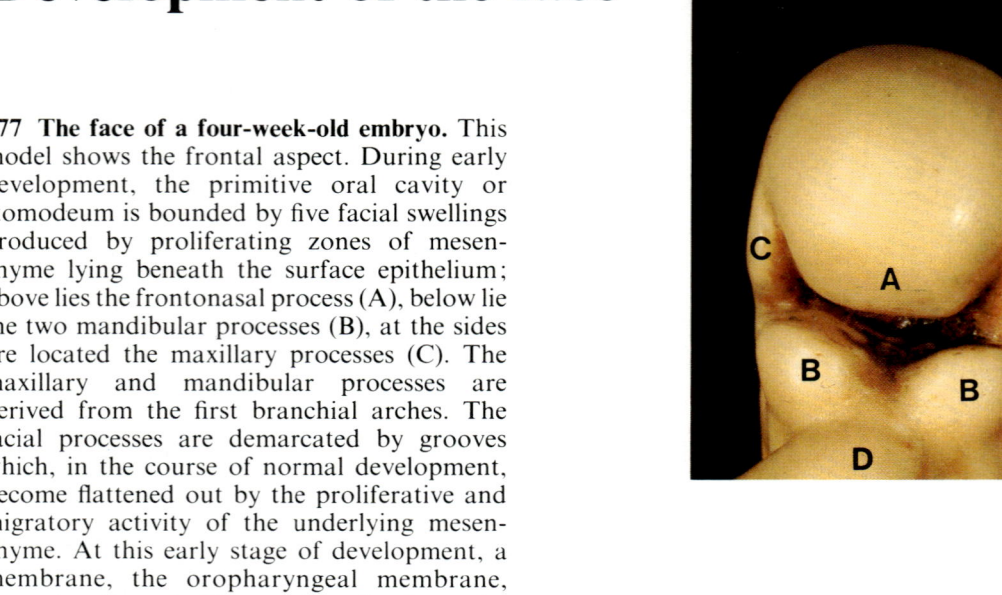

377 The face of a four-week-old embryo. This model shows the frontal aspect. During early development, the primitive oral cavity or stomodeum is bounded by five facial swellings produced by proliferating zones of mesenchyme lying beneath the surface epithelium; above lies the frontonasal process (A), below lie the two mandibular processes (B), at the sides are located the maxillary processes (C). The maxillary and mandibular processes are derived from the first branchial arches. The facial processes are demarcated by grooves which, in the course of normal development, become flattened out by the proliferative and migratory activity of the underlying mesenchyme. At this early stage of development, a membrane, the oropharyngeal membrane, separates the primitive oral cavity from the developing pharynx. The oropharyngeal membrane is bilaminar, being composed of an outer ectodermal layer and an inner endodermal layer. This membrane soon breaks down to establish continuity between the ectodermally-lined oral cavity and the endodermally-lined pharynx. Though not detectable in the adult, the demarcation zone between mucosa derived from ectoderm and endoderm corresponds to a region lying just behind the third permanent molar. (D), pericardial swelling.

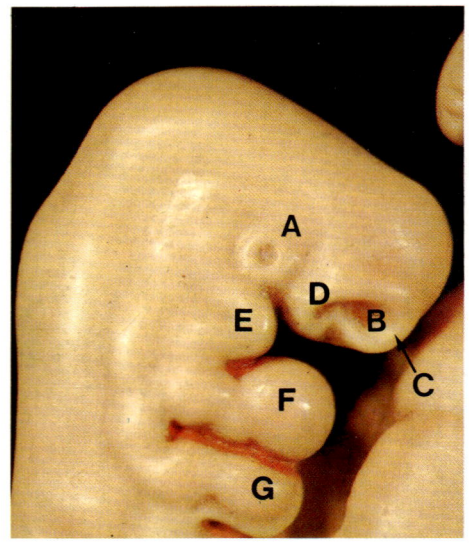

378 The face of a five-week-old embryo. This model shows the lateral aspect. Localised thickenings of ectoderm give rise to the nasal and optic (A) placodes. These placodes will form the olfactory epithelium and lens of the eyes. The nasal placodes sink into the underlying mesenchyme, forming two blind-ended nasal pits (B), the primitive nasal cavities. Proliferation of mesenchyme from the frontonasal process around the openings of the nasal pits produces the medial (C) and lateral (D) nasal processes. Also shown on the model is a maxillary process (E), a mandibular process (F) and the second branchial arch (G).

The nasal pits continue to deepen until eventually they approach the roof of the primitive oral cavity, being partitioned from it by bucconasal membranes. By the end of the fifth week these membranes rupture, thus producing communications between the developing nasal and oral cavities. Before the bucconasal membrane ruptures, a sheet of epithelium, the nasal fin, may be seen in front of each nasal pit.

The nasal fin does not, as was once thought, form an epithelial partition between the maxillary and medial nasal processes. A bridge of mesenchyme, the maxillary isthmus, joins the two processes in front of the nasal fin.

379 Sagittal section through the developing nasal (A) and oral (B) cavities. This shows the position of the nasal fin (C), the bucconasal membrane (D), and the maxillary isthmus (E) at the end of the fifth week of development. The nasal fin is eventually incorporated into the walls of the nasal pit or into the bucconasal membrane. However, should the fin become enlarged, it may constitute a line of weakness between the mesenchyme of the maxillary and medial nasal processes and eventually lead to a cleft in this region.

380 The face of a six-week-old embryo. This model shows the lateral aspect. The two mandibular processes (A) fuse in the midline to form the tissues of the lower jaw. Rarely, persistence of a midline groove in this region produces a mandibular cleft. The mandibular and maxillary (B) processes meet at the angles of the mouth, thus defining its outline. Disturbances in this process may give rise to macrostomia or microstomia or rarely an astomia. From the corners of the mouth, the maxillary processes grow inwards beneath the lateral nasal processes (C) towards the medial nasal processes (D) of the upper lip. Between the merging maxillary and the lateral nasal processes lie the naso-optic furrows (E). From each furrow a solid ectodermal rod of cells sinks below the surface and canalises to form the nasolacrimal duct. Persistence of the naso-optic furrow may produce an oblique facial cleft.

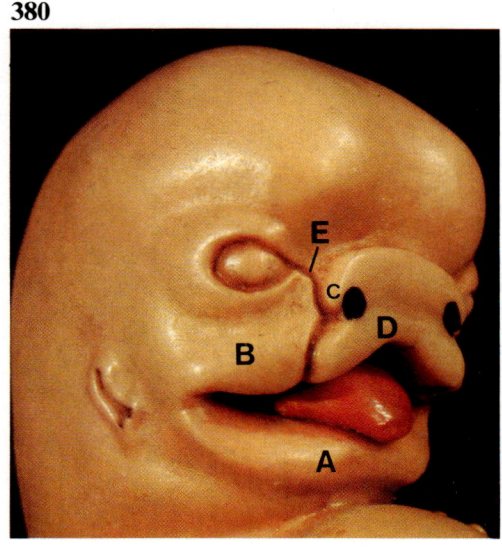

Two differing accounts have been given for the development of the upper lip. One view suggests that the maxillary processes overgrow the medial nasal processes to meet in the midline and thus contribute all the tissue for the upper lip. This is based upon an appreciation of the innervation of the fully formed upper lip (i.e. the infraorbital branch of the maxillary division of the trigeminal nerve), the maxillary processes being supplied by the maxillary nerve, the frontonasal process by the ophthalmic nerve. Alternatively, it has been suggested that the maxillary processes meet the medial nasal processes without such overgrowth, the middle third of the upper lip being derived from the frontonasal process. While histological evidence favours this explanation, at present, little is known about the behaviour of the mesenchyme of the facial processes after the initial fusion to exclude the possibility of subsequent migration of tissue derived from the maxillary processes towards the midline. Failure of the maxillary and medial nasal processes to fuse produces the common congenital malformation of cleft lip; this may present as a unilateral or bilateral cleft lip. Failure of the medial nasal processes to merge may be responsible for the formation of the median cleft lip. The facial muscles are derived from the mesenchyme of the second branchial arch which migrates into the substance of the lips.

381 Contributions to the adult face from the embryonic facial processes.
A Maxillary process.
B Mandibular process.
C Medial nasal process.
D Lateral nasal process.

This diagram is based upon the suggestion that the middle third of the upper lip is derived from the frontonasal process. The facial derivatives shown are therefore at odds with the sensory distribution of the adult face for, as previously mentioned, the fully developed lip is supplied only by the maxillary division of the trigeminal and has no contribution from the ophthalmic division.

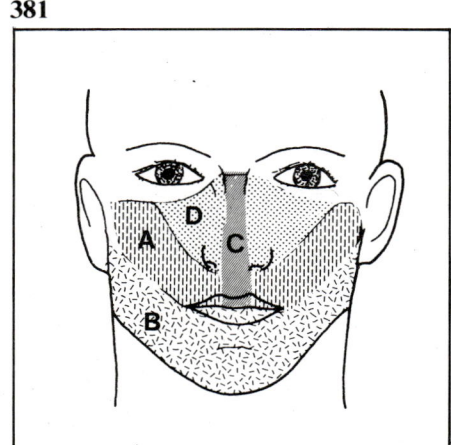

Development of the palate

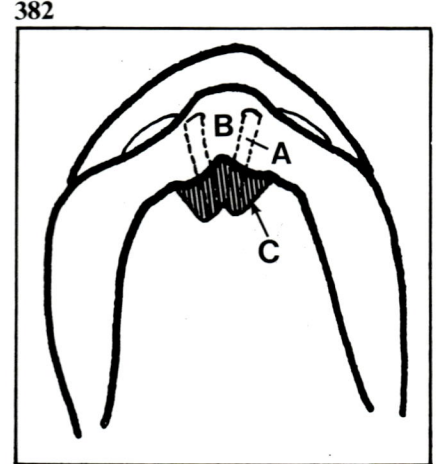

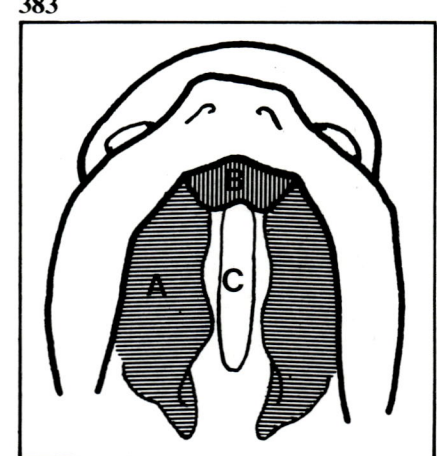

382 By the sixth week of development, the primitive nasal cavities (A) are separated by a primary nasal septum (B) and are partitioned from the primitive oral cavity by a primary palate (C). Both the primary nasal septum and primary palate are derived from the fronto-nasal process. The stomodeal chamber is divided at this stage into the small primitive oral cavity beneath the primary palate, and the relatively large oro-nasal cavity behind the primary palate.

383 During the sixth week of development, two lateral palatal shelves (A) develop behind the primary palate (B). From the maxillary processes a secondary nasal septum (C) grows down from the roof of the stomodeum behind the primary nasal septum, thus dividing the nasal part of the oro-nasal cavity into two.

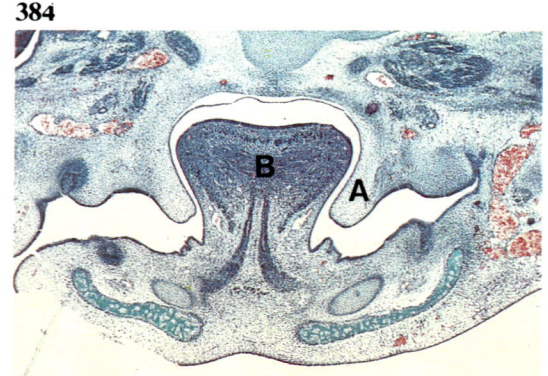

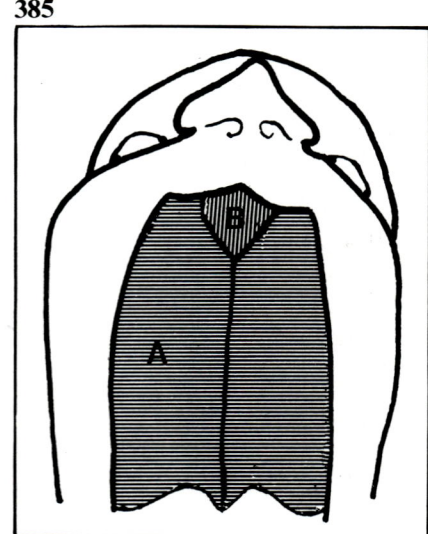

384 Decalcified, coronal section through the developing head during the seventh week of development showing the lateral palatal shelves (A) of the maxillae. Note that the oral part of the oro-nasal cavity becomes completely filled by the developing tongue (B). Growth of the lateral palatal shelves continues such that they come to lie in the only available space on either side of the tongue, being vertically inclined. (*Masson's trichrome, × 30*)

385 During the eighth week of development, the stomodeum enlarges, the tongue 'drops' and the vertically-inclined lateral palatal shelves become horizontal. It has been suggested that the descent of the tongue is related to mandibular growth and/or a change in the shape of the tongue. On becoming horizontal, the lateral palatal shelves contact each other and the secondary nasal septum in the midline to form the secondary palate. The shelves contact the primary palate anteriorly so that the oro-nasal cavity becomes subdivided into its constituent oral and nasal cavities. B, primary palate. A, lateral palatal shelves forming secondary palate.

Several mechanisms have been proposed to account for the rapid movement of the lateral palatal shelves from the vertical to the horizontal position including: rapid differential mitotic growth, variations in blood flow, the presence of an intrinsic shelf force, biochemical changes in the connective tissue, reflex jaw activity, pressure differences between the oral and nasal cavities.

386 Decalcified, coronal section through developing oro-nasal regions following contact of the lateral palatal shelves (A) and secondary nasal septum (B). The epithelium (C) which initially separates the processes begins to break down commencing at a point approximately one-third of the way from the front of the lateral palatal shelves, subsequently spreading both anteriorly and posteriorly. Epithelial degeneration is thought to be brought about by programmed cell death. Fusion of the palatal processes is complete by the twelfth week of development. Behind the secondary nasal septum, the lateral palatal shelves fuse to form the soft palate and uvula. D, developing bone of maxilla. (× 30)

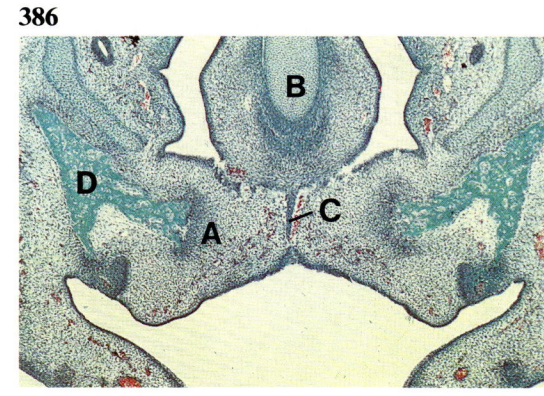

The hard palate ossifies intramembranously from four centres of ossification, one in each developing maxilla and one in each developing palatine bone. The maxillary ossification centre lies above the developing deciduous canine tooth germ and appears in the sixth week of development. The palatine centres of ossification are situated in the region forming the future perpendicular plate and appear in the eighth week of development. Incomplete ossification of the palate from these centres defines the median and transverse palatine sutures. There does not appear to be a separate centre of ossification for the primary palate (the premaxilla).

387 Coronal section through the developing hard palate showing early ossification. A, developing body of maxilla. B, bone extending from body into palate. C, nasal cavity. The expansion of the nasal cavities is reflected in resorption of bone at the upper border of the palate and deposition at its lower border. Note the osteoclasts on the nasal surface and osteoblasts on the oral surface of the palatal bone. (*Masson's trichrome*, × 80)

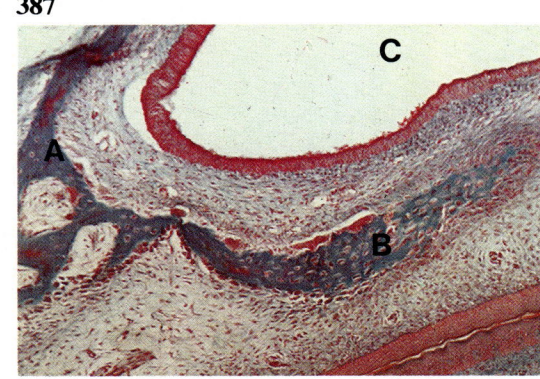

Though relatively flat at birth, subsequent growth (especially related to the eruption of the teeth) gives the palate its arched shape.

Interference with normal palate formation may result in a cleft palate. Clefts of the palate, like those of the lip, are polygenic or multifactorial malformations. The mildest form of cleft is that affecting the uvula, such a disturbance occurring relatively late in the process of palatal fusion. Greater disturbance, occurring during the early phases of palatal fusion, results in a more extensive cleft involving most of the secondary palate. Should the cleft involve the primary palate, it may extend either to the right and/or the left of the incisive foramen to include the alveolus, passing between the lateral incisor and canine teeth. Cleft palate may be associated with cleft lip, though the two conditions are independently determined. Dental malformations are commonly associated with a cleft involving the alveolus.

Development of the jaws

The mandible

388 Meckel's cartilage (A) around which the bone of the mandible (B) is forming in membrane. This is a horizontal section through the developing mandible. C, tongue. D, mandibular symphysis. Meckel's cartilage, the cartilage of the first branchial arch, extends from the cartilaginous otic capsule to the midline symphysis where initially it is separated from its fellow of the opposite side by mesenchyme. (*Masson's trichrome*, ×12)

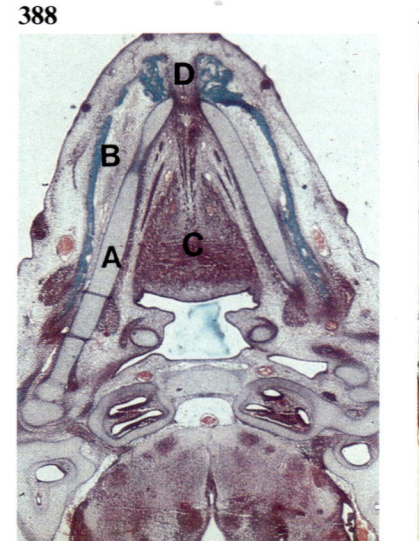
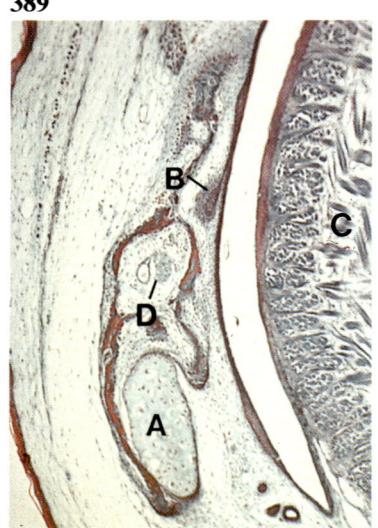

Meckel's cartilage makes little contribution to the adult mandible but provides a framework around which the bone of the mandible forms. The mandible first appears as a band of dense fibrous tissue on the anterolateral aspect of Meckel's cartilage. During the seventh week of intra-uterine life, a centre of ossification appears in this fibrous tissue at a site related to the future mental foramen. From this centre, bone formation spreads rapidly backwards, forwards and upwards around the inferior dental nerve and its terminal branches, the incisive and mental nerves. Further spread of the developing bone in a forward and backward direction produces a plate of bone on the lateral side of Meckel's cartilage which corresponds to the future body of the mandible and which extends towards the midline where it comes to lie in close relationship with the bone forming on the opposite side. However, the two plates of bone remain separated at the mandibular symphysis by fibrous tissue.

389 Decalcified, transverse section through the early developing mandible (eighth week of development). At this stage, only a small amount of mandibular bone has formed intramembranously on the lateral aspect of Meckel's cartilage (A). Note the beginnings of tooth development in this region indicated by the dental lamina (B). C, tongue. D, neurovascular bundle. (*Masson's trichrome*, ×60)

390 A later stage in the development of the body of the mandible. The alveolar process (A), grows to surround the developing tooth germ. The developing teeth share the same common crypt as the neurovascular bundle (B). Note that Meckel's cartilage (C) is now comparatively small though it still lies medial to the developing mandibular bone. D, developing tongue. (*Masson's trichrome*, ×25)

391 Even later stage in the development of the body of the mandible. Meckel's cartilage has been resorbed. The neurovascular bundle (B) is now contained within its own bony canal and there has been considerable development of the alveolar processes (A). C, developing tongue. (*Masson's trichrome*, ×25)

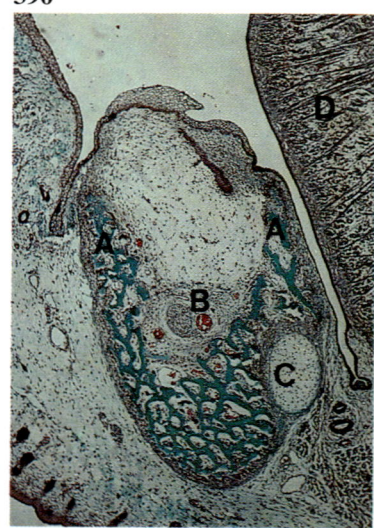
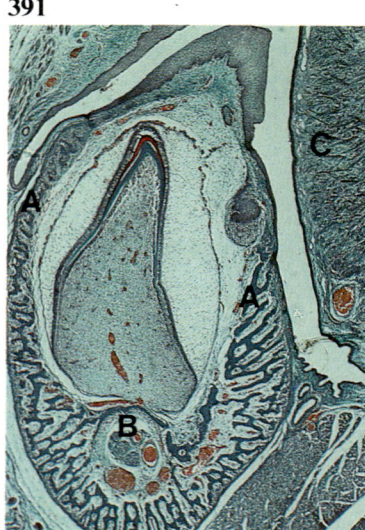

Though Meckel's cartilage contributes no significant tissue to the developing mandible, in the region of the symphysis, nodular remnants of cartilage may be seen up till birth, and in its most dorsal part it ossifies to form the ear ossicles, the malleus and incus. Behind the body of the mandible, the perichondrium of Meckel's cartilage persists as the sphenomandibular and sphenomalleolar ligaments. The sphenomandibular ligament ossifies at its sites of attachment to form the lingula of the mandible and the spine of the sphenoid bone.

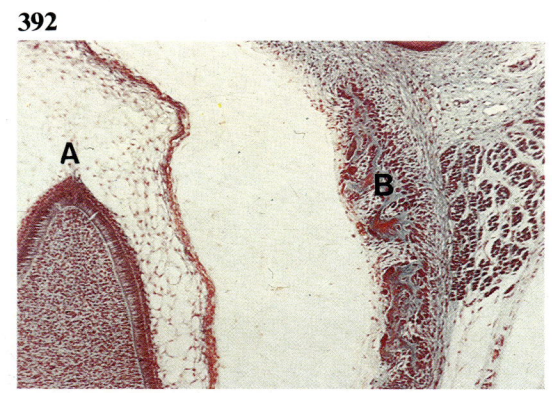

392 Development of the mandibular alveolus, shown in a decalcified, transverse section of a jaw in the region of a developing tooth (A). As the developing tooth germ reaches the early bell stage, developing bone becomes closely related to it to form the alveolus (B). The size of the alveolus is dependent upon the size of the growing tooth germ. Note that resorption is occurring on the inner wall of the alveolus (indicated by osteoclasts lying in Howship's lacunae) while on the outer wall of the alveolus, bone is being deposited (indicated by osteoblasts lining an osteoid seam). The developing teeth therefore come to lie in a trough of bone. Later, the teeth become separated from each other by the development of interdental septa. With the onset of root formation, interradicular bone develops in multirooted teeth. (Some shrinkage has occurred within the tissues of the dental follicle during preparation of this specimen, producing a space between the developing tooth germ and alveolus.) (*Masson's trichrome, ×60*)

The ramus of the mandible is first mapped out as a condensation of fibrocellular tissue which, though continuous with the developing body of the mandible, is positioned some way laterally from Meckel's cartilage. Further development of the ramus is associated with a backward spread of ossification from the body and by the appearance of a number of secondary cartilages. Between the tenth and fourteenth week *in utero*, three secondary cartilages develop within the growing mandible. The largest and most important of these is the condylar cartilage which, as its name suggests, appears beneath the fibrous articular layer of the future condyle. By proliferation and subsequent ossification of the cartilage, it is thought to serve as an important centre of growth for the mandible, functioning up to about the 20th year of life. Less important, transitory, secondary cartilages are seen associated with the coronoid process and in the region of the mandibular symphysis.

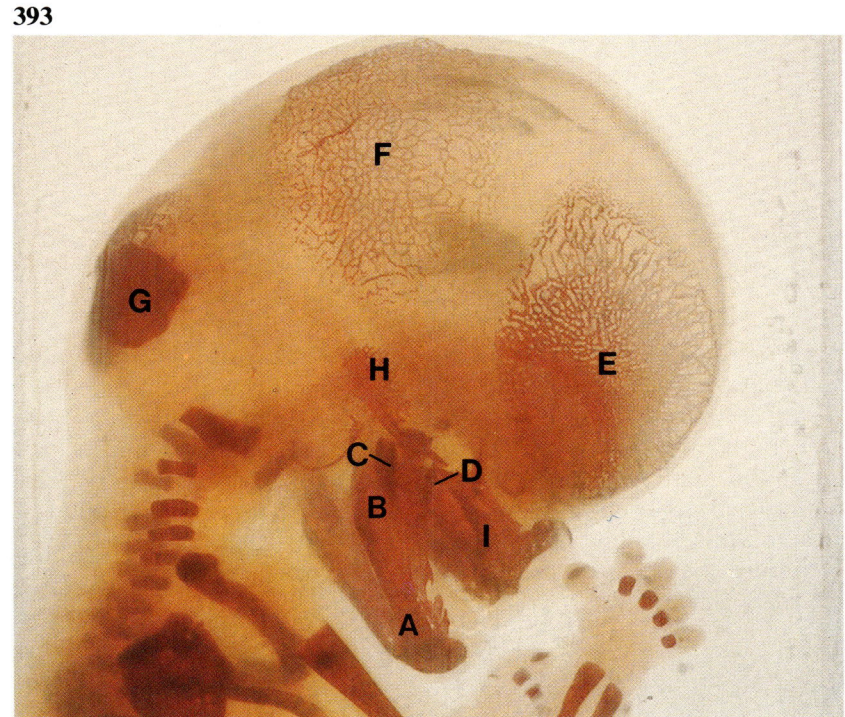

393 The appearance of the developing jaws of a human foetus (14 weeks i.u.).
A Body of mandible.
B Ramus of mandible.
C Secondary condylar cartilage.
D Secondary coronoid cartilage.
E Frontal bone.
F Parietal bone.
G Occipital bone.
H Squamous portion of temporal bone.
I Maxilla.
(*Cleared, alizarin red preparation, ×5*)

394 Decalcified, transverse section through the early developing condyle showing the condylar cartilage (A). B, Meckel's cartilage. C, developing bone of glenoid fossa. D, part of developing articular disc of temporomandibular joint. (*Masson's trichrome, × 20*)

The temporomandibular joint develops from mesenchyme lying between the developing mandibular condyle below and the temporal bone above, which develop intramembranously. During the twelfth week of intrauterine life, two clefts appear in the mesenchyme producing the upper and lower joint cavities, the remaining intervening mesenchyme becoming the intra-articular disc. The joint capsule develops from a condensation of mesenchyme surrounding the developing joint. At birth, the articular fossa is flat and there is no articular eminence, the latter only becoming prominent following the eruption of the deciduous dentition.

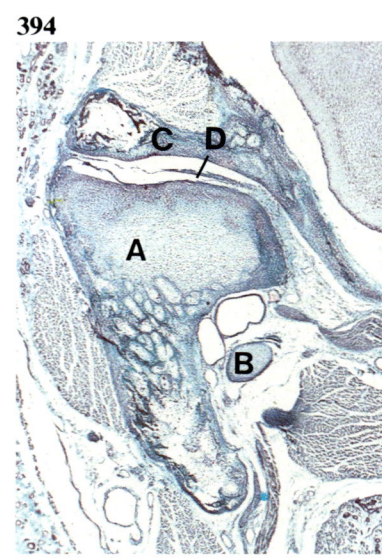

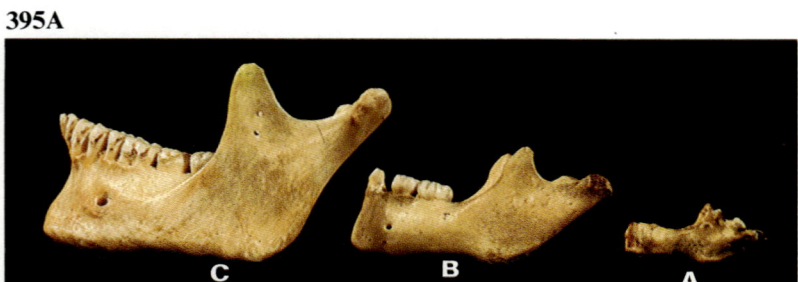

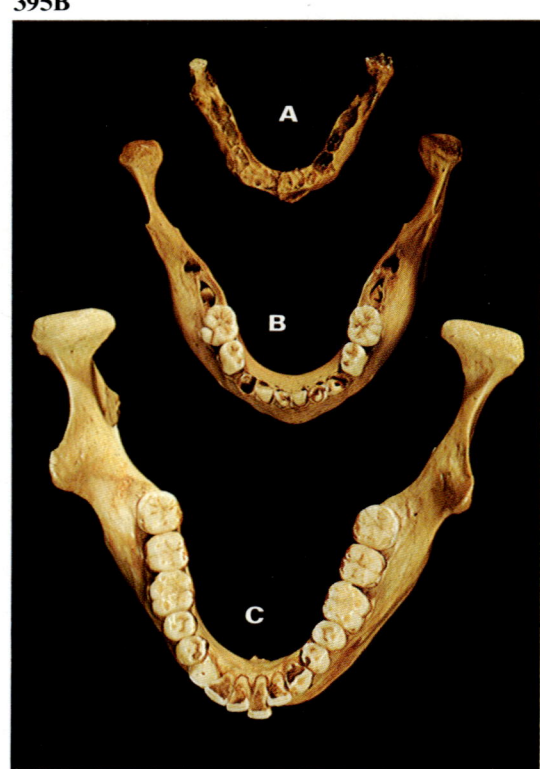

395 The postnatal development of the mandible illustrated by lateral and occlusal views of the mandible at birth (A), at six years (B) and in an adult (C). The ratio of body to ramus is greater at birth than in the adult, indicating a proportional increase with time in the development of the ramus. At birth, there is no distinct chin and the two halves of the mandible are separated by the mandibular symphysis. Ossification of the symphysis is complete during the second year, the two halves of the mandible uniting to form a single bone. The chin becomes most prominent after puberty.

Growth of the mandible occurs by remodelling of bone. Increase in the height of the body occurs primarily by formation of alveolar bone, though some bone is also deposited along the lower border of the mandible. Increase in the length of the mandible is accomplished by bone deposition on the posterior surface of the ramus with compensatory resorption on its anterior surface, accompanied by deposition of bone on the posterior surface of the coronoid process and resorption on the anterior surface of the condyle. Increase in width of the mandible is produced by deposition of bone on the outer surface of the mandible and resorption on the inner surface.

There is some controversy concerning the rôle of the condylar cartilages in mandibular growth. One view states that continued proliferation of this cartilage is primarily responsible for the increase in both the mandibular length and the height of the ramus. Alternatively, it has been suggested that proliferation of the condylar cartilage is a response to growth, this view being supported by experiments showing that mandibular growth is relatively unaffected following condylectomy, providing normal mandibular function is maintained.

Though the mandible is a single bone, it may be thought of as a number of skeletal units each associated with one or more soft tissue 'functional matrices'. The behaviour of these matrices primarily determines the growth of each skeletal unit. For example, the coronoid process forms a skeletal unit acted upon by the temporalis muscle. Sectioning of the temporalis muscle during early mandibular development may result in atrophy or complete absence of a coronoid process in the adult mandible. Similarly, the alveolar process is influenced by the teeth, the condyle by the lateral pterygoid muscle, the ramus by the medial pterygoid and masseter muscles and the body by the neurovascular bundle.

The maxilla

The maxilla ossifies in membrane within the mesenchyme of the maxillary process of the first branchial arch. Its centre of ossification appears close to the site of the deciduous canine.

396 Decalcified, transverse section through the early developing maxilla in the region of the developing deciduous canine. From this site, ossification spreads throughout the developing maxilla into its growing processes (i.e. palatine zygomatic, frontal and alveolar processes). See figure **387** for the ossification of the palatine processes, and figure **393** for the appearance of the developing maxilla seen in a cleared alizarin red preparation. (× 35)

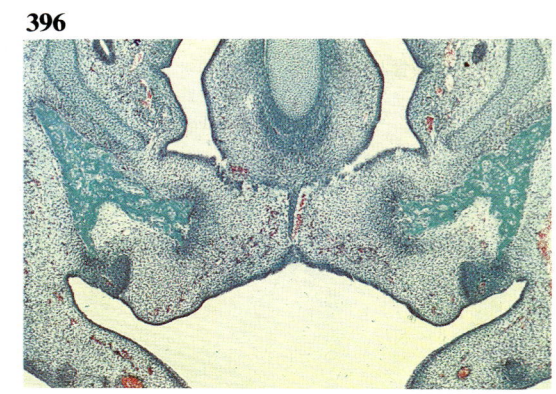

At one time it was thought that the incisor-bearing part of the maxilla which develops from the frontonasal process, the premaxilla, had a separate centre of ossification. However, it is now clear that ossification spreads from the body of the maxilla into its incisor-bearing component.

Growth of the maxilla occurs by surface deposition of bone with associated resorption and by sutural growth. Among the agencies which provide the forces separating the maxilla from the adjacent bones – thus permitting growth at the sutures – are the growing eyeballs, cartilaginous nasal septum and orbital pad of fat. Thus, growth of the maxilla is not an isolated phenomenon but occurs in association with the development of the orbital, nasal and oral cavities. It has recently been suggested that the growing nasal septum pulls the maxilla forward by means of a septo-premaxillary ligament which runs from the anterior border of the nasal septum postero-inferiorly towards the anterior nasal spine and interpremaxillary suture. As in the lower jaw, growth in height of the maxilla is related to the development of the alveolar process.

The maxillary sinus appears as an outpocketing of the mucosa of the middle meatus of the nose at the beginning of the fourth month of intra-uterine life. Though small at birth, the maxillary sinus is identifiable radiologically. After birth, the maxillary sinus enlarges with the growing maxilla though it is only fully developed following the eruption of the permanent dentition.

397 Growth trends of the skull. Since every single bone in the skull of the growing child shows some degree of growth at some period, no point can strictly be considered fixed. However, a reasonable idea of the overall increase in size and direction of the growth of the face of an individual can be obtained when tracings of a series of lateral skull radiographs, taken at varying ages using a cephalostat are superimposed at the registration points with the Bolton planes parallel (see figure **123**). Such studies show that the general trend is for the facial complex to grow forwards under the cranium. Note that, with differential growth, the face to neurocranium ratio by volume increases. R= registration point.

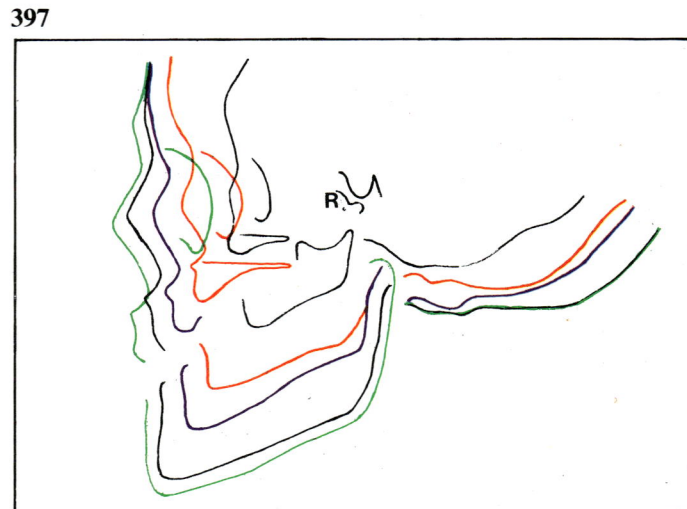

Development of the tongue

398 The schema of tongue primordia. The model is of the ventral wall of the pharynx at the fourth week of intrauterine life. The anterior two-thirds of the tongue develop from three swellings, the lateral lingual swellings (A) and the midline tuberculum impar (B). Each is formed by proliferation of mesenchyme beneath the endodermal lining of the first branchial arch. The posterior third of the tongue develops from a single midline swelling, the cupola (C) which is derived mainly from the third branchial arch with a small contribution from the fourth arch. The cupola overgrows the second arch to merge with the first arch swellings.

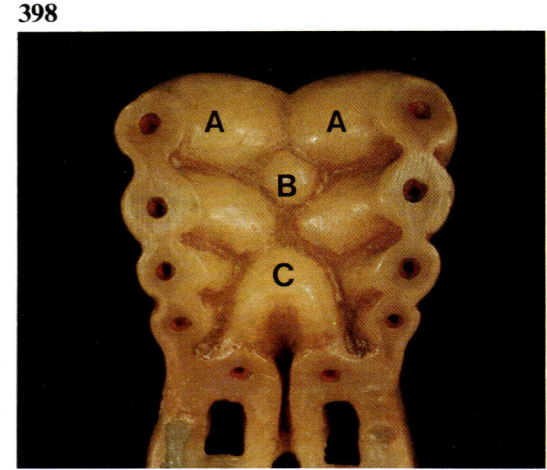

The diverse embryological origin of the tongue explains its diverse sensory supply (see figure **98**). General sensation to the anterior two-thirds of the tongue is supplied by the lingual nerve, a nerve of the first branchial arch. General sensation and taste to the posterior third of the tongue is supplied by the glossopharyngeal and superior laryngeal nerves, the nerves of the third and fourth arches. The perception of taste in the anterior two-thirds of the tongue is associated with the chorda tympani nerve. The chorda tympani is a branch of the facial nerve, the nerve of the second branchial arch. Since this arch does not contribute tissue to the anterior part of the tongue, in this situation it is termed a pretrematic nerve. The muscles of the tongue develop primarily from occipital somites which migrate into the developing tongue carrying their nerve supply, the hypoglossal nerve, with them.

The thyroid gland develops between the tuberculum impar and the cupola. On the fully formed tongue, this site is demarcated by a small pit, the foramen caecum (see figure **9**).

Early tooth development

The first detectable signs of tooth development are the appearance of a condensation of mesenchymal tissue and capillary networks beneath the presumptive dental epithelium of the primitive oral cavity. Evidence suggests that this mesenchyme is of neural crest origin. By the sixth week of development, the oral epithelium invaginates into this mesenchyme to form the primary epithelial band. By the seventh week, this band gives rise to two processes, the vestibular and the dental laminae. It is not known whether invagination of the primary epithelial band and the vestibular and dental laminae is genetically determined or induced by the underlying mesenchyme.

399 The vestibular lamina (A) and the dental lamina (B). This is a transverse section through the primitive oral epithelium. The vestibular lamina contributes to the development of the vestibule, delineating the lips and cheeks from the tooth-bearing regions. It lies buccal to the dental lamina which contributes to the development of the teeth. (*H&E*, × 120)

400 Further development of the dental lamina (A) is characterised by an increase in length, though it is not known whether this results from active invagination of the lamina or upward proliferation of the mesenchyme. (*Masson's trichrome*, × 130)

401 By the eighth week, a series of swellings develop on the deep surface of the dental lamina. On the model, the complete dental lamina of the lower jaw is shown as the green structure and the epithelial swellings are arrowed. Note that the dental lamina appears as a concentric arch-shaped band of tissue following the line of the vestibular fold (A). Though not shown on the model, each epithelial swelling is almost completely surrounded by a mesenchymal condensation.

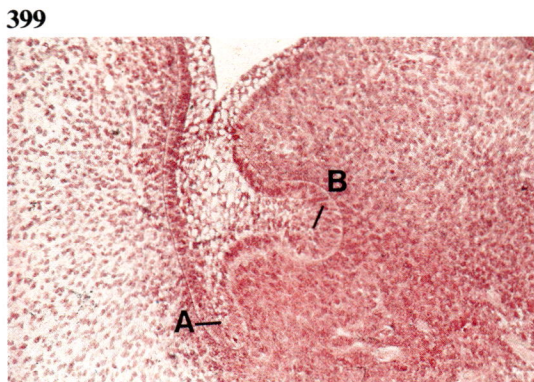

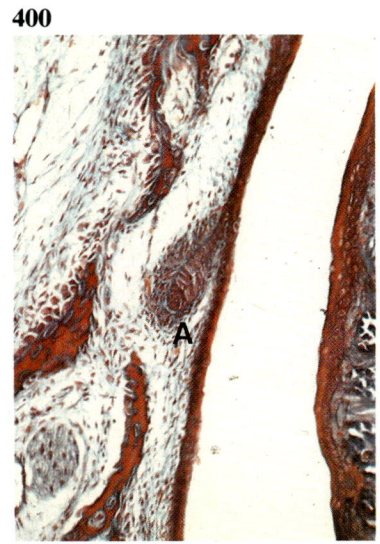

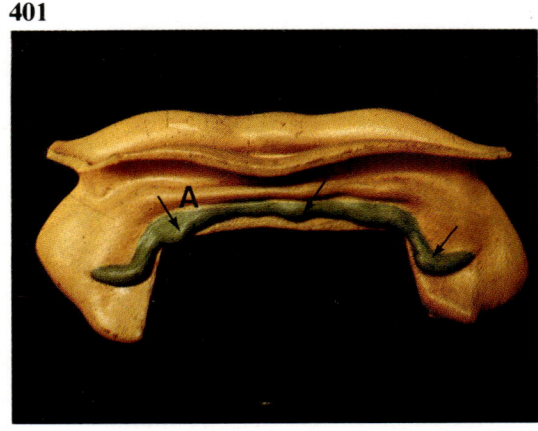

For descriptive purposes, tooth germs are classified into bud, cap and bell stages according to the degree of morphodifferentiation and histodifferentiation of their epithelial components (enamel organs).

402 Bud stage. The enamel organ (A) in the bud stage appears as a simple, spherical to ovoid, epithelial condensation which is relatively poorly morphodifferentiated and histodifferentiated. Compared with the overlying oral epithelium, however, the cells of the tooth bud have a higher RNA content, a lower glycogen content and an increased oxidative enzyme activity. Note the mesenchymal condensation (B). As yet, it has not been established whether the epithelial bud is induced by the underlying mesenchyme. Nevertheless, the successful development of the tooth germ relies upon a complex interaction of the mesenchymal and epithelial components since, should these be separated and cultured individually, neither component will differentiate further. (*Masson's trichrome,* ×60)

403 Early cap stage. By the eleventh week, morphogenesis has progressed, the deeper surface of the enamel organ invaginating to form a cap-shaped structure. In this section, both maxillary and mandibular cap stages are shown, each enamel organ appearing relatively poorly histodifferentiated. However, a greater distinction develops between the more rounded cells in the central portion of the enamel organ and the peripheral cells which are becoming arranged to form the external and internal enamel epithelia. Also shown are Meckel's cartilage (A), developing tongue (B) and developing bone of the upper and lower jaws. (*Masson's trichrome,* ×32)

404 Late cap stage. By about twelve-and-a-half weeks, the central cells of the enlarging enamel organ have become separated though maintaining contact by desmosomes. The resulting intercellular spaces contain significant quantities of glycosaminoglycans. The resulting tissue is termed the stellate reticulum (A), though it is not fully developed until the later bell stage. The cells of the external enamel epithelium (B) remain cuboidal whereas the internal enamel epithelial cells (C) become more columnar. The cells of the internal enamel epithelium show an increase in RNA content and hydrolytic and oxidative enzyme activity as they become taller. The mesenchymal cells continue to proliferate and surround the enamel organ. The part of the mesenchyme lying beneath the internal enamel epithelium is termed the dental papilla (D) while that surrounding the tooth germ forms the dental follicle (E). (*H&E,* ×75)

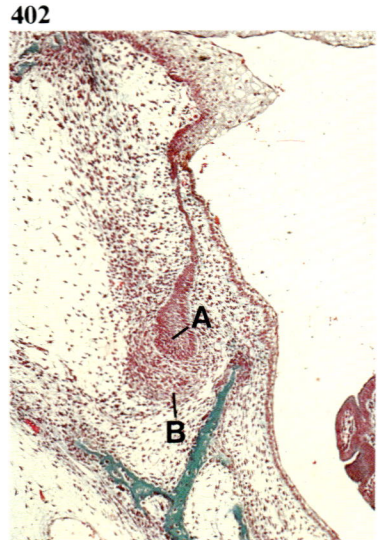
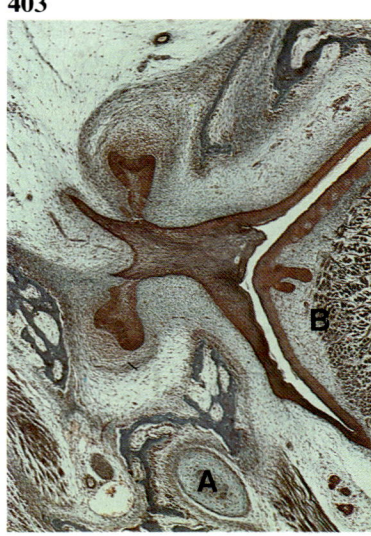
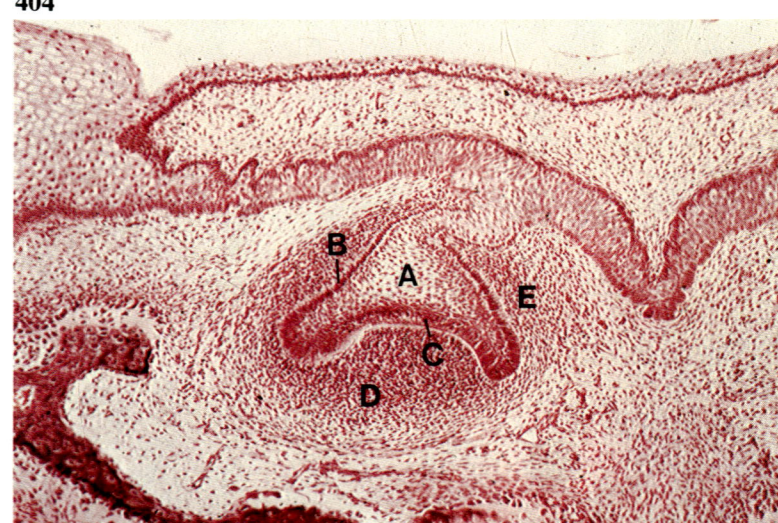

405 The arrangement of deciduous tooth germs at 13 weeks on the dental lamina of the lower jaw (model). The dental lamina is represented by the green, arch-shaped band on which the tooth germs (red structures) are aligned, five in each quadrant. At this time, most of the tooth germs are at the cap stage. The labelling identifies the developing deciduous teeth according to the Zsigmond system (page 18). V, vestibular fold.

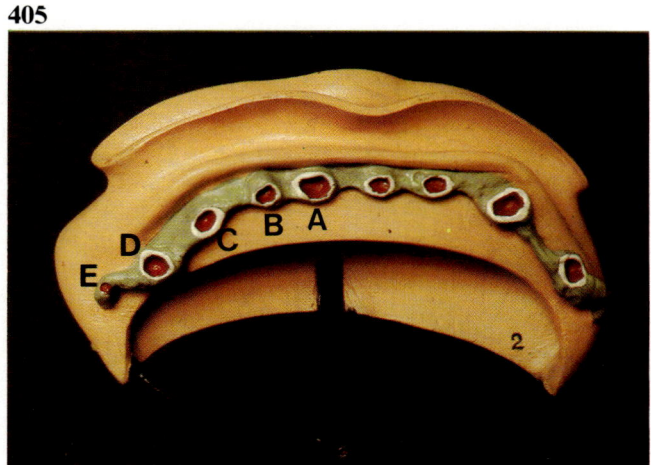

406 Bell stage. By the fourteenth week, further morphodifferentiation and histodifferentiation of the tooth germ leads to the bell stage. The configuration of the internal enamel epithelium broadly maps out the occlusal pattern of the tooth. This folding is related to differential mitosis along the internal enamel epithelium. The future cusps and incisal margins are sites of precocious cell maturation associated with cessation of mitosis, while areas corresponding to the fissures and margins of the tooth remain mitotically active. Thus, cusp height is related more to continued downward growth at the margins and fissures rather than to upward extension of cusps. Recent experiments suggest that, at this stage, the dental papilla and not the enamel organ is the morphogenetic 'organiser' for, should the dental papilla of a mouse molar be cultured with the enamel organ of a mouse incisor, the resulting chimera will be molariform. A rôle in morphogenesis has been attributed to the basement membrane which separates the dental papilla from the enamel organ. Should the collagenous basis of the membrane be disrupted using lathyritic agents, then morphogenesis of tooth germs cultured *in vitro* is severely disrupted.

During the bell stage of development, the enamel organ loses its connection with the oral epithelium as the dental lamina breaks down. At the same time the dental lamina between tooth germs also degenerates. Remnants of the dental lamina may remain as clumps of resting cells in the adult mucosa and may be involved in the aetiology of cysts.

Interposed between the enamel organ and the wall of the developing bony crypt is the mesenchymal tissue of the dental follicle which is generally considered to have three layers. The inner layer (A) is a vascular, fibrocellular condensation, three to four cells thick, immediately surrounding the tooth germ; the nuclei of the cells tend to be elongated circumferentially. Beyond this layer is the outer layer of the dental follicle (B), represented by a vascular mesenchymal layer which lines the developing alveolus. Between the two layers the intervening tissue is made up of loose connective tissue with no marked concentration of blood vessels. There is evidence to suggest that the cells of the inner layer of the dental follicle may be derived from cells of the neural crest. (*Masson's trichrome, × 40*)

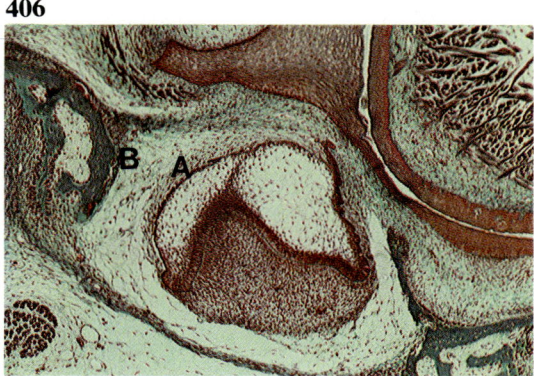

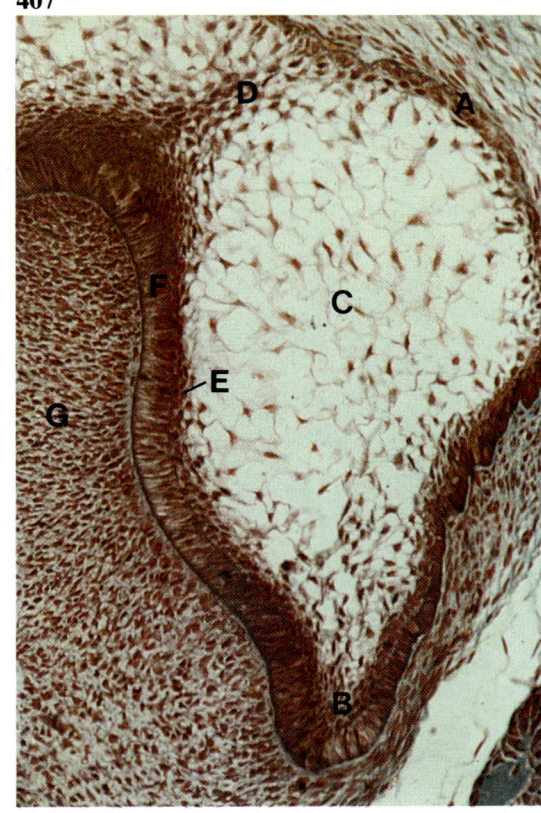

407 A high power view of the bell shows the high degree of histodifferentiation which has been achieved. The enamel organ shows four distinct layers:

1 The external enamel epithelium (A). As its name suggests, this forms the outer layer of cuboidal cells which limits the enamel organ. It is thought to be involved in the maintenance of shape of the enamel organ and in the exchange of substances between the enamel organ and the environment. Where the external enamel epithelium is continuous with the internal enamel epithelium lies the cervical loop (B) at which there is considerable mitotic activity.

2 Stellate reticulum (C). This tissue is most fully developed at the bell stage. The interstitial spaces become fluid-filled, presumably related to osmotic effects arising from the high concentration of glycosaminoglycans. The cells contain alkaline phosphatase but only small amounts of RNA and glycogen. Within the stellate reticulum can be seen a 'structure' termed the enamel cord (D) (see also figure **412**).

Two main functions have been ascribed to the stellate reticulum, mechanical and nutritive:

Mechanical. This relates to the protection of the underlying dental tissues against physical disturbance and the maintenance of tooth shape. It has been suggested that the hydrostatic pressure generated within the stellate reticulum is in equilibrium with that of the dental papilla, thus ensuring the integrity of the shape of the internal enamel epithelial layer during crown morphogenesis.

Nutritive. This relates to the utilisation of glycosaminoglycans during enamel formation.

3 Stratum intermedium (E). This layer makes its appearance at the bell stage and consists of two or three layers of flattened cells lying over the internal enamel epithelial cells and their derivatives. The cells of the stratum intermedium resemble those of the stellate reticulum, though the intercellular spaces are smaller. However, the alkaline phosphatase content of the stratum intermedium is considerably greater than that of the stellate reticulum and this feature is thought to be important during the development of enamel.

4 Internal enamel epithelium (F). The cells of this layer are columnar in shape. Beginning at the tips of the cusps (i.e. the sites of initial enamel formation), the cells become elongated. The cells of the internal enamel epithelium are rich in RNA but, unlike the stratum intermedium and stellate reticulum, do not contain alkaline phosphatase.

The differentiation of the dental papilla (G) is less striking than that of the enamel organ. Up until the late bell stage, the dental papilla consists of closely packed mesenchymal cells with only a few delicate extracellular fibrils. Histochemically, the dental papilla becomes rich in glycosaminoglycans. (*Masson's trichrome, ×120*)

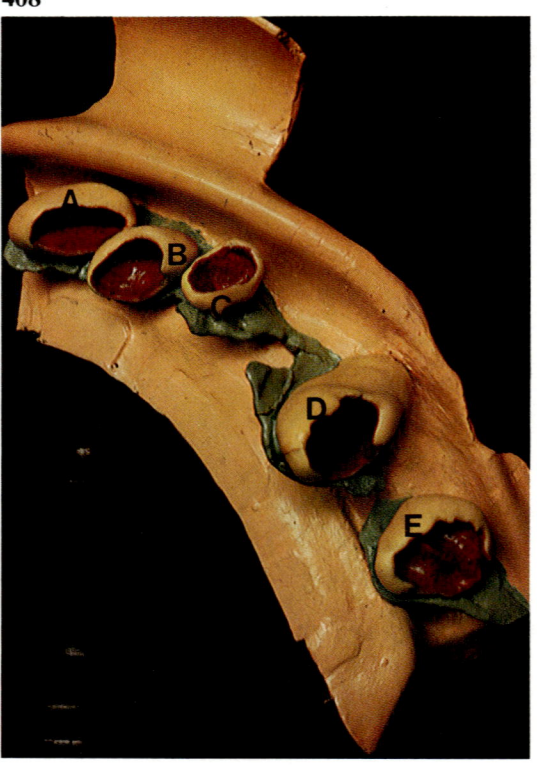

408 The arrangement of deciduous tooth germs at 17 weeks on the dental lamina of a lower jaw quadrant (model). The dental lamina is represented in green. Note the beginnings of its loss of continuity. The labelling identifies the developing deciduous teeth which are at the bell stage according to the Zsigmond system (page 18).

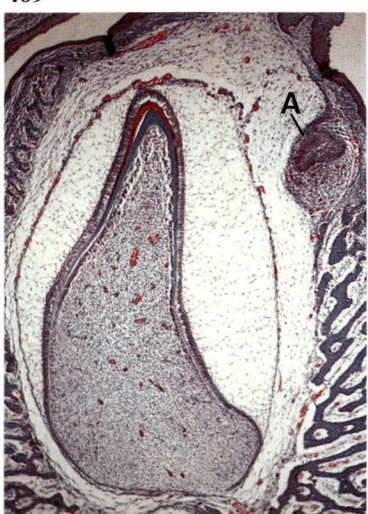

409 Late bell stage. This stage is associated with the formation of the dental hard tissues commencing at about the eighteenth week. Dentine formation always precedes enamel formation. Detailed accounts of dentinogenesis and amelogenesis are given on pages 164–7 and 158–63 respectively. In the section shown, developing enamel is stained red and dentine blue. Downgrowths of the remaining dental lamina appear on the lingual side of enamel organs. In deciduous teeth, these lingual downgrowths gives rise to the tooth germs of the permanent successors. In enamel organs of permanent teeth, however, these downgrowths eventually disappear. In this section, the permanent tooth (A) has reached the bud stage of development. (*Masson's blue trichrome, ×40*)

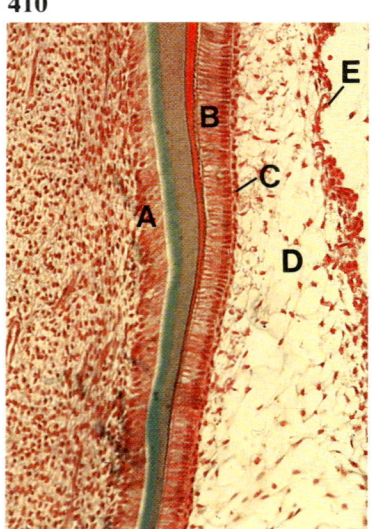

410 High power view of region showing enamel and dentine formation. Under the inductive influence of developing ameloblasts the adjacent mesenchymal cells of the dental papilla become columnar and differentiate into odontoblasts (A). The odontoblasts then become involved in the formation of dentine. In this decalcified section, the matrix of the calcified dentine is stained pale green while the uncalcified predentine nearer the odontoblasts is a darker green. The presence of dentine induces the ameloblasts (B) to secrete enamel. The developing enamel is stained red. C, stratum intermedium. D, stellate reticulum. E, external enamel epithelium. (*Masson's trichrome, ×100*)

During the early stages of tooth development, three transitory structures may be seen: the enamel knot, enamel niche and enamel cord.

411 The enamel knot (A) is a localised mass of cells produced by a rapid multiplication of cells in the centre of the internal enamel epithelium. Characteristically, the enamel knot forms a bulge into the dental papilla at the centre of the tooth germ. It was once thought that the enamel knot played a role in the formation of crown pattern by outlining the central fissure. This has not been substantiated and its role is unknown, though the enamel knot appears to contribute cells to the enamel cord. (*H&E, ×120*)

412 The enamel cord (A) is a strand of cells seen in the bell stage of development which extends from the stratum intermedium into the stellate reticulum generally reaching the external enamel epithelium. Where present, the enamel cord overlies the incisal margin of a tooth or the apex of the first cusp to develop (primary cusp). When it completely divides the stellate reticulum into two, it is termed the enamel septum. Where the enamel cord meets the external enamel epithelium a small invagination termed the enamel navel (B) may be seen. The cells of the enamel cord are distinguished from the surrounding stellate reticulum cells by their elongated nuclei. It has been suggested that the enamel cord may be involved in the process by which the cap stage is transformed into the bell stage, acting as a mechanical tie and/or that it is a focus for the origin of stellate reticulum cells. (*Masson's trichrome, ×120*)

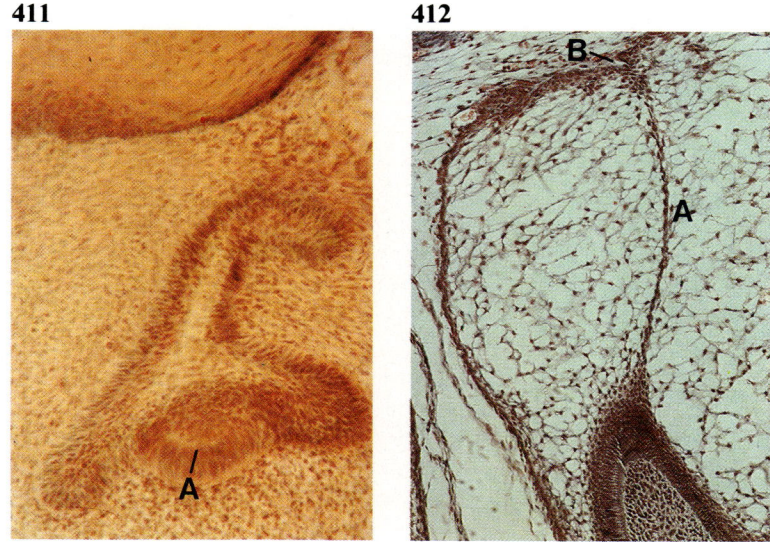

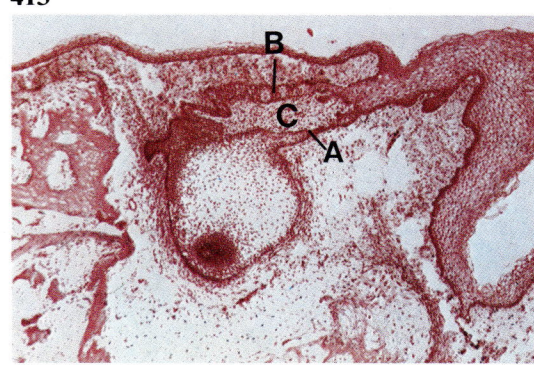

413 Enamel niche. The tooth germ may appear to have a double attachment to the dental lamina, the lateral (A) and medial (B) enamel strands. These strands enclose a funnel-shaped depression containing connective tissue which is termed the enamel niche (C). Its significance is unknown. (*H&E, ×40*)

The enamel cord and the double attachment of the tooth germ were once regarded as evidence supporting the view that the complex crown form of mammalian teeth evolved from fusion of a number of individual, simpler elements though this view is not now generally accepted.

Amelogenesis

The development of enamel begins at the late bell stage shortly after dentinogenesis has commenced. As in the formation of other hard tissues, amelogenesis involves the synthesis and secretion of an organic matrix and its subsequent mineralisation with hydroxyapatite crystals. Unlike other hard tissues, however, the cells responsible for the secretion and organisation of the organic matrix of enamel, the ameloblasts, are ectodermally derived and the matrix is not collagenous but is protein unique to enamel. Furthermore, much of the organic matrix is removed from the tissue during its maturation phase.

At the early bell stage of tooth development, before dentine or enamel are secreted, the internal enamel epithelium forms a layer of low, columnar cells whose nuclei are not uniformly arranged and which may show mitotic figures (see figure **407**).

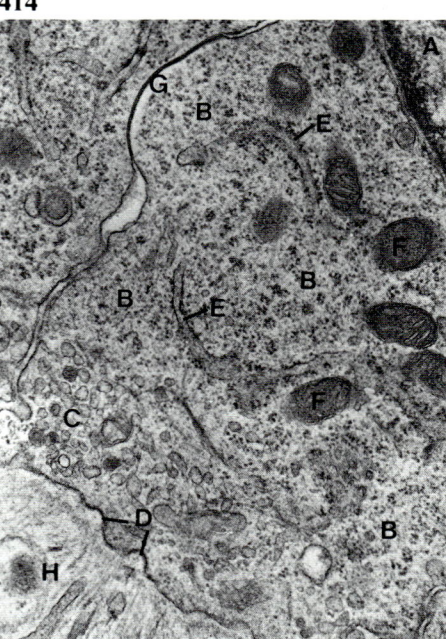

414 The distal cytoplasm of an early differentiating ameloblast. Internal enamel epithelial cells and early differentiating ameloblasts possess a large ovoid nucleus (A) and a small Golgi complex which lies in the basal end of the cell adjacent to the stratum intermedium. In the distal cytoplasm neighbouring the dental papilla, there are a few organised membranous structures but large numbers of free ribosomes (B). Numerous vesicles (C) are present and the surface membrane shows invaginations (D) typical of pinocytosis. E, rough endoplasmic reticulum. F, mitochondria. G, gap junction. H, dental papilla. The differentiating ameloblasts induce the adjacent mesenchymal cells of the dental papilla to differentiate into odontoblasts. (*Electron micrograph, × 21,000*)

Differentiation of ameloblasts follows an orderly sequence of changes which results in the formation of a highly developed, secretory cell. The cells become columnar, the cell height increasing to about 40μm. Directional guidance for the elongation of the cells is thought to be associated with the development in the distal cytoplasm of large numbers of microtubules orientated parallel to the long axis of the cell. The nuclei of the differentiating ameloblasts become uniformly located at the basal region of the cell. The Golgi complex migrates from its former position at the basal end of the cell to lie in the distal half (reversal of polarity) where there is an increasing amount of free ribosomes and smooth and rough endoplasmic reticulum. Mitochondria mainly occupy the basal end of the cell.

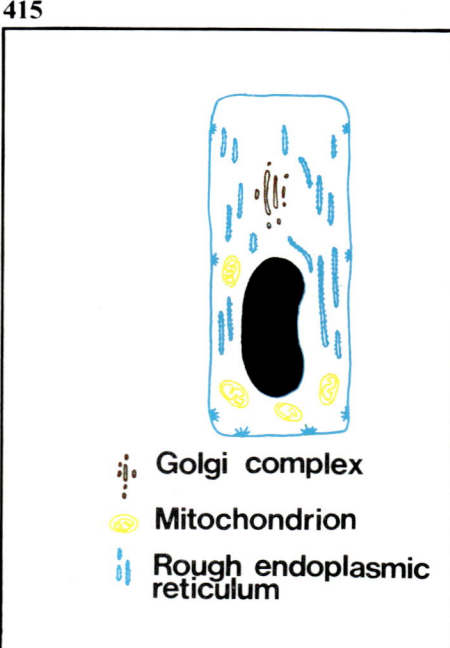

415 Diagram of a newly-differentiated ameloblast.

Initially a basal lamina separates the early ameloblasts from the differentiating odontoblasts. It is only after this basal lamina is disrupted that calcification of predentine occurs and amelogenesis begins. The onset of amelogenesis is thought to be under the inductive influence of the first formed dentine.

416 The distal ends of early secretory ameloblasts. Immediately prior to the onset of amelogenesis there is a marked aggregation of vesicles, some containing stippled material, at the distal end of the ameloblast. A, secretory vesicles. The material contained within the vesicles is thought to be the organic matrix of enamel. By reverse pinocytosis, the contents of the vesicles are discharged into the extracellular space. Enamel matrix (B) can be seen in this section between adjacent ameloblasts. As the enamel matrix is secreted the ameloblasts are pushed outwards away from the dentine surface (C). A distinct zone of uncalcified organic matrix, corresponding to osteoid of bone and predentine of dentine, is rarely seen since hydroxyapatite crystals begin to form when the enamel matrix is only about 50nm thick. In the illustration, the early calcified enamel (D) shows thin, needle-like hydroxyapatite crystals. Recent evidence suggests that the initial foci for enamel crystals may be crystallites in the adjacent mantle dentine. Note that at this early stage of amelogenesis, the distal ends of the ameloblasts form a relatively flat surface and that no prismatic structure can be discerned in the developing enamel. (*Electron micrograph, × 11,200*)

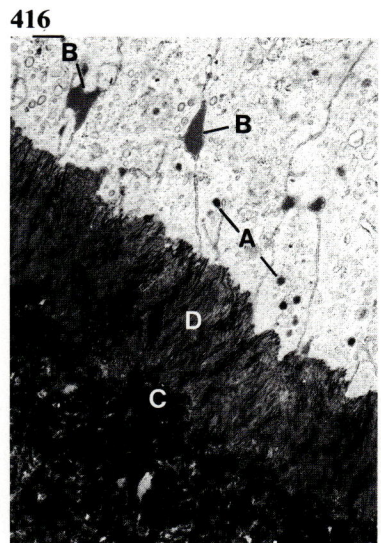

417 Part of a secretory ameloblast showing two large, dense vesicles or secretory granules (A). The stippled material within the vesicles is thought to be the future organic matrix of enamel. B, rough endoplasmic reticulum. C, Golgi vesicles. D, Golgi units. (*Electron micrograph, × 30,500*)

418 Decalcified, longitudinal section through a tooth germ during the initial stages of amelogenesis and dentinogenesis.
A Ameloblasts.
B Odontoblasts.
C Developing enamel.
D Developing dentine.
E Stratum intermedium.
F Stellate reticulum.

The cells of the stratum intermedium and stellate reticulum are believed to play a role in enamel formation. Ameloblasts are rich in RNA and have a high oxidative enzyme activity. However, they lack the enzyme alkaline phosphatase which is present in large amounts in the cells of the stratum intermedium. It has been suggested that the stratum intermedium may be concerned with the synthesis of proteins, with the transport of materials to and from the ameloblast or with the concentration of materials. The stellate reticulum is rich in glycosaminoglycans, a substance which may be utilised during amelogenesis. (*Masson's trichrome, × 100*)

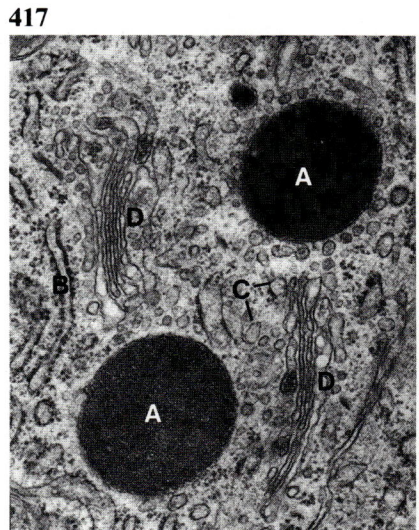

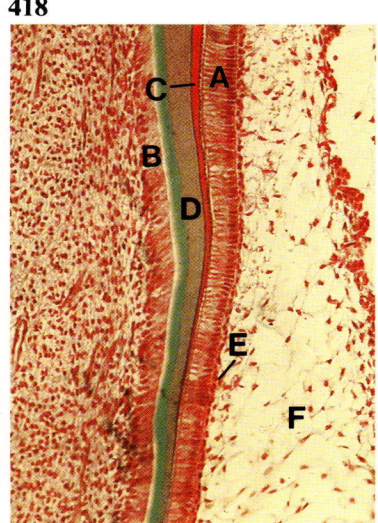

After the initial stages of amelogenesis, the secretory end of the ameloblast becomes conical in shape forming the so-called Tomes' process.

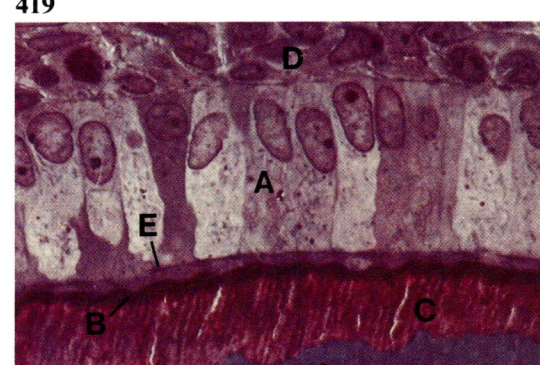

419 Decalcified, longitudinal section through developing enamel showing the cone-shaped Tomes' process at the distal end of each ameloblast.
A Ameloblasts.
B Enamel matrix.
C Dentine.
D Stratum intermedium.

Note that in this section, taken from a developing human tooth, Tomes' processes are present after only a small amount of enamel has been laid down. The Tomes' processes are demarcated at their bases by junctional complexes. The alignment of these complexes gives the appearance of a terminal bar (E) running through the ameloblast layer. At the electron microscope level, the terminal bars appear as desmosomes with associated tonofilaments. The tonofilaments pass only a short distance into the cell to form an incomplete septum between the Tomes' process and the rest of the ameloblast. A similar terminal bar apparatus is found at the basal end of the ameloblast. Other desmosomes and tight junctional complexes may be discerned at a variety of sites linking adjacent ameloblasts. (*Toluidine blue, ×1,000*)

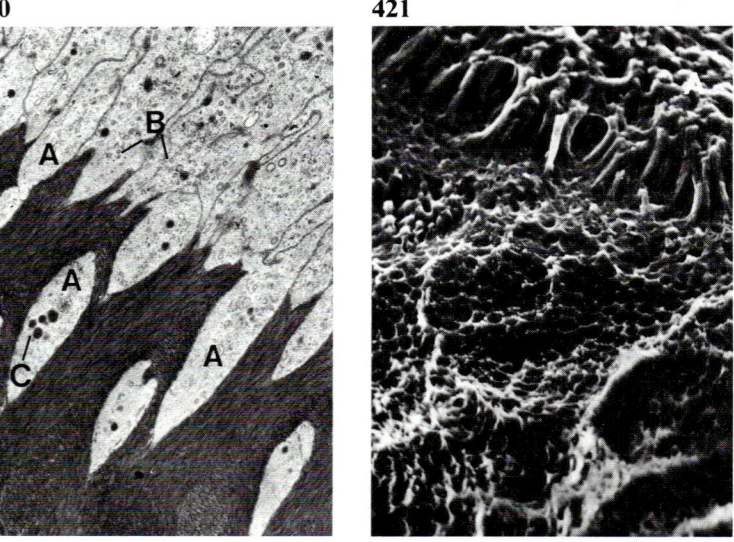

420 Advanced secretory ameloblasts showing Tomes' processes (A). B, vesicles. C, secretory granules. (*Electron micrograph, ×10,000*)

421 Pits in the developing enamel surface each of which was occupied by a Tomes' process. Some of the ameloblasts (A) have been retained. (*Scanning electron micrograph, ×500*)

It has been suggested that the presence of prisms is related to the configuration of the Tomes' processes.

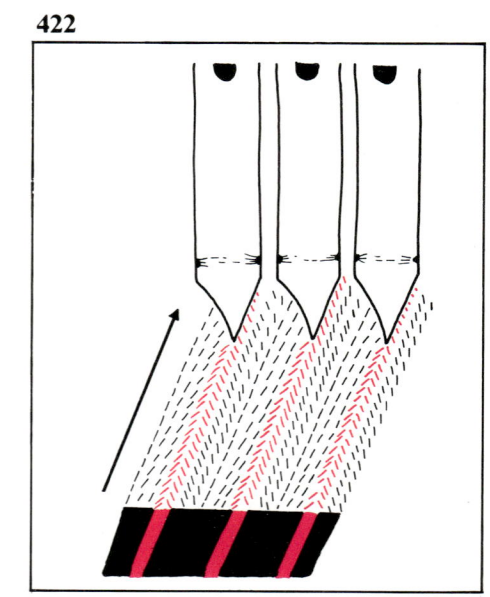

422 The relationship between crystallite orientation, the shape of the mineralising front and the direction of movement of ameloblasts. Note that the crystals are aligned with their long axes approximately perpendicular to the surface of the Tomes' process. Thus, the wedge-shaped appearance of the Tomes' process will produce abrupt changes in crystallite orientation and this, as previously shown (see page 82), may explain the appearance in light microscopy of the prism core and prism boundaries. It would seem, therefore, that more than one ameloblast contributes to the formation of a single prism and that each ameloblast is involved in the development of more than one prism.

The orientation of crystallites is possibly related to the tendency of crystallites to be orientated perpendicular to the mineralising front. Growth of apatite crystals is rapid along their C-axes and since the source of essential ions is the Tomes' process, it is possible that crystals will grow preferentially along the concentration gradient. It is assumed that once formed, the crystallites continue to grow in the same direction. An additional 'stroking' orientating factor may occur in regions where there is a relative sliding movement between the ameloblast cell (Tomes' process) surface and the mineralising front, the crystallites being orientated slightly in the direction of this movement.

Other views suggest that the orientation of crystallites is related to flow patterns set up by shearing forces within the enamel matrix as the ameloblast retreats at an angle from the developing enamel front, or to the directional influence of microvilli at the surface of the Tomes' process.

Amelogenesis is a rhythmic process, periods of activity alternating with periods of quiescence. This rhythmic activity is reflected in the presence of two incremental markings, the cross-striations (figure **176**) and the striae of Retzius (figure **179**). Hunter-Schreger bands (figure **172**) result from optical interference produced by alternating planes of prisms, but the migratory activity of the ameloblasts required to produce these alternating planes has not been fully explained, to date.

It is generally accepted that enamel formation occurs in two main phases. During the first phase the full thickness of enamel matrix is laid down. This matrix is only partially mineralised, having a mineral content of 25 to 30 per cent by weight. The second phase, termed maturation, involves the final mineralisation of the enamel. Maturation not only involves a rapid increase in the rate of mineralisation, but also changes in the quality and quantity of the organic matrix. Though there are a number of difficulties in the analysis of the composition of young enamel matrix during the first phase of amelogenesis, it seems that its constituent proteins have a unique amino-acid composition, possessing an unusually high content of proline, a low content of cysteine, and a histidine, lysine and arginine ratio, of 3:1:1. The protein is not fibrous but is in the form of an amorphous gel.

During maturation there is a withdrawal of water and a selective withdrawal of protein. The protein withdrawn differs in composition from that which remains. Thus the amino-acid composition of mature enamel differs from that of 'young' enamel, containing relatively more glycine and less histidine and proline. In addition, the removal of matrix which occurs when the crystallites are expanding from their early dimensions of 1.5nm thick to their mature thickness of 25nm may be aided by the thixotropic properties of the matrix i.e. its ability to flow under pressure. Its thixotropic properties may also explain the selective withdrawal of protein, the more thixotropic proteins being removed more easily. An alternative but more unlikely explanation for the degradation of the enamel matrix involves the extracellular secretion of hydrolytic enzymes. The resorption of material may not just be confined to the later maturation stages of development. Indeed, morphological differences between the cuspal and cervical surfaces of the Tomes' processes has been used as evidence in favour of the view that one surface may primarily be concerned with absorptive activity, while the other surface may be concerned with secretion. Thus, the ameloblast may simultaneously be capable of secreting and resorbing.

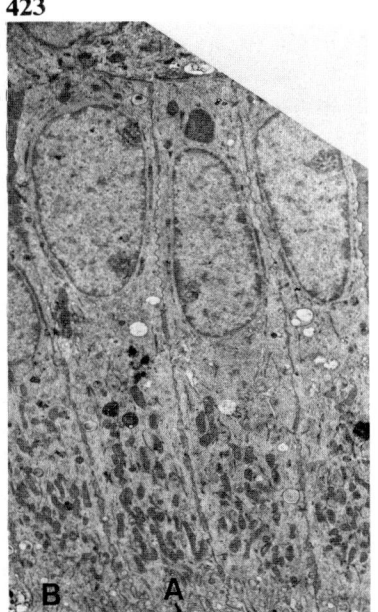

423 A decalcified section showing ameloblasts at the early maturation stage (A, enamel space). Compared with the ameloblast during its secretory phase, the cell shortens and loses its Tomes' process to be replaced by a striated border (B) consisting of an infolded cell membrane. Mitochondria, though scattered throughout the cell, are arranged in two major clusters, one at the basal end of the cell, the other at the distal end near the striated border. There is a great reduction in the amount of rough endoplasmic reticulum. Associated with the loss of Tomes' processes, the surface layer of enamel may be prism free (figure **175**). (*Electron micrograph,* × 2,700)

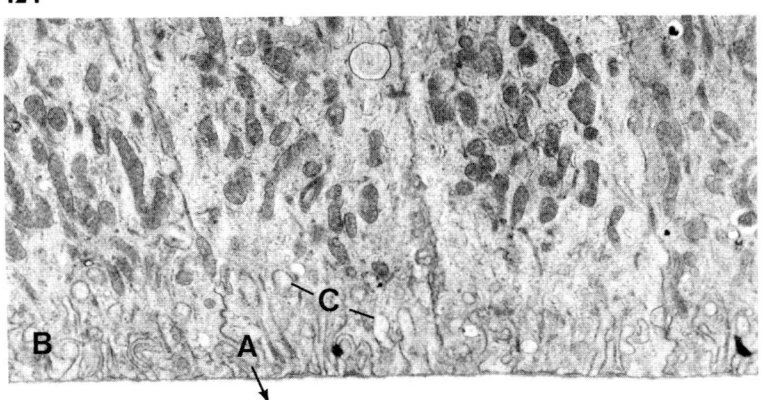

424 High power view of figure 423 showing striated border (B). A, enamel space. In undemineralised material, the projections from the distal end of the cell are separated from the mineralised mass of the enamel by a narrow interval containing dense, finely granular material. It is assumed that such material is being absorbed into the ameloblast within absorption granules (C). Within the cell there is increased acid phosphatase and amino-peptidase activity. (*Electron micrograph,* × 6,700)

During late maturation, a striated border is no longer present, the distal cell membrane lying parallel to the enamel surface. Absorption granules are no longer present but large numbers of mitochondria are distributed throughout the cytoplasm. Filaments are also found.

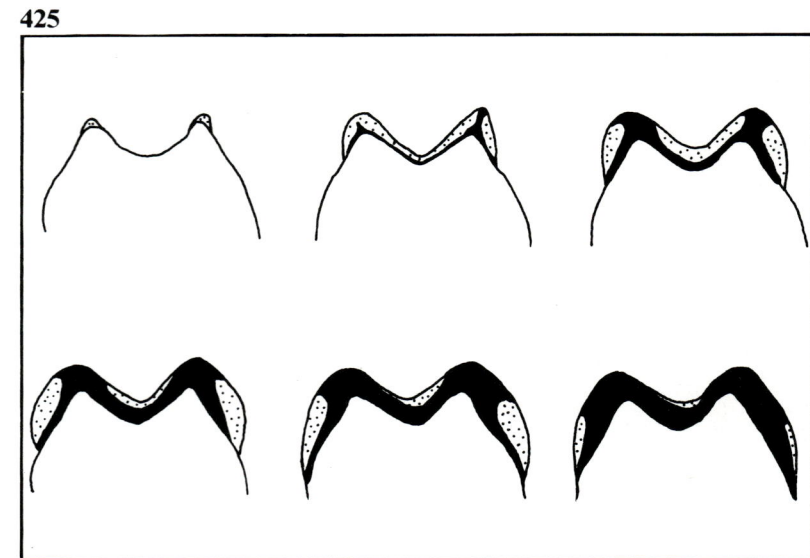

425 Pattern of mineralisation in a molar tooth during maturation Stippled zones represent partially mineralised matrix. The dark shaded areas indicate the advance of the final mineralisation from the amelodentinal junction to the tip of the cusps and then throughout the remaining enamel towards the cervix. Thus, the occlusal (and incisal) regions reach maturity ahead of the cervical regions.

At the end of amelogenesis, the ameloblasts become almost indistinguishable from the outer cells of the enamel organ, their nuclei being frequently crenulated. At this stage, they become part of the reduced enamel epithelium.

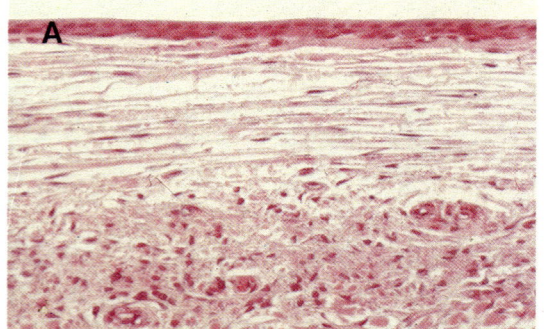

426 Decalcified section of the reduced enamel epithelium (A). (*H&E, × 160*)

The cells of the reduced enamel epithelium appear to be separated from the enamel surface by an amorphous layer, approximately 1μm thick, the primary enamel cuticle. Although this cuticle is considered by some to be the last product of the ameloblast, it may also represent enamel matrix which has been extruded from enamel during maturation. For further details of the reduced enamel epithelium and the enamel cuticle see pages 89–91 and 173.

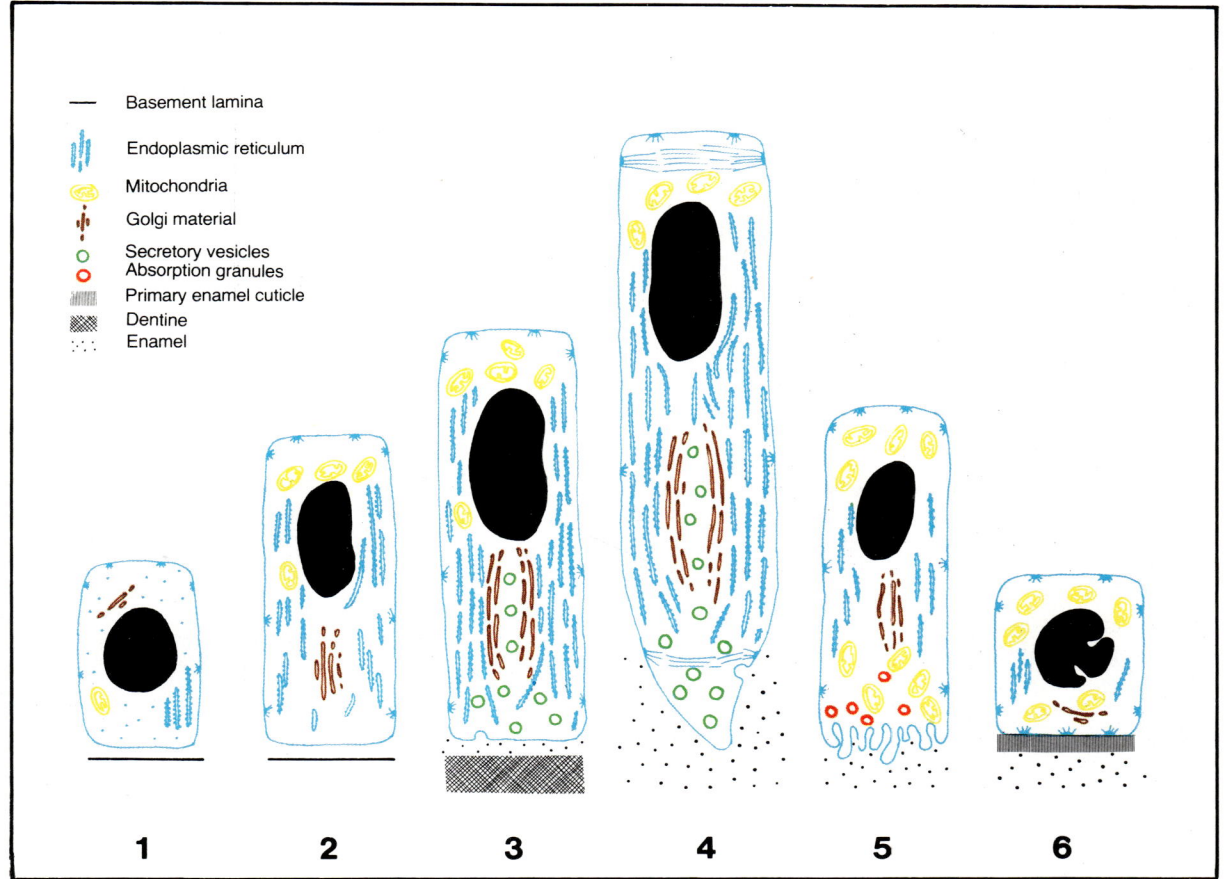

427 Diagram summarising the morphological and cytological changes in the ameloblast during its life cycle.
1 Internal enamel epithelial cell.
2 Newly differentiated ameloblast prior to the secretion of enamel.
3 Early secreting ameloblast before the appearance of a Tomes' process.
4 Secreting ameloblast with a Tomes' process.
5 Early maturing ameloblast with a striated border.
6 Reduced enamel epithelial cell with hemidesmosomes. A primary enamel cuticle separates the cell from the enamel surface.

The development of circumpulpal dentine differs from mantle dentine in the following respects:
1 The matrix of circumpulpal dentine is synthesised principally by odontoblasts while that of mantle dentine is formed at least in part by subodontoblastic cells.
2 The collagen fibres of circumpulpal dentine are preferentially orientated parallel to the amelodentinal junction while those of mantle dentine lie perpendicular to the amelodentinal junction.
3 Mineralisation of circumpulpal dentine appears to proceed in the absence of matrix vesicles, probably by growth from pre-existing calcification centres.

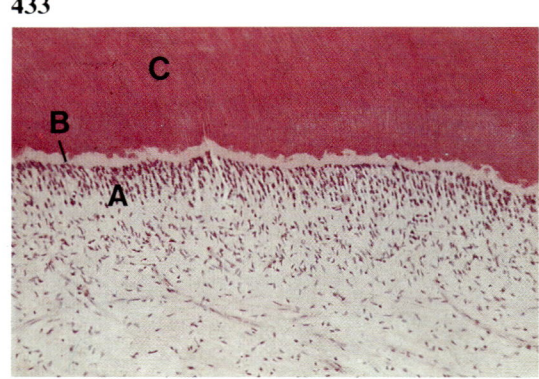

433 Decalcified section through developing circumpulpal dentine. During the formation of circumpulpal dentine the odontoblasts mature, becoming larger and containing more intracytoplasmic organelles. As they migrate pulpwards they become crowded, giving the appearance of a pseudo-stratified layer of columnar odontoblasts (A) several cells deep (see also figure **251**). Matrix is deposited around the processes of the retreating odontoblasts, thereby defining the dentinal tubules. The matrix, consisting of collagen fibres embedded in a gel presumably secreted by the odontoblast, is only mineralised after a certain thickness has been laid down. Thus, a layer of unmineralised matrix, the predentine (B), is always present between the odontoblasts and the mineralised part of the dentine (C). The irregular boundary between the matrix of the mineralised circumpulpal dentine and the predentine results from the shape of calcospherites. At the mineralising front above the predentine, complex, little-understood reactions take place involving the glycosaminoglycans of the ground substance. (*H&E, ×80*)

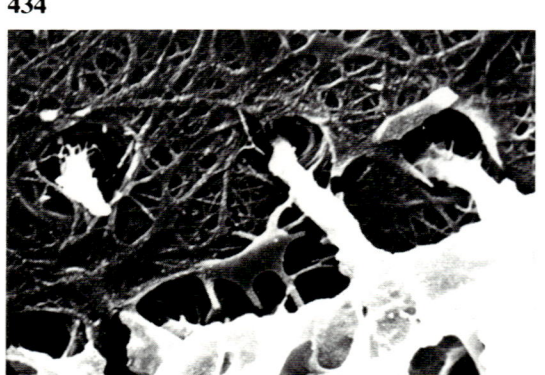
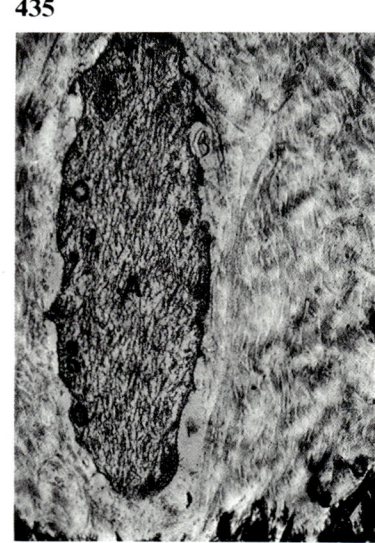

434 Predentine surface in circumpulpal dentine showing arrangement of collagen fibres. In circumpulpal dentine, von Korff type fibres are either much rarer than in mantle dentine or are absent. The collagen fibres, as previously indicated, are arranged as a network with the majority lying parallel with the forming front, perpendicular to the tubules. Odontoblast processes are seen entering the dentinal tubules. (*Scanning electron micrograph, ×2,700*)

435 Predentine, showing collagen fibres arranged as a network around an odontoblast process (A). (*Electron micrograph, ×15,000*)

Mineralisation of circumpulpal dentine occurs either along an advancing linear front and/or by the fusion of discrete globules of calcified material, the calcospherites.

436 Circumpulpal predentine showing calcospherites (*arrowed*). The crystals within the calcospherites are arranged radially. The calcospherites grow by the addition of calcified material to their outer surfaces until they contact and fuse with each other. Where fusion does not occur, hypomineralised interglobular areas may remain (see page 100). (*Electron micrograph*, × 1,450)

437 Calcospherites. The predentine surface has been cleared of organic debris with sodium hypochlorite solution to show the calcospherites. Note the tubules running through the calcospherites. (*Scanning electron micrograph*, × 500)

438 The calcospheritic pattern of mineralisation. This is a longitudinal, ground section of dentine viewed in polarised light. Spherical outlines can be seen in the circumpulpal dentine representing junctional zones between calcospherites. These are seen in polarised light because of differences in orientation of both the collagen and mineral. The mantle zone (A) in this section appears black. (× 25)

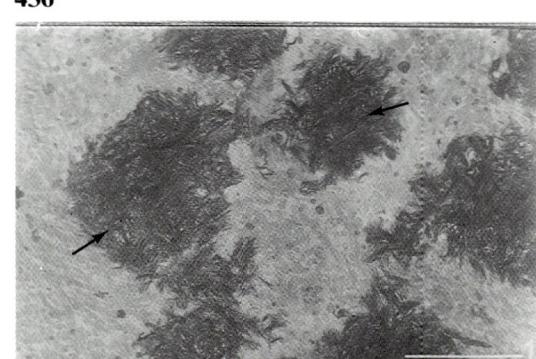
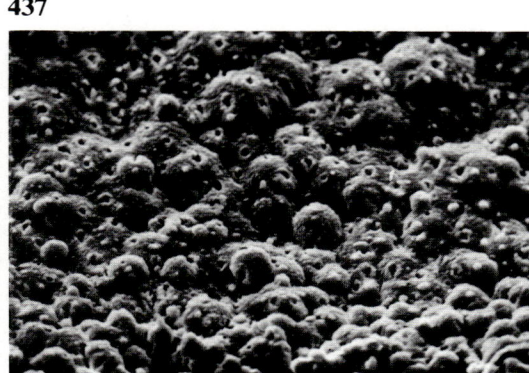
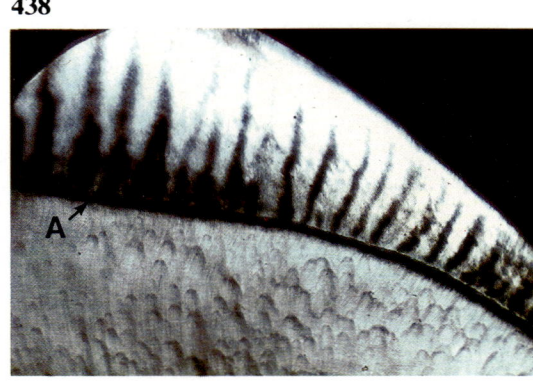

Dentinogenesis is a rhythmic process which proceeds with alternating periods of activity and quiescence. The periods of inactivity or decreased activity are associated with incremental lines. Some of these structural markings are associated with the deposition of the matrix, others with its mineralisation (see pages 99–100).

The bulk of the root dentine is of the circumpulpal variety; its formation differs little from that in the crown. The odontoblasts which form the root dentine are induced to differentiate by the internal enamel epithelial cells of the root sheath (see pages 169–70). The formation of the outer granular and hyaline layers is poorly understood. There is some evidence that the hyaline layer, which contains few tubules, mineralises centrifugally unlike circumpulpal dentine which mineralises centripetally.

Dentine formation does not cease once the primary dentine has been fully formed, regular secondary dentine (pages 100–101) and peritubular dentine (pages 93–94) being deposited throughout the life of the tooth.

Development of the pulp

As the superficial cells of the dental papilla differentiate into odontoblasts and begin to deposit dentine, the central region of the dental papilla begins to differentiate into pulp tissue. The cells of the papilla, initially small and undifferentiated, become more widely dispersed and the great majority develop into active fibroblasts. Their cytoplasm increases and organelles associated with protein synthesis and secretion become more abundant. The fibroblasts secrete collagen into the extracellular space throughout development of the tooth. In the young pulp, the collagen is dispersed evenly in the form of fine fibre bundles. Coarse fibre bundles only appear at about the time the tooth reaches maturity. In the adult tooth, there is a tendency for the collagen in the pulp to become increasingly concentrated with age. Glycosaminoglycans increase in amount until the time of eruption and then decrease.

At the time of eruption a cell-rich zone becomes apparent underneath the odontoblast layer. The formation of this zone appears to be accomplished by cell migration. The mature pulp contains macrophages, pericytes and lymphoid cells in addition to fibroblasts. These probably enter the pulp with the invading blood vessels, though the defence cell population of the developing tooth has not been adequately studied.

Vascularisation of the developing pulp starts during the bell stage.

439 The vascular pattern within the dental papilla at the late bell stage of development. To highlight the vasculature, Indian ink has been introduced into the vascular system. Note that as the developing central pulp vessels reach the future cusp regions, they give off numerous small branches which form a plexus of venules, arterioles and capillaries. (*H&E*, ×40)

440 The vascular plexuses in the region of the developing cusp. Beneath the odontoblast layer (A) lies the subodontoblastic plexus (B) from which vessels pass between the odontoblast cells to form an odontoblastic vascular plexus. The vascularity around the odontoblast layer increases as dentine is progressively laid down, probably as the result of the odontoblasts retreating inwards through the vascular bed. Eventually, some capillaries are found immediately next to the predentine surface. (×100)

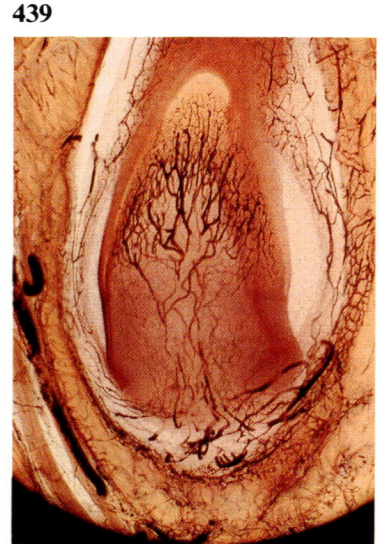
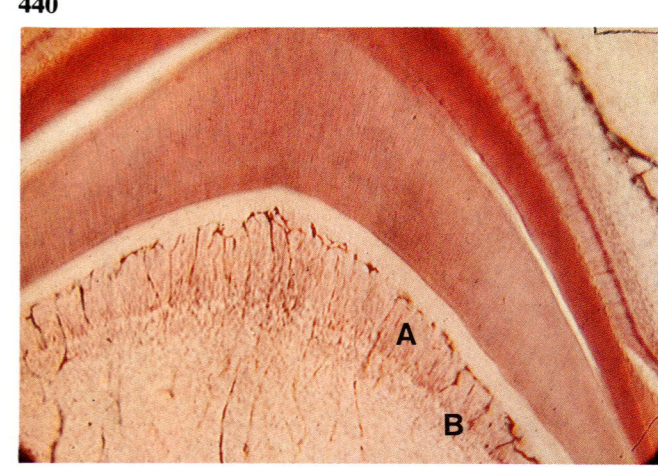

The first nerve fibres to enter the pulp accompany the blood vessels. They are non-myelinated and are presumed to be autonomic. Much later, when root formation is well advanced, sensory branches grow out from the dental nerves supplying the jaws and enter the root canals as pulpal nerves. These course towards the cuspal regions and give off branches to the subodontoblastic region. The plexus of Raschkow is not fully established until root formation is nearly complete. With the formation of dentine and the retreat of odontoblasts, some nerve fibres become trapped in predentine or dentine.

Development of the root and periodontal ligament

Root development proceeds some time after the crown has formed and involves interactions between the dental follicle, the apical tissues of the enamel organ (epithelial root sheath of Hertwig) and the dental papilla. The onset of root development coincides with the onset of the axial phase of tooth eruption.

441 Longitudinal, decalcified section through a developing root. At the late bell stage when amelogenesis and dentinogenesis are well advanced, the external and internal enamel epithelia at the cervical edge of the enamel organ form a double-layered epithelial root sheath (A) which is said to proliferate apically to map out the shape of the future root (though studies indicate that it shows little mitotic activity). Growth of the epithelial root sheath occurs to enclose the dental papilla (B) except for an opening at the base, the primary apical foramen (C). Beneath the dental papilla, the epithelial sheath usually appears angled to form the root diaphragm. Note that between the two epithelial layers there is no stellate reticulum or stratum intermedium. The dental follicle (D) lies external to the root sheath and forms cementum, periodontal ligament and part of the alveolar bone. E, developing root dentine. F, odontoblast layer. (H&E, ×32)

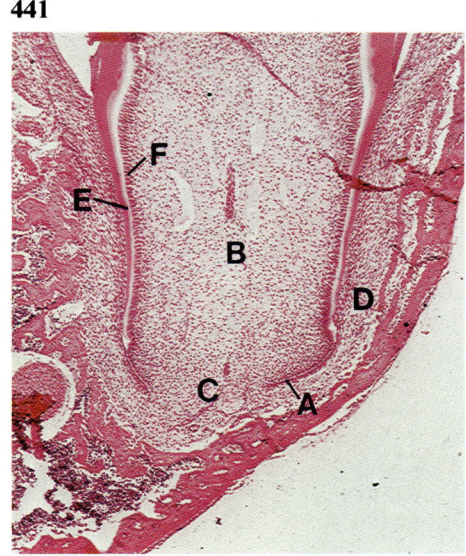

442 The configuration of the epithelial root sheath in the formation of a single-rooted tooth (A), a two-rooted tooth (B) and a three-rooted tooth (C). Root morphogenesis is associated with the dynamic activity of the epithelial root sheath, though it may be under the inductive control of the dental papilla. The primary apical foramen subdivides into a number of secondary apical foraminae by the ingrowth of epithelial shelves from the margins of the root sheath which subsequently fuse near the centre of the root. The number and location of these epithelial shelves correspond to the number and location of the definitive roots of the tooth. It has been suggested that the ingrowth of the epithelial shelves takes place along paths of low vascularity.

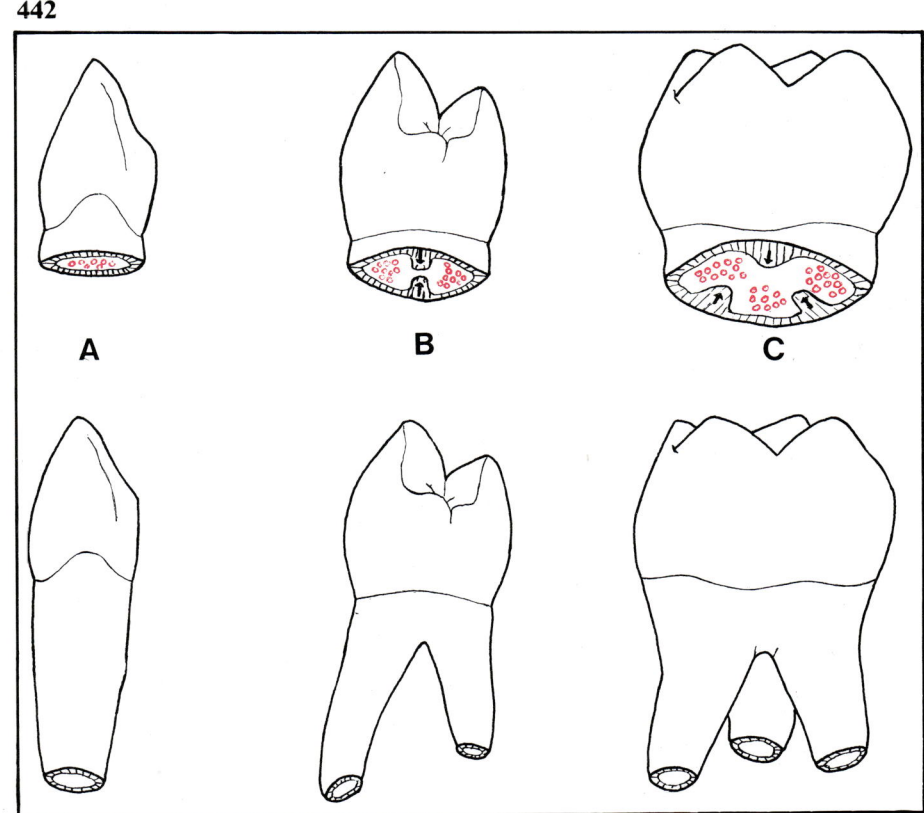

443 Further development of the root illustrated by a schematic drawing of the apical region of the epithelial root sheath. In the region of the root diaphragm, the epithelial root sheath (A) is a continuous sheet of tissue sandwiched between the undifferentiated mesenchyme of the dental papilla (B) and dental follicle (C). Above the root diaphragm, towards the developing crown, the cells of the internal layer of the epithelial sheath induce the peripheral cells of the dental papilla to differentiate into odontoblasts (D). Following the onset of dentinogenesis in the root, the epithelial cells of the root sheath lose their continuity, becoming separated from the surface of the developing root dentine to form epithelial rests (E) in the developing periodontal ligament (see figure 304). The mesenchymal cells of the dental follicle adjacent to the root dentine now differentiate into cementoblasts (F) and cementogenesis commences. In the diagram, G represents developing alveolar bone, H, developing cementum and J, developing periodontal ligament. K, root dentine.

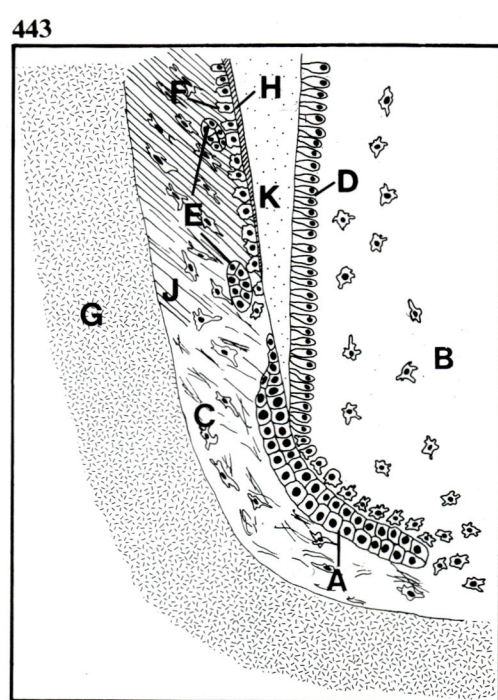

444 Longitudinal, decalcified section through the apical region of the developing root, periodontal ligament and alveolus.
A Epithelial root sheath.
B Dental papilla.
C Odontoblasts.
D Dentine of root.
E Predentine layer.
F Cementoblasts.
G Developing cementum.
H Developing alveolar bone.

At this stage the tissues of the dental follicle at the developing root apex can be subdivided into three layers. Adjacent to the epithelial root sheath is the inner layer (I) of the dental follicle which is said to be derived from the neural crest. Adjacent to the developing alveolar bone is the outer layer (J) of the dental follicle which is separated from the inner layer by an intermediate layer (K). Unlike the tissues of the inner layer, the outer and intermediate layers are thought to be mesodermal in origin; their cells contain few cytoplasmic organelles and the extracellular compartment appears relatively structureless. Cells of the inner layer of the dental follicle differentiate into the cementoblasts which form a layer of cuboidal cells on the surface of the root dentine. The cementoblasts secrete an organic matrix of collagen and ground substance which eventually calcifies to form cementum. Once cementogenesis has begun some of the cells of the remaining dental follicle become obliquely orientated along the root surface (*arrowed*) and show an increased content of intracellular organelles, becoming the fibroblasts of the periodontal ligament. These fibroblasts secrete collagen into the extracellular compartment. (*H&E, × 150*)

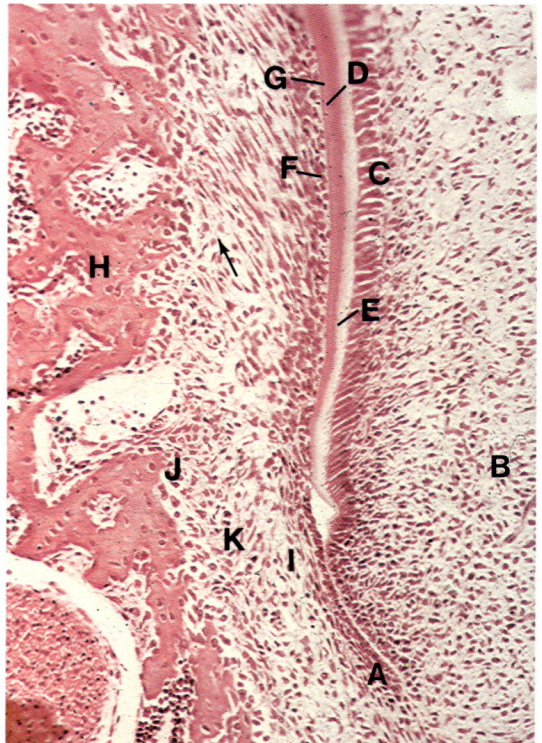

445 Decalcified, longitudinal section through a developing root apex to show the pulp-limiting membrane. The loose proliferative connective tissue of the dental follicle passes beneath the growing root apex to form a pulp-limiting membrane (*arrowed*). This structure has erroneously been described as being attached at its margins to the walls of the bony alveolar crypt, forming the so-called 'cushioned hammock ligament'. This ligament was thought to play a role in the process of tooth eruption. (*Mallory's trichrome, × 30*)

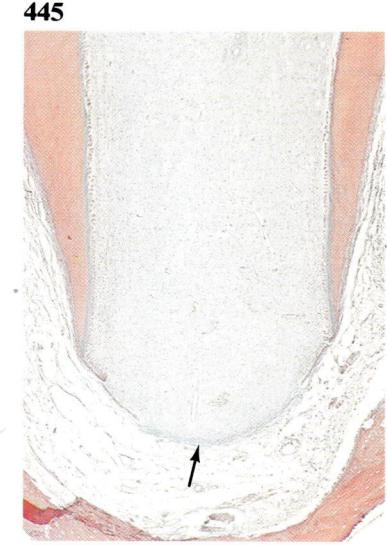

An indication of the important rôle played by the inner layer of the dental follicle in the formation of the periodontal ligament can be deduced from experiments in which developing tooth germs, surrounded only by the inner layer of the dental follicle, are removed from the jaws and transplanted to other sites. Such tooth germs continue developing to produce a root, periodontal ligament and alveolar bone. Using techniques for labelling the transplanted cells, it can be shown that the inner layer of cells of the dental follicle give rise to cementoblasts, periodontal ligament fibroblasts and osteoblasts forming alveolar bone. The periodontal ligament of such transplants has well organised principal fibre groups, which may suggest preadaptation to function. Despite these findings, however, contributions from the outer layer of the dental follicle to the periodontal ligament and alveolar bone in the normal developmental situation cannot be precluded.

The mechanisms responsible for the orientation of the principal fibres of the periodontal ligament are unknown, though it has been suggested that they may be arranged along lines of stress set up at the growing end of the root.

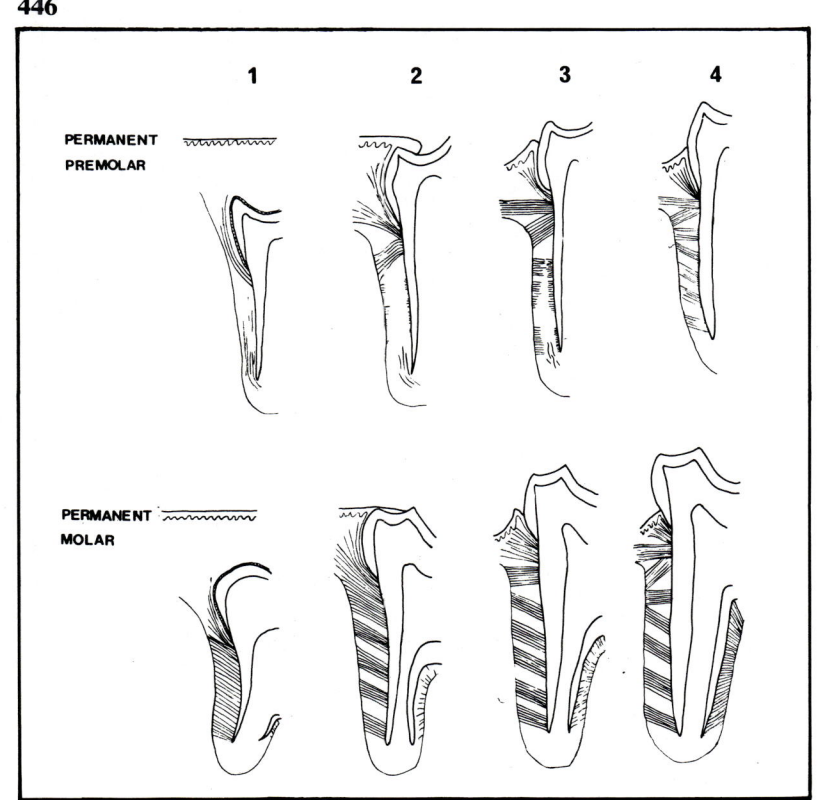

446 Significant differences in the development of the principal fibres have been described between teeth without successors (i.e. permanent molars) and successional teeth (i.e. permanent premolars), the fibres of successional teeth being organised more slowly.

Stage 1 Prior to eruption, the dento-gingival and oblique dento-alveolar fibres are well-developed in the permanent molar. In the permanent premolar only the dento-gingival fibres are organised, the developing periodontal ligament being composed of loosely structured collagenous elements.

Stage 2 As the tooth emerges into the oral cavity, the periodontal ligament of the permanent molar is well-differentiated, the oblique fibres being most conspicuous. However, at this stage in the permanent premolar only the fibres in the region of the alveolar crest are becoming organised. In the periodontal ligament itself, though collagen fibres are developing, they do not yet span the periodontal space.

Stage 3 On reaching occlusion, the fibre groupings in the cervical region of the permanent molar now become organised. In the permanent premolar, while the fibre groups cervically appear prominent, those in the apical part of the root appear relatively undeveloped.

Stage 4 After a period in function, the fibres of both the permanent molar and premolar show the classical organisation of the principal fibres.

Thus, permanent premolar teeth erupt into their functional position without a well-organised arrangement of collagen fibres in the periodontal ligament.

Cementogenesis begins following the breakup of the epithelial root sheath. The factors responsible for the differentiation of cementoblasts are poorly understood. The organic matrix of the first-formed cementum is derived both from cementoblast activity and from the connective tissue of the inner layer of the dental follicle. At a later stage, it is derived almost entirely from the cementoblasts. Once sufficient matrix has been formed, it is mineralised. The initial foci of calcification is thought to be crystallites of the adjacent dentine. At first, the cementoblasts migrate from the developing front of cementum. This primary cementum is termed acellular cementum to indicate its lack of cellular inclusions. At a later stage, the cementoblasts may be incorporated within their own secretions to become cementocytes, this secondary cementum being termed cellular cementum.

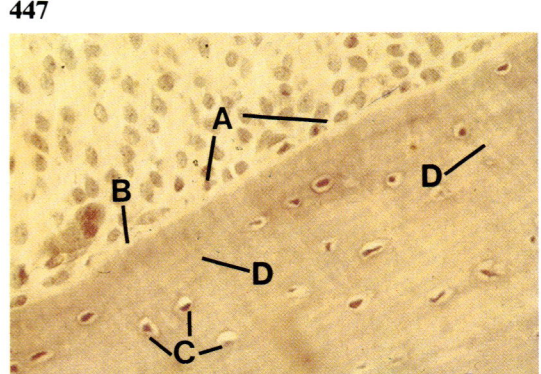

447 Developing cellular cementum. This is a decalcified section through the root. A, cementoblasts. B, precementum (unmineralised matrix). C, cementocytes within the mineralised cellular cementum. Note that in addition to the collagen fibres secreted by cementoblasts, cementum also contains collagen fibres derived from the periodontal ligament, the Sharpey fibres (D). Since cementum is being continuously deposited newly-synthesised collagen fibres of the periodontal ligament can be attached to the tooth under changing functional situations. (*H&E, ×300*)

448 The surface of developing cementum. A, cementoblast. During cementogenesis, the cementoblast has the ultrastructural characteristics typical of cells actively synthesising proteins and protein-polysaccharide complexes, i.e. a well-developed Golgi apparatus, an abundant endoplasmic reticulum and numerous mitochondria (see figure **301**). The dark zone (B) indicates the calcifying surface of the cementum. Hydroxyapatite crystals are deposited within, and on the surface of, collagen fibrils, the long axes of the crystals being parallel to the long axes of the collagen fibres. C, precementum. D, Sharpey's fibres. (*Electron micrograph, ×4,000*)

Cementogenesis occurs rhythmically, periods of activity alternating with periods of quiescence. The periods of inactivity or decreased activity are associated with incremental lines (see figure **275**) which are believed to have a higher content of ground substance and mineral and a lower content of collagen than adjacent cementum.

Development of alveolar bone is described with the development of the jaws (pages 149, 151).

Development of the dentitions

When the crowns of the teeth are complete and the roots have begun to develop, the teeth start to move through the tissues of the jaws to erupt eventually into the oral cavity.

Tooth eruption has conventionally been divided into three phases – the pre-eruptive, prefunctional and functional phases. During the pre-eruptive phase, the enamel organ lying within the developing jaw reaches its full size. The prefunctional phase begins with root formation and is completed when the tooth reaches the occlusal plane. During this phase, the crown penetrates the overlying oral mucosa to appear in the oral cavity. The functional phase refers to movement of a tooth once it has reached the occlusal plane. Though the main component of eruptive movement is an axial one, a tooth may tilt, rotate or move in a horizontal plane (drift) in order to attain its functional position. During the pre-eruptive phase, there is little axial movement, though areas of bone deposition on the walls of the crypts may indicate drift in tooth position. Whether patterns of bone activity are the cause of such tooth movements or simply represent the response to movement produced by another mechanism has not been established. It is during the prefunctional phase of the eruptive cycle that the most rapid rate of axial movement occurs. As the tooth approaches the oral cavity, the overlying bone is resorbed and a number of changes take place in the overlying soft tissues.

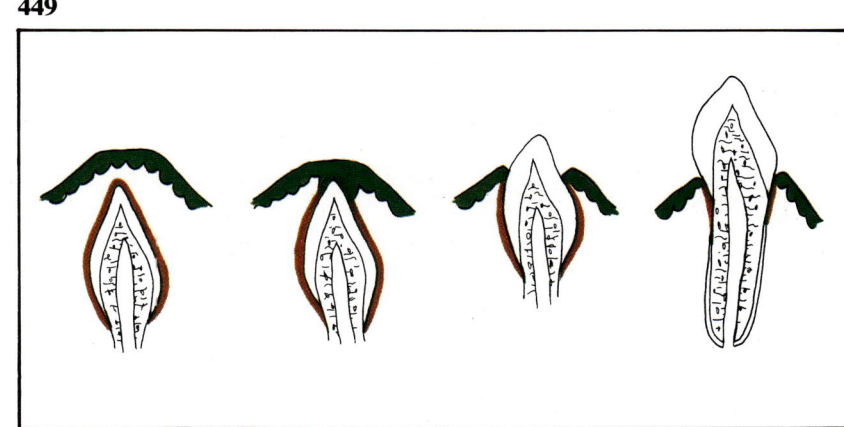

449 The development of the dento-gingival junction during the eruption of a tooth. The green outline delineates the oral epithelium, the red outline delineates the reduced enamel epithelium.

Before the tooth erupts, the enamel surface is covered by the reduced enamel epithelium (see figure **201**) which is a vestige of the enamel organ. This epithelium is separated from the overlying oral epithelium by connective tissue. As the tooth erupts, the outer cells of the reduced enamel epithelium actively proliferate into the connective tissue lying between the cusp tip and oral epithelium. It has been suggested that these proliferating epithelial cells secrete enzymes which break down collagen. Many of the fibroblasts in the resorbing connective tissue overlying erupting teeth cease fibrillogenesis; they actively take up extracellular material and synthesise acid hydrolysis. Eventually, the cells degenerate.

Reduced enamel epithelial cells may also be concerned with the removal of breakdown products resulting from resorption of connective tissue. Depolymerisation of ground substance has been detected in the connective tissue overlying erupting teeth. Though a relationship between the degeneration of the connective tissue and the pressure exerted by the underlying erupting tooth has not been established, ischaemia is thought to be a contributory factor to such changes.

Though the changes in the connective tissue overlying erupting teeth do not appear to contribute actively to the eruptive mechanism, they may allow a tooth to erupt along a path of least resistance. Furthermore, it is possible that abnormal changes within such a tissue could increase the resistance to eruption.

As the tooth approaches the oral epithelium, the cells of the outer layer of the reduced enamel epithelium and the basal layer of the oral epithelium actively proliferate so that the two epithelia join. The epithelium covering the tip of the tooth now degenerates at its centre, thus enabling the crown to emerge through an epithelial-lined pathway into the oral cavity.

Further emergence of the tooth into the oral cavity results both from active eruptive movements and passive separation of the oral epithelium from the crown surface. When the tooth first erupts into the oral cavity, the reduced enamel epithelium is attached to the unerupted part of the crown, thus forming an epithelial seal, the junctional epithelium. The subsequent stages in the development of the junctional epithelium is a matter of controversy. One view suggests that the reduced enamel epithelium persists, another suggests that with time it is replaced by oral epithelium. With continued eruption, as more of the crown is exposed, the region above the junctional epithelium forms the gingival crevice.

As the tooth erupts, the root develops. However, the root is not completely formed until about two years after the tooth has reached a functional position. The bony crypt around the erupting tooth is modified by resorption and deposition of bone so that it is finally shaped to accommodate the roots and becomes the socket.

450 An erupting deciduous molar prior to its emergence into the oral cavity. This is a decalcified, transverse section through the jaw. A, enamel space. B, developing roots. C, developing alveolar crypt. D, oral epithelium. E, vestiges of enamel organ. A high power view of the region above the erupting crown is seen in figure **201**. (*H&E, ×4*)

451 Decalcified, buccolingual section through an erupted deciduous canine (A) and its erupting successor (B). Initially, each deciduous tooth and its developing permanent successor share a common alveolar crypt, the permanent tooth germ being situated lingually to the developing deciduous tooth. With continued growth and eruption of the deciduous tooth, the permanent tooth comes to lie near to the root apex of the deciduous tooth within its own bony crypt. However, the alveolar crypt of the permanent tooth is not complete, there being an opening in its roof through which the dental follicle of the tooth germ communicates with, and is attached to, the overlying oral mucosa. This opening has been termed the gubernacular canal (C). (*H&E, ×4*)

452 A gubernacular canal and its contents. The gubernacular canal contains strands of vascular connective tissue (the gubernacular cords) and epithelial remains of the dental lamina (A). The gubernacular cords are thought by some to play an important part in the movements of the developing teeth through the growing jaws. During tooth eruption, the gubernacular cords decrease in length but increase in thickness, producing a widening of their canals. The gubernacular tissue also becomes less dense. Whether the gubernaculum provides a duct, a path of least resistance or is actively engaged in pulling the tooth during the early prefunction phase of eruption has not been established. (*H&E, ×25*)

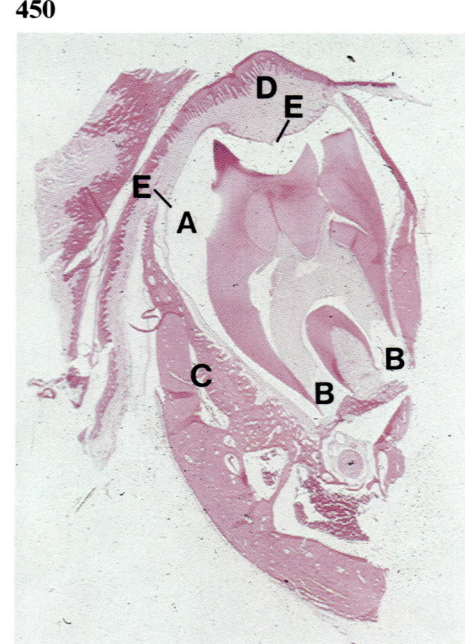

450

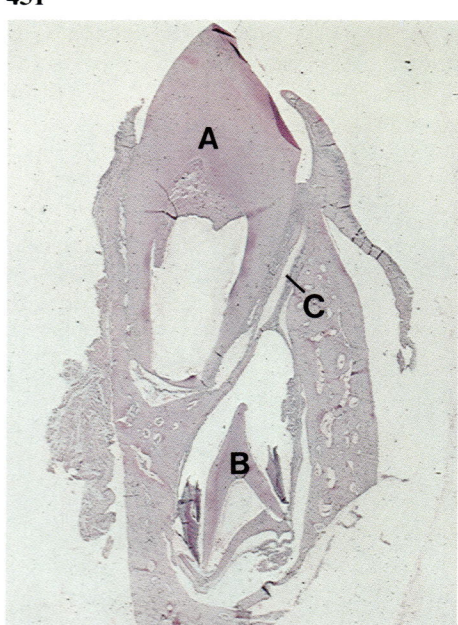

451

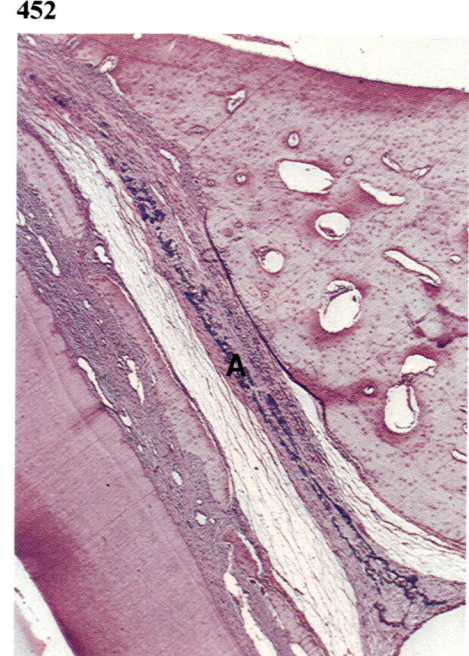

452

Before the permanent incisors, canines and premolars erupt into the mouth, the overlying deciduous teeth are usually resorbed and shed.

453 Decalcified, buccolingual section through a resorbing deciduous tooth (A) and its erupting successor (B). During the early eruptive stages of the permanent tooth the bone separating it from its deciduous predecessor is resorbed (*arrow*). Following this, resorption of the hard tissues of the deciduous tooth takes place, beginning at the apical part of the lingual root surface of the deciduous incisors and canines and at the interradicular root surfaces of the deciduous molars. The vascular, resorbing tissue has been termed the resorbing organ of Tomes. Continued resorption of the root usually results in the permanent tooth coming to lie immediately beneath the deciduous tooth. However, it is possible for the permanent tooth to erupt at some distance from its deciduous predecessor so that it appears behind the deciduous tooth which is still in its functional position. Resorption of a deciduous tooth can also take place in the absence of its successor. (*H&E, ×12*)

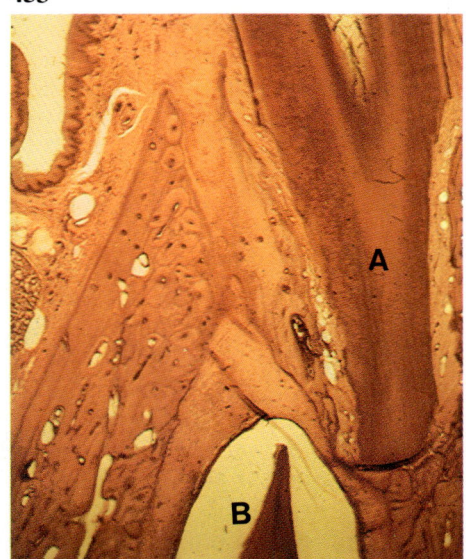

The shedding of deciduous teeth is the result of progressive resorption of their roots by osteoclast-like cells. The initiation of resorption may be an inherent developmental process or it may be related to pressure from the permanent successor against the overlying bone or tooth.

454 Resorbing dentine. Note the multinucleated osteoclast-like cells within resorption lacunae (Howship's lacunae). These cells have been termed odontoclasts. Odontoclasts differentiate from the connective tissue of the periodontal ligament. They are vacuolated and have long cytoplasmic processes. In an electron micrograph, the cytoplasmic projections form a brush border with the tooth surface. The odontoclasts have an abundance of ribosomes and a large number of mitochondria. (*H&E, ×300*)

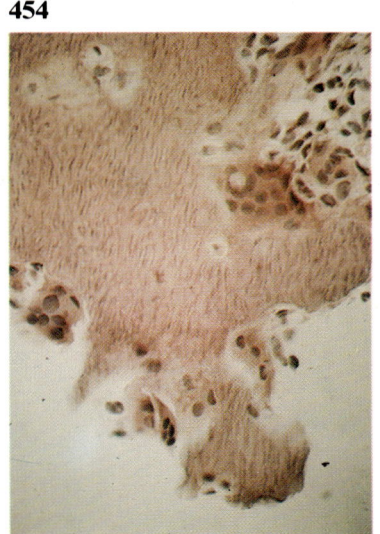

Resorption of deciduous teeth is not a continuous process. During rest periods, reparative tissue may be formed leading to a reattachment of the periodontal ligament. The tissue of repair is cementum-like and the cells responsible for its formation are similar in appearance to cementoblasts. If the repair process prevails over the resorption for long periods of time then the tooth may become ankylosed to the surrounding bone.

455 Fusion between dentine (A) and bone (B). This is a decalcified section through an ankylosed root. Ankylosis may also be related to trauma and/or infection of a tooth. Where a deciduous tooth becomes ankylosed, its position within the jaw remains constant so that, with increasing height of the alveolar bone, it appears to sink gradually below the level of the adjacent teeth. Such ankylosed teeth are referred to as 'submerged' teeth. The submergence may continue to such an extent that the teeth become completely buried within bone. The section is viewed in blue light. (*×150*)

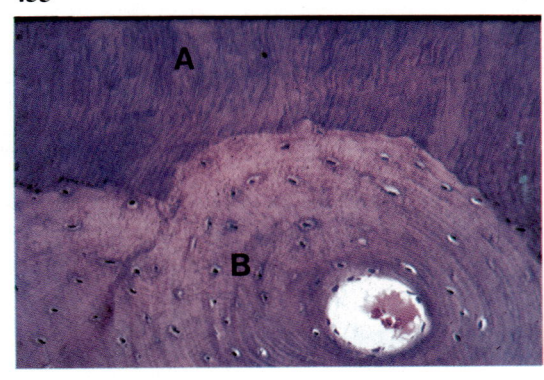

Tooth eruption is traditionally considered to be a developmental process whereby the tooth moves in an axial direction from its position within the alveolar crypt of the jaw into a functional position within the oral cavity. However, eruption can be regarded as a lifelong process since a tooth will often move axially in response to changing functional situations, e.g. overeruption resulting from the removal of an antagonist, and compensatory eruption related to attrition.

The rate of eruption represents a balance between forces tending to move the tooth into the mouth (eruptive force) and forces tending to prevent this movement (resistive force). Resistance may be produced by overlying soft tissues and alveolar bone, the viscosity of the surrounding periodontal ligament and occlusal forces. Thus, changes in the rate of tooth movement may be brought about by changes in either the eruptive forces and/or the resistive forces. At present, little is known about the nature, source and magnitude of either the eruptive or resistive forces. Furthermore, it is not known whether the forces are of the same nature and value at various stages of the eruptive cycle. By and large, this situation results from difficulties encountered in producing experimental systems which isolate for study single possible agents associated with the eruptive process.

All tissue within the vicinity of the tooth thought capable of generating a force have, at one time or another, been implicated in the eruptive process. The theories advanced to explain the mechanism of tooth eruption can be divided into two main groups. One view suggests that the tooth is pushed out as a result of forces generated beneath and around it, either by alveolar bone growth, root growth, blood-pressure/tissue fluid pressure or cell proliferation. Alternatively, the tooth may be pulled out as a result of tension within the connective tissue of the periodontal ligament. Though some are of the opinion that the force effecting eruption is derived primarily from a single source or prime mover, others believe that more than one agent has important contributions to the overall force. No one theory is yet supported by sufficient experimental evidence.

Some observations have been made on the rate of emergence of human teeth into the oral cavity. Initially, there is a period of slow eruption when the crown is carried towards the oral mucosa. For permanent teeth, this period may be between two and four years. A tooth erupts most rapidly as it enters the oral cavity, at which time the length of its root is about two-thirds complete. Eruption then slows as the tooth approaches the occlusal plane. Once the tooth has emerged into the oral cavity, it may take one to two years to reach the occlusal plane. As previously mentioned, the emergence of the crown is partly due to axial movement of the tooth (active eruption) and partly due to retraction of the adjacent soft tissues (passive eruption). For human maxillary incisors, the maximum eruption rate at the time of crown emergence is about 1mm per month. For maxillary third molars, the maximum rates are seen in spaced dentitions and are less than half that recorded for incisors. In crowded dentitions, the rates are even lower (less than 1mm in six months).

Chronology of tooth development and the order of eruption

Chronology of the deciduous dentition

Tooth	*First evidence of calcification (months I.U.)*	*Crown completed (months)*	*Eruption (months)*	*Root completed (years)*
Maxillary				
A	3–4	4	7	1½–2
B	4½	5	8	1½–2
C	5	9	16–20	2½–3
D	5	6	12–16	2–2½
E	6–7	10–12	21–30	3
Mandibular				
A	4½	4	6½	1½–2
B	4½	4½	7	1½–2
C	5	9	16–20	2½–3
D	5	6	12–16	2–2½
E	6	10–12	21–30	3

I.U. = *In utero*. Unless otherwise indicated all dates are *post-partum*. The teeth are identified according to the Zsigmond System.

Chronology of the permanent dentition

Tooth	*First evidence of calcification*	*Crown completed (years)*	*Eruption (years)*	*Root completed (years)*
Maxillary				
1	3–4 months	4–5	7–8	10
2	10–12 months	4–5	8–9	11
3	4–5 months	6–7	11–12	13–15
4	1½–1¾ years	5–6	10–11	12–13
5	2–2½ years	6–7	10–12	12–14
6	Birth	2½–3	6–7	9–10
7	2½–3 years	7–8	12–13	14–16
8	7–9 years	12–16	17–21	18–25
Mandibular				
1	3–4 months	4–5	6–7	9
2	3–4 months	4–5	7–8	10
3	4–5 months	6–7	9–10	12–14
4	1¾–2 years	5–6	10–12	12–13
5	2¼–2½ years	6–7	11–12	13–14
6	Birth	2½–3	6–7	9–10
7	2½–3 years	7–8	12–13	14–15
8	8–10 years	12–16	17–21	18–25

All dates are *post-partum*. Teeth are identified according to the Zsigmond System.

456 Development of the human dentition

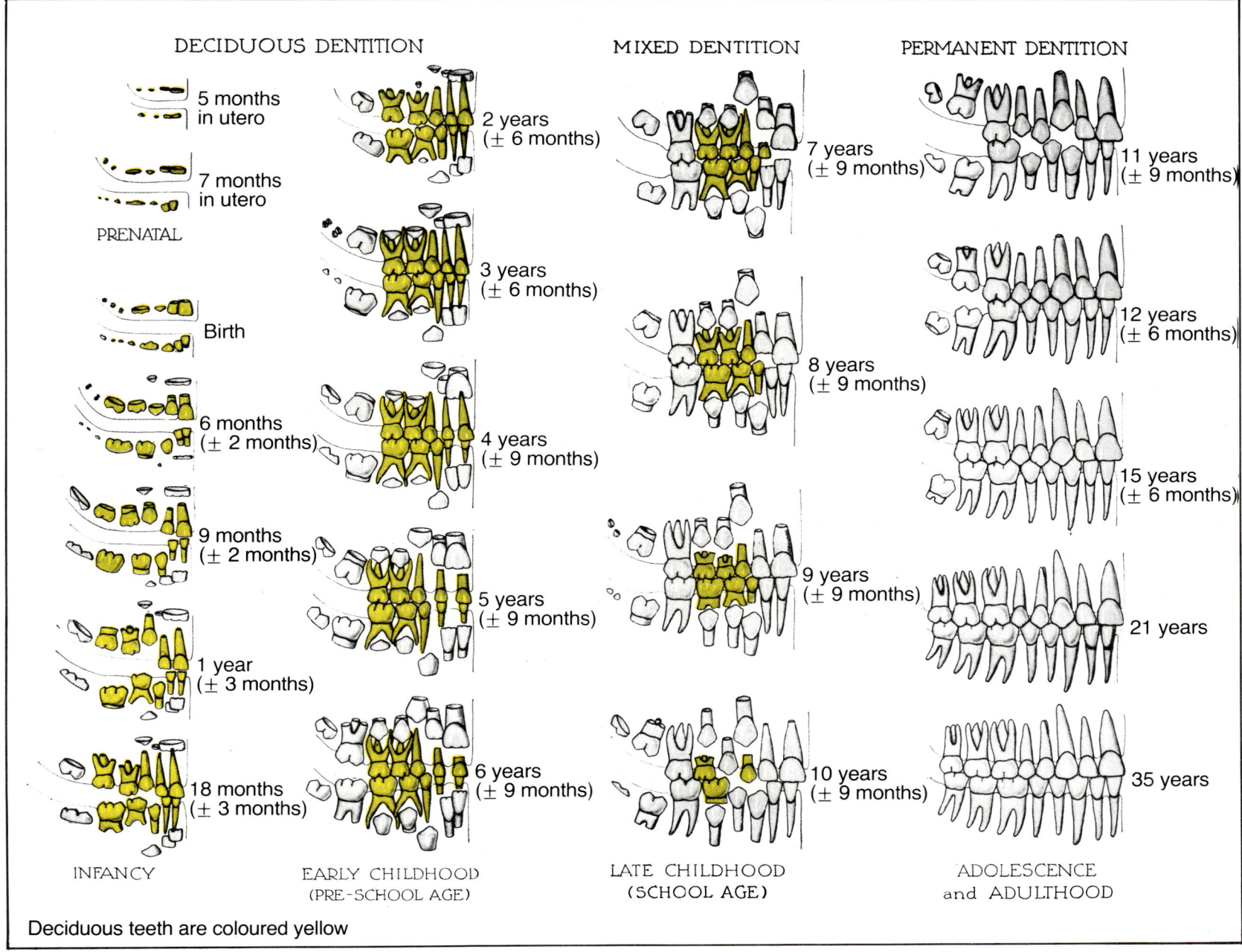

Deciduous teeth are coloured yellow

Because no individuals are exactly alike in their development, the times given in the above tables are approximate. Variations of six months either way are not unusual, but the tendency is for teeth to erupt late rather than early. By and large, the development of the permanent dentition is more advanced in girls. There does not appear to be any sex difference in the development of the deciduous dentition.

Since the sequence of development and eruption of teeth is under genetic control, and since chronological age is an unreliable guide to the progress of development of an individual child, dental age is a useful index of maturity, especially when used in conjunction with skeletal age. Dental age may be estimated clinically by a visual assessment of the stage of eruption of the dentition or, more satisfactorily, by a radiographic assessment of both the stages of development of the crowns and roots and the stages of eruption.

Once a tooth reaches its functional position it is believed to occupy a position of equilibrium between the soft tissues of the cheeks and lips externally and the tongue internally.

The movement which has attracted the most attention during the functional phase of tooth eruption is mesial drift. Mesial drift may involve considerable bodily movement of the tooth. It has been reported that between the ages of 6 and 18 years the first permanent molar drifts approximately 4mm in a mesial direction. Four hypotheses have been postulated to account for this movement:

1 that the mesial inclination of teeth produces a resultant force during biting favouring mesial drift;
2 that the action of certain jaw muscles, particularly the buccinator, 'propel' the teeth forwards;
3 that bone deposited preferentially on the distal surface of the sockets pushes the teeth mesially.
4 that contraction of the transseptal fibre system pulls the teeth mesially.

The radiographic appearance of the dentitions at varying ages

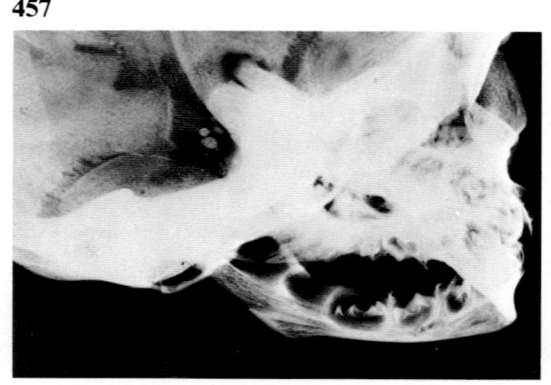
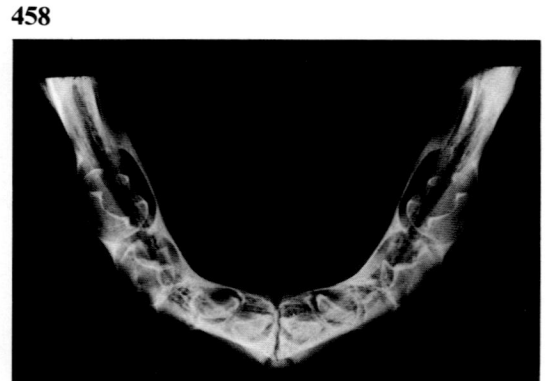

457 The dentition at birth, a lateral oblique view of the skull.

458 The dentition at birth, an occlusal view of the mandible.

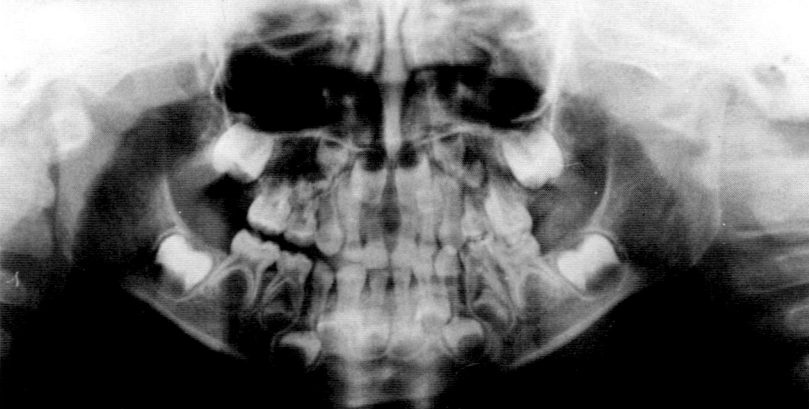

459 Dental age 2½ years.

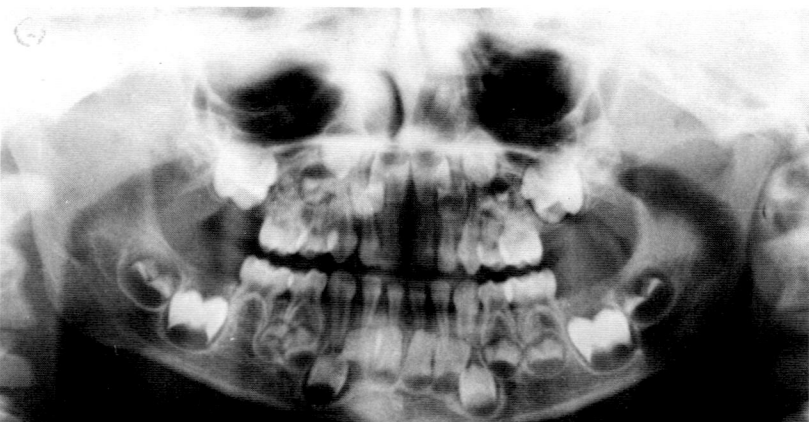

460 Dental age 4 years.

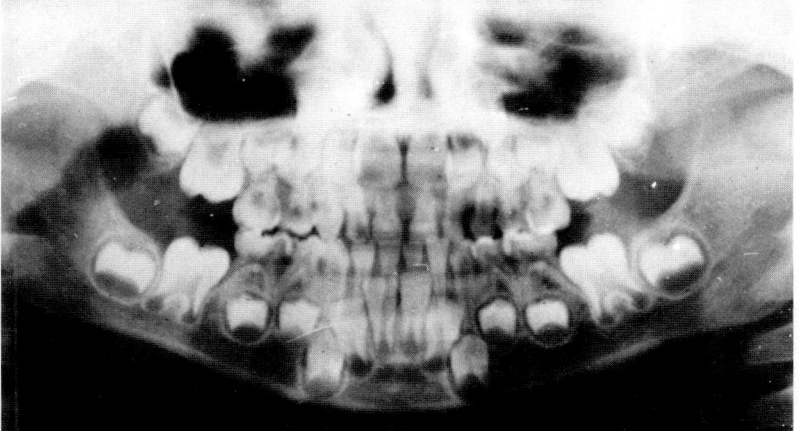

461 Dental age 5½ years.

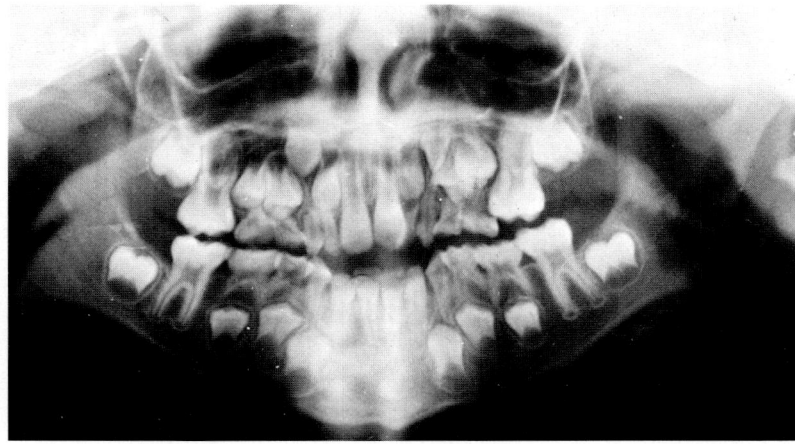

462 Dental age 7 years.

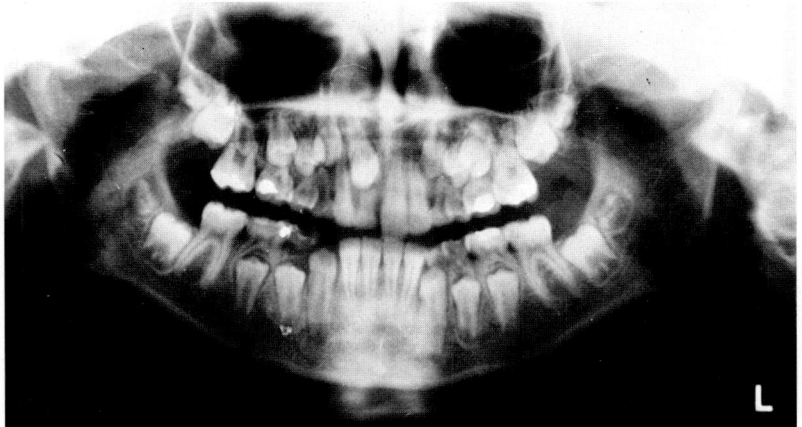

463 Dental age 9 years. Note the unerupted upper right central incisor and an associated unerupted supernumerary tooth.

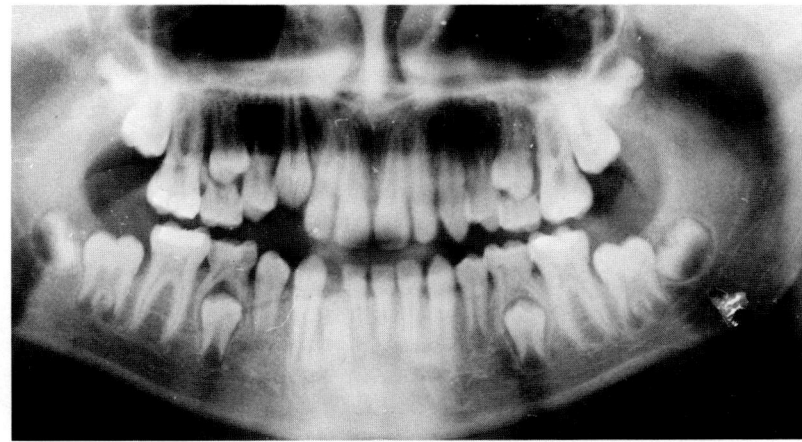

464 Dental age 11 years. 2| is unerupted.

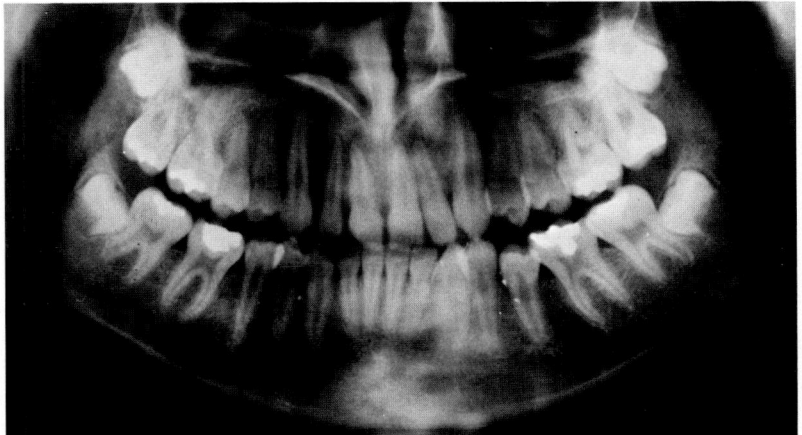

465 Dental age 14 years.

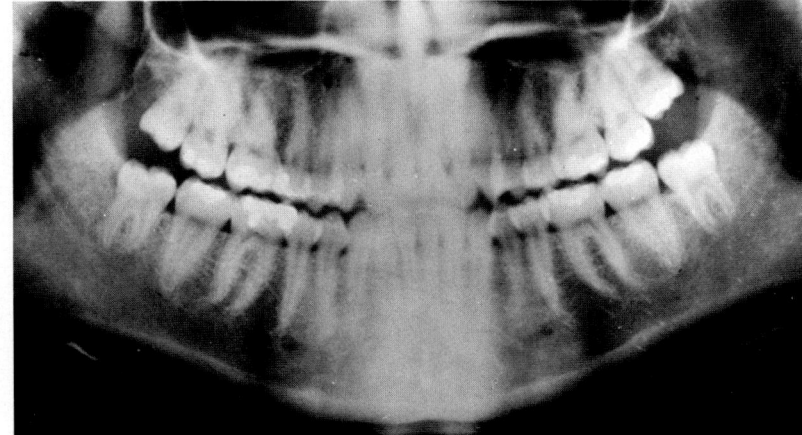

466 Dental age 19 years.

Development of occlusion

At birth, the oral mucosa over the developing alveoli is greatly thickened to form the maxillary and mandibular gum pads. They show a series of elevations each of which corresponds to an underlying deciduous tooth. The elevations associated with the second deciduous molars do not however become prominent until about the sixth month. The gum pads rarely come into occlusion, the space left between them being occupied by the tongue. The maxillary gum pad overlaps the mandibular gum pad both buccally and labially, the overjet usually being considerable. Beneath the gum pads there is generally considerable crowding of the developing teeth, especially the incisors. However, during the first year of life the gum pads grow rapidly, especially in lateral directions, thus providing space for the developing teeth. The deciduous teeth start to erupt at about the sixth month and the deciduous dentition is complete by the third year. At this time, the occlusion of the deciduous dentition differs from that of the permanent dentition in the following respects:

1 The incisors are more vertically positioned within the alveolus and are often spaced.
2 The overbite is usually greater.
3 There may be significant spacings distal to the lower canines and mesial to the upper canines (the anthropoid or primitive spaces).
4 Although the anteroposterior relationships of the deciduous arches have not been adequately assessed, it appears that the distal edges of the upper and lower deciduous molars are flush and the mesiobuccal cusps of the upper first and second deciduous molars occlude in the buccal grooves of the lower first and second deciduous molars respectively.

Several changes now occur in the deciduous occlusion before the appearance of the permanent teeth. These result from changes in the dental bases. As the dental arches become wider and longer, so the deciduous teeth become more spaced. Since there is a greater forward growth of the mandible compared to the maxilla, the lower arch moves forwards relative to the upper so that an edge-to-edge incisor relationship is obtained. As a further consequence, the distal surfaces of the deciduous second molars may now show a slight mesial step from maxilla to mandible, the mesiobuccal cusp of the upper second deciduous molar lying distal to the buccal groove of the lower second deciduous molar. As the deciduous teeth approach the end of their functional lives, they may show signs of considerable wear.

After the age of six years, the dentition is said to be mixed, comprising both deciduous and permanent teeth.

The first molars are the first permanent teeth to erupt. Initially, they have a cusp-to-cusp relationship which is governed by the position of the deciduous second molars. The first molars take up their normal adult relationship once the deciduous second molars are shed. The permanent incisors erupt between the ages of six and nine years. Since the permanent incisors are much larger than their deciduous predecessors, they are accommodated into the dental arches not just by the utilisation of the space left by the deciduous predecessors, but also by lateral growth of the alveolar arches and the greater proclination of the permanent incisors. In their developmental positions, the lateral incisors are overlapped by the central incisors, being positioned more palatally. As a rule, space is made for the lateral incisors as the central incisors erupt. However, should there be insufficient growth of the alveolus, the lateral incisors may continue to lie in their developmental, palatal positions. Frequently, when the permanent incisors erupt, they fan out (incline distally) so that there may be a significant space or diastema between the central incisors. This appearance has been termed the 'ugly duckling' stage and is said to result from pressure on the roots of the permanent incisors from the developing permanent canines. The diastema usually closes following eruption of the permanent canines. The canines and premolars which usually erupt between the ages of nine and 12 years are readily accommodated into the dental arches, since the combined mesiodistal diameters of the deciduous canines and molars is generally greater than that of their permanent successors. Any leeway space which remains is usually taken up by forward movement of the first permanent molars. By the age of 12 years, all the deciduous teeth have been shed to be replaced by permanent teeth and henceforth the occlusion appears similar to that in the adult (see pages 35–39). Space is provided for the permanent molar teeth by continued growth of the mandible and maxilla.

Although there is a tendency for the mandible to grow slightly further forward than the maxilla after the age of 12 years, usually there is no appreciable occlusal change. During the later stages of facial growth there may be an accompanying uprighting of the incisors with the result that they become more crowded. It has been suggested that mesial drift may take up any remaining space in the arches or even be responsible for some late crowding.

Comparative dental anatomy

Simplified classification of living vertebrates

Class	Subclass	Examples
Agnatha	Cyclostomata	Hagfishes, lampreys
Chondrichthyes	Elasmobranchii	Sharks, rays
	Holocephali	Chimaeras
Osteichthyes	Actinopterygii	Majority of bony fish
	Sarcopterygii	Lung-fishes, coelocanths
Amphibia	Lissamphibia	Frogs, toads, newts, salamanders
Reptilia	Anapsida	Turtles, tortoises
	Lepidosauria	Lizards, snakes
	Archosauria	Crocodiles, alligators
Aves		Birds
Mammalia	Prototheria	Platypus
	Theria—Metatheria	Marsupials
	—Eutheria	Placental mammals

Evolution of the jaws and teeth

Evolution of jaws

467

A The earliest vertebrates were small, fish-like animals without jaws (Class – *Agnatha*). They were filter feeders and possessed 5 to 15 pairs of gill slits supported by skeletal gill bars.

B A significant advance in vertebrate evolutionary history was the development of jaws from gill arch elements. It is probable that one or two anterior gill arches gradually disappeared with the expansion of the mouth cavity so that the gill arch which developed phylogenetically into the jaws of ancestral gnathostomes was not the first of the series. The upper jaw elements in these early 'jawed' vertebrates (Class – *Placodermi*) were the palatoquadrate cartilages which articulated posteriorly with the lower jaw elements, the mandibular (Meckel's) cartilages. In the placoderm illustrated in B, the upper part of the hyoid gill arch immediately behind the jaws, the hyomandibula, was unspecialised. The jaws were attached to the chondrocranium only by ligaments. Where the hyomandibula is non-functional as a supporting structure and where the upper jaw is self-supporting, the jaw suspension is termed autostylic.

C, E & F At a later stage, the hyomandibula became involved in the jaw support mechanism, being braced above against the otic region of the braincase and below by ligaments to the jaws. The gill slit between the jaws and hyoid arch became reduced to a tube or spiracle which, subsequently, became involved in the evolution of the ear. In a few sharks, where there is a direct articulation of the upper jaw and braincase as well as support from the hyomandibula, the jaw articulation is termed *amphistyly* (C). In most modern fish (E & F), the upper jaw has no direct connection with the braincase and the jaw joint is braced entirely by the hyomandibula. This type of articulation is termed *hyostyly*. In bony fish (F & G), the chondrocranium is surrounded by dermal bones. A number of replacement bones form in the upper jaw, the most important being the quadrate bone which forms the upper part of the hinge of the jaw. In the lower jaw, dermal bones support the teeth and Meckel's cartilage regresses, its only replacement bone being the articular bone which forms the lower part of the jaw hinge. The hyomandibula usually supports the jaw, the articulation therefore being hyostylic. In the lung fishes (G), however, the upper jaw is fused directly to the braincase to produce a modified autostyly termed *holostyly*. The same is true of the chimaeroids (D).

467

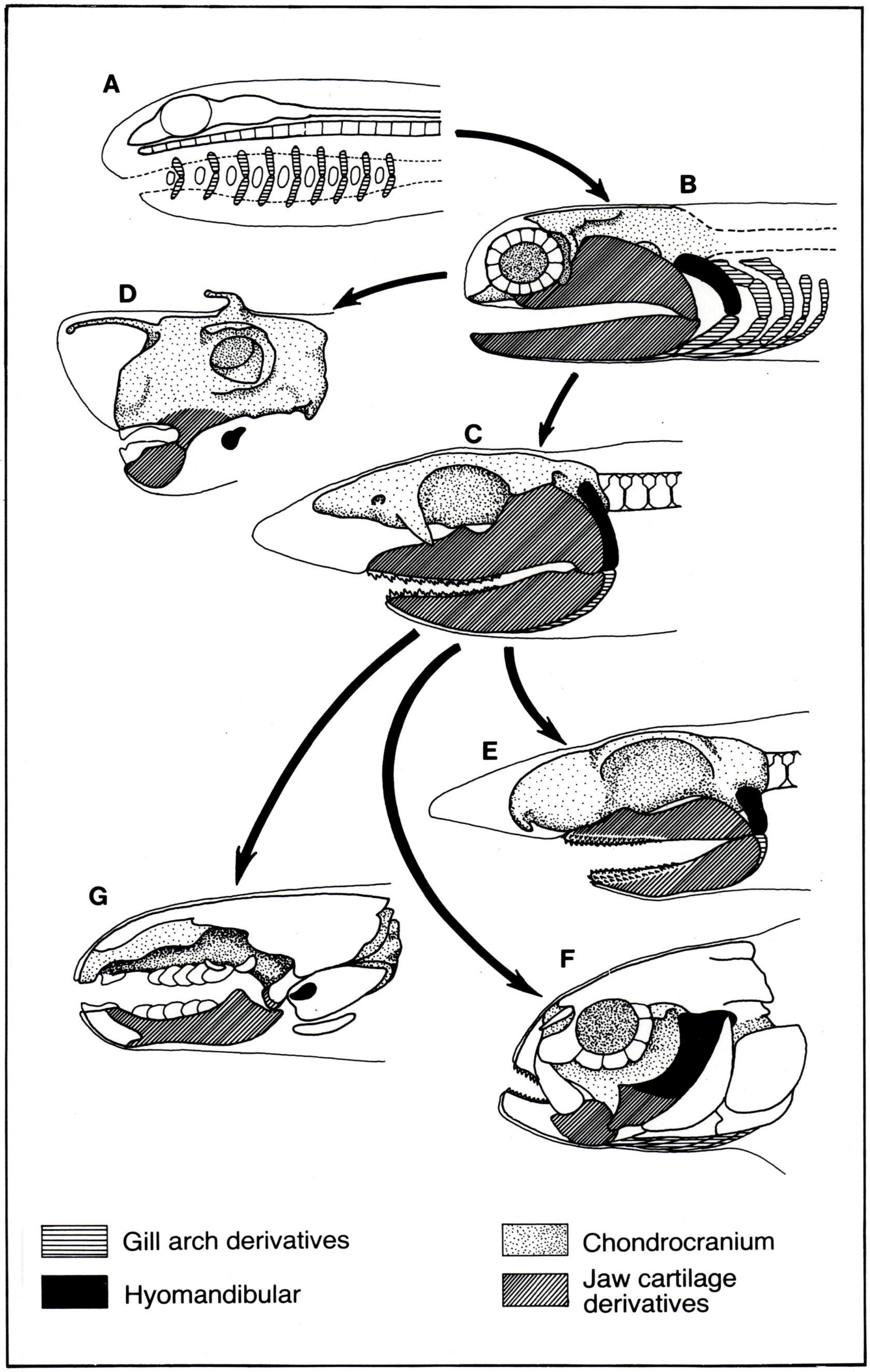

A
B
C
D
E
F
G
Gill arch derivatives
Hyomandibular
Chondrocranium
Jaw cartilage derivatives

468

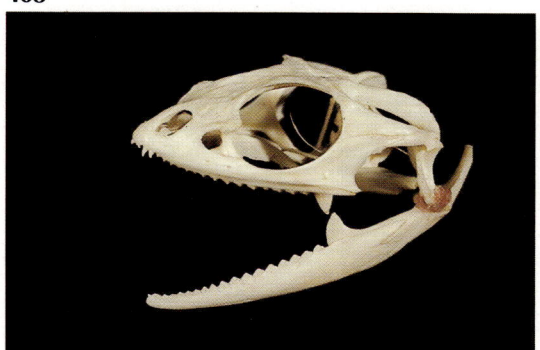

468 A number of significant changes occurred in the skull during the evolution of the amphibians and reptiles. These changes may be appreciated by the study of the skull of a bearded lizard (*Amphibolurus barbatus*). The upper jaw becomes firmly united to the skull. The quadrate of the upper jaw articulates with the squamosal bone of the skull without the participation of the hyomandibula. The jaw suspension is thus a modified autostyly. The hyomandibula becomes incorporated into the evolving auditory system as an ear ossicle, the columella (or stapes in mammals). The spiracular pouch of the embryo never breaks through to the surface and gives rise to the middle ear cavity and Eustachian tube. The lower jaw consists of a number of bones, the dentary being tooth-bearing.

pm
n
na
fr
pa
prf
pof
sf
l
o
po
mx
sq
j
q
c
sa
d
an

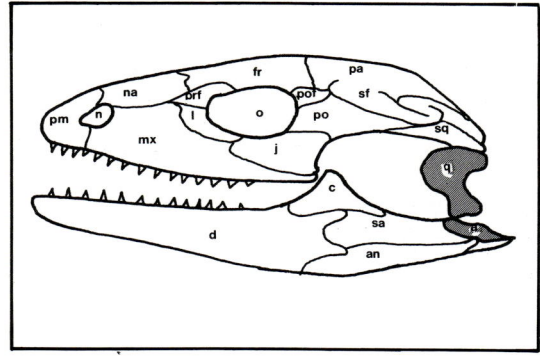

pm, premaxilla. (n, external nostril.) na, nasal. mx, maxilla. fr, frontal. prf, prefrontal. l, lacrimal. o, orbit. j, jugual. pof, post-frontal. po, post-orbital. pa, parietal. sf, superior temporal fossa. sq, squamosal. q, quadrate. a, articular. d, dentary. c, coronoid. an, angular. sa, surangular. The characteristic quadrate-articular jaw articulation is hatched.

469 Evolutionary changes in the lower jaw of mammal-like reptiles. 1 *Dimetrodon*. 2 *Cynarioides*. 3 *Cynognathus*. sp, splenial. a, angular. sa, surangular. ar, articular. Hatched area designates the dentary. The trend is for an increase in size of the dentary which extended backwards to a position beneath the squamosal of the upper jaw close to the quadrate-articular joint. These evolutionary changes eventually led to the typical mammalian lower jaw which consists of a single bone, the dentary, articulating directly with the squamous part of the temporal bone. The articular and quadrate bones became ear ossicles, the malleus and incus respectively.

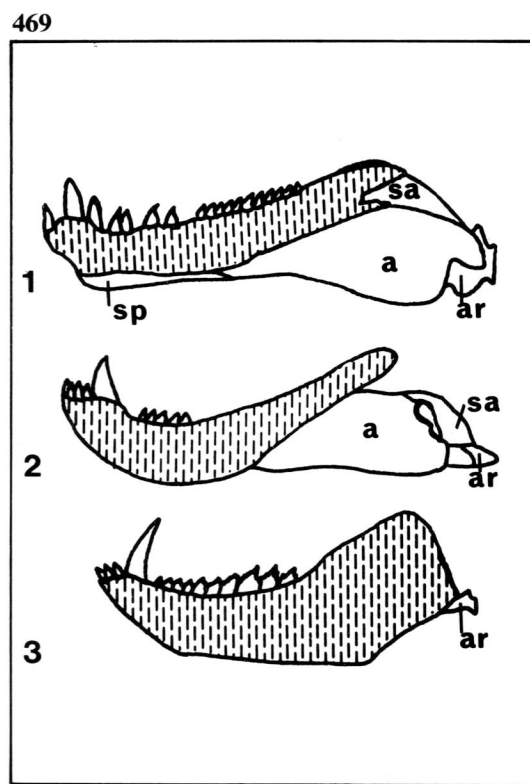

The mechanism whereby the typically mammalian squamosal-dentary articulation enlarged at the expense of the typically reptilian quadrate-articular articulation is not fully understood. *Probainognathus* is a carnivorous cynodont of the mid-Triassic period which is intermediate in form, having both a squamosal-dentary articulation and a quadrate-articular connection.

470 The jaw joint of *Probainognathus* viewed medially. sq, squamosal. q, quadrate. a, articular. c, incipient condyle of mandible. f, incipient articular fossa of squamosal. san, surangular. pra, prearticular. d, dentary (hatched).

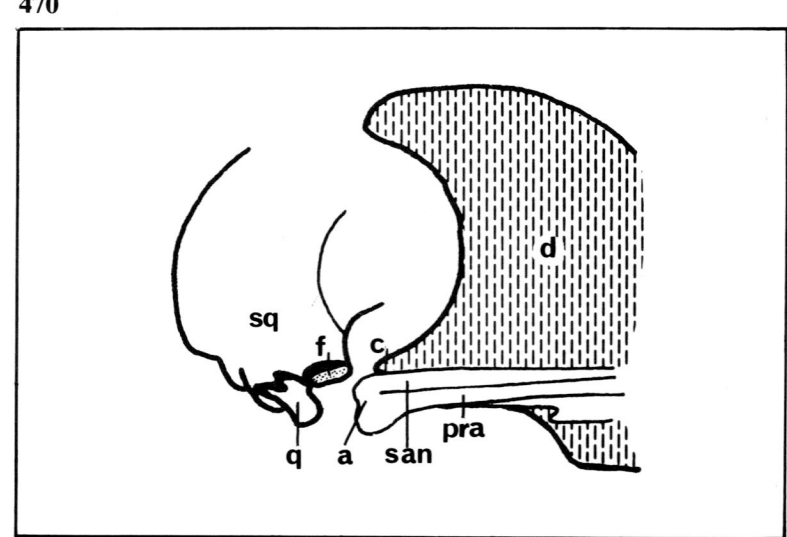

It has been generally assumed that as the quadrate-articular joint decreased in size in advanced cynodonts, the posterior tip of the dentary gradually grew backwards until it established contact with the squamosal. At that point in time, the jaw articulation must have been fragile. However, recent work has suggested another interpretation, namely that a subsidiary articulation between the surangular and squamosal was present which, together with the quadrate-articular, formed a substantial articulation. According to this interpretation, the squamosal-surangular articulation was the predecessor of the squamosal-dentary articulation. As the dentary grew backwards to form a condyle, it occupied the former squamosal-surangular articulation, the surangular part decreasing in size and ultimately disappearing.

Evolution of teeth

Primitive agnathans had extensive dermal armour protecting the underlying tissues. This armour consisted of a bony layer surmounted by a dentine-like tissue. The surface of this dentine was sculptured, being covered with numerous tubercles. Since this armour was subepidermal, it should be considered a mineralised dermis. During evolution there was a tendency for the dermal armour to break up into smaller units, but it survives in modern elasmobranchs in the form of large numbers of small, tooth-like, placoid scales or dermal denticles which protrude through the skin. Some of these placoid scales retain bone-like subdermal basal plates. Teeth are thought to have evolved from dermal denticles of this type. It is believed that denticles in the region of the mouth enlarged and became attached to the jaw elements. The phylogenetic development of the many varieties of dental hard tissues and tooth forms seen in vertebrates from these early denticles is controversial.

Comparative histology of the dental tissues

Enameloid

Covering the dentine of the teeth of fish is tissue known as enameloid. It is hypercalcified with respect to the underlying dentine.

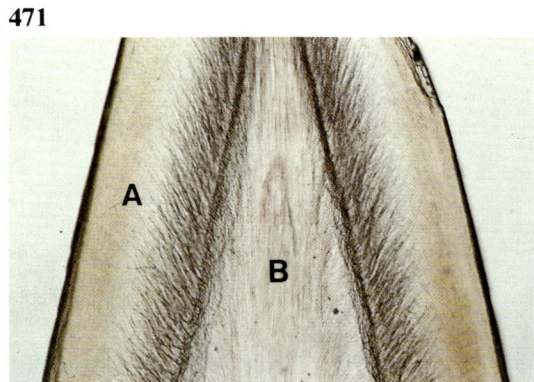

471 Longitudinal, ground section through a tooth of a piranha (*Serrasalmus rhombeus*). This shows enameloid (A) covering an inner core of dentine (B). Enameloid may be limited to a small cap of tissue overlying the tip of a tooth, as in the eel (*Anguilla anguilla*) or, as shown here, may cover most of the tooth surfaces. Enameloid appears as a relatively structureless, nonprismatic layer. Within the inner enameloid numerous dark lines may be seen which are continuations of the dentinal tubules. Some fish (e.g. sheeps-head fish, *Sargus ovis*) also have tubules running from the surface of the tooth into the enameloid for varying distances. ($\times 80$)

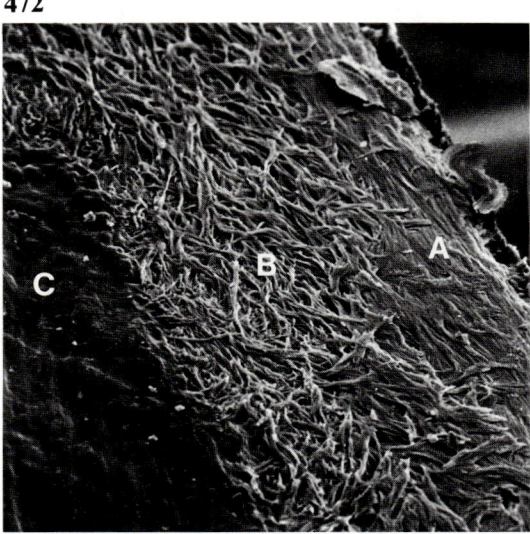

472 Longitudinal section of enameloid from the tooth of a piranha (*Serrasalmus rhombeus*). The surface of the section has been etched with dilute acid in order to more clearly demonstrate the crystallite bundles. Note the differences in crystallite orientation between the outer (A) and inner (B) zones of the enameloid. C, dentine. It has been suggested that the varying arrangement of crystallites may help counteract stresses and strains set up within the enameloid during feeding. (*Scanning electron micrograph*, $\times 400$)

Enameloid differs in many respects from ectodermally-derived enamel and should be regarded as a hypercalcified layer of specialised dentine.

473 Decalcified, longitudinal section through the developing tooth of a wrasse (*Labrus bergylta*). This shows the enameloid matrix (A). The developing matrix of enameloid is partly collagenous and is secreted by the odontoblasts (B). There is evidence, however, that some matrix protein is also secreted by the internal enamel epithelial cells (C) of the tooth germ. Unlike the mammalian tooth germ, those of fish teeth lack a definite stellate reticulum and stratum intermedium. Enameloid formation occurs before that of the true dentine. (*H&E, ×100*)

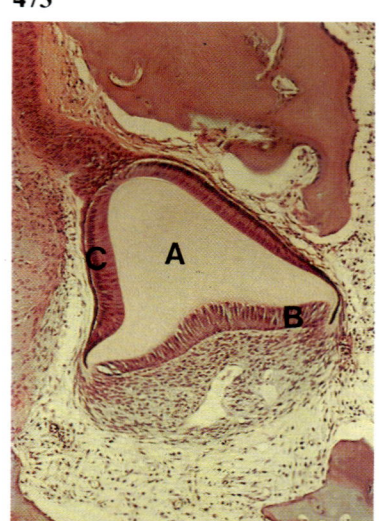

474 Developing enameloid in the eel (*Anguilla anguilla*). The matrix of the enameloid (A) is, as yet, uncalcified and contains many collagen fibres. The internal enamel epithelial cells (B) contain rough endoplasmic reticulum, Golgi material and secretory vesicles. These intracytoplasmic organelles suggest that these cells are involved in protein synthesis and may therefore contribute material to the enameloid matrix. Similar organelles are seen in the odontoblasts (C). Note the odontoblast processes (*arrowed*) in the developing enameloid. (*Electron micrograph, ×8,000*)

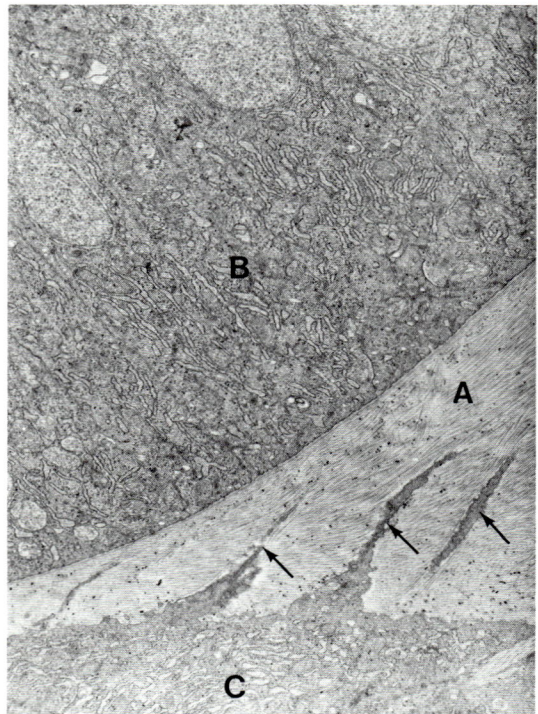

475 View through mineralising enameloid in the tooth of a dogfish (*Scyliorhinus canicula*). Fluorapatite crystals are being formed within the collagenous matrix of enameloid. The characteristic banding of the collagen can be seen. (*Electron micrograph, ×11,000*)

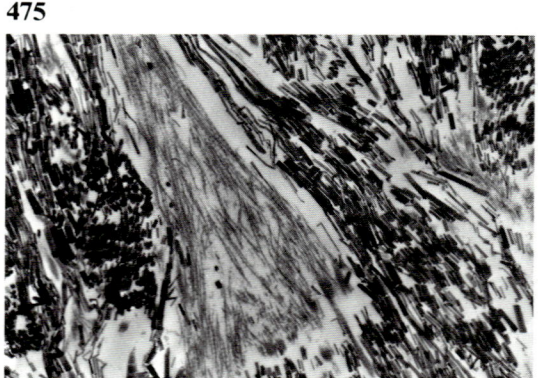

476 View through mature enameloid in a tooth of a dogfish (*Scyliorhinus canicula*). During maturation of enameloid, the labile collagen fibres disappear, the tooth germ perhaps assisting in its final removal. The fluorapatite crystals have been cut transversely, showing their hexagonal habit. Thus, although the matrix of developing enameloid is partly collagenous, chemical analysis of mature enameloid shows that its protein content is similar to ectodermally derived mammalian enamel. (*Electron micrograph, ×34,000*)

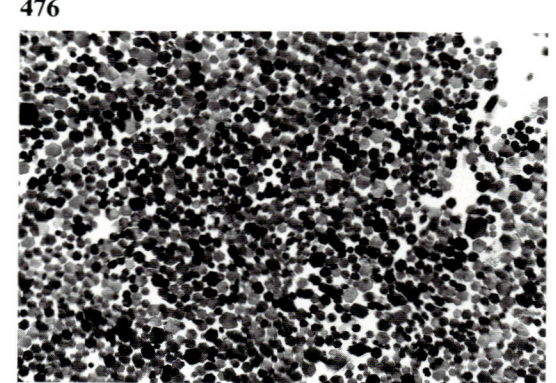

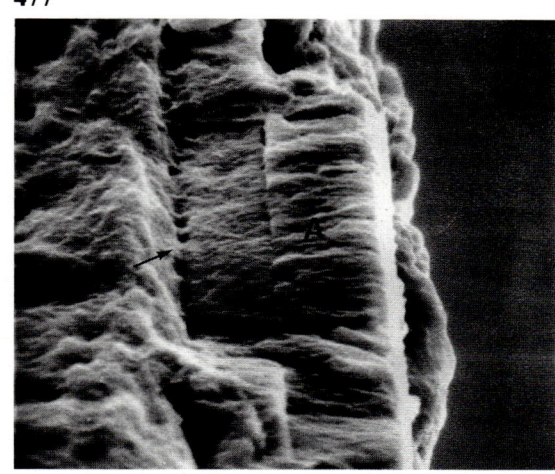

477 Fractured coelacanth tooth (*Latimeria chalumnae*). Although the outer covering of fish teeth is mesodermally derived, that of the teeth of the lobe-finned fish, the coelacanth, is thought to be ectodermally derived, non-prismatic enamel (A). Note the alignment of the enamel crystallites parallel to the surface. Ectodermal enamel may also be present on the tooth plates of the lung-fishes, creatures distantly related to the coelacanth. The arrow indicates the enamel-dentine junction. (*Scanning electron micrograph,* × 3,800)

Aprismatic enamel

The outer covering of reptilian and adult amphibian teeth is a thin layer of ectodermally derived enamel which appears relatively structureless.

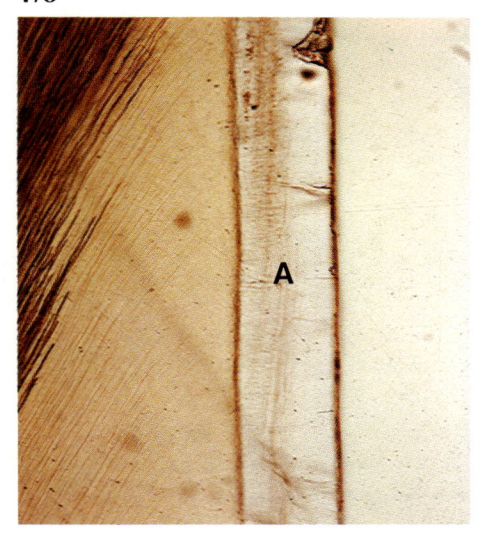

478 Longitudinal, ground section of a crocodile tooth (*Crocodilus niloticus*) showing aprismatic enamel (A). Some incremental lines may be seen running parallel with the enamel surface. (× 130)

The aprismatic nature of this enamel results from the parallel arrangement of all the crystallites at right angles to the enamel surface, there being no sudden changes in crystallite orientation. The parallel orientation of the crystallites is thought to be associated with the flattened secretory ends of the ameloblasts.

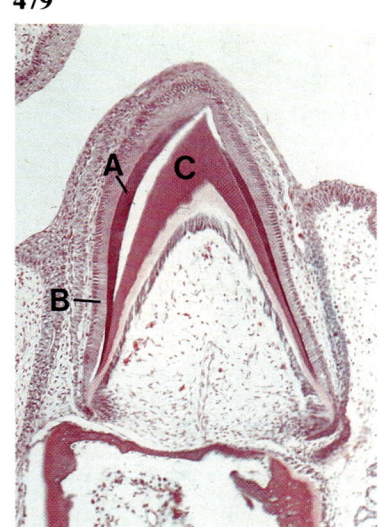

479 Decalcified, longitudinal section through a developing tooth of the green lizard (*Lacerta viridis*). The enamel matrix (A) is secreted by the ameloblasts (B). Dentine (C) formation precedes enamel formation. (*H&E,* × 80)

Though the aprismatic enamel of adult amphibians is of ectodermal origin, the teeth of the larval forms of Urodeles (e.g. axolotls, newts, salamanders) have a covering of *enameloid*.

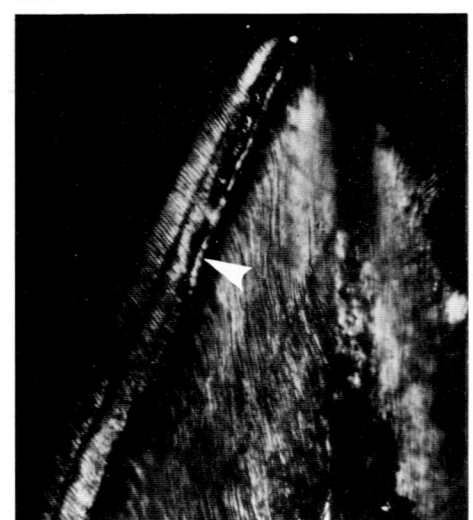 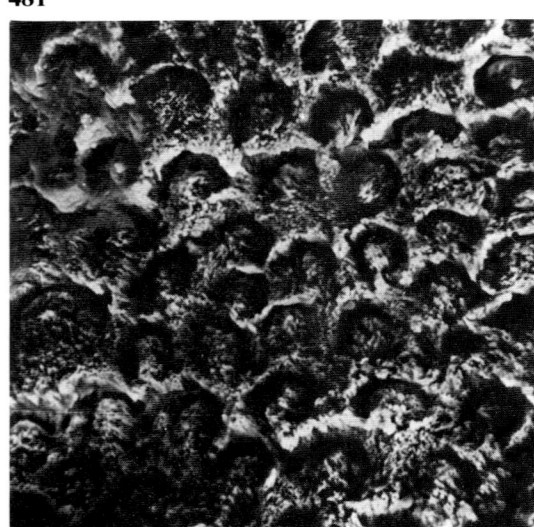

480 Longitudinal ground section of a tooth of the spiny-tailed lizard (*Uromastyx hardwicki*). Unlike all other reptiles, the enamel covering the teeth of a spiny-tailed lizard is prismatic. The section shown is viewed under polarised light between crossed polars which have been rotated towards extinction position. The amelodentinal junction is arrowed. (×50)

481 Cross-sectional view of enamel prisms in the spiny-tailed lizard (*Uromastyx hardwicki*). The enamel has been treated with a complexing agent which has preferentially dissolved the peripheral parts of the prisms, thereby highlighting the prismatic nature of the enamel. (*Scanning electron micrograph,* ×1,700)

Prismatic enamel

The evolutionary change from aprismatic to prismatic enamel appears to have occurred in the early mammals of the Cretaceous period.

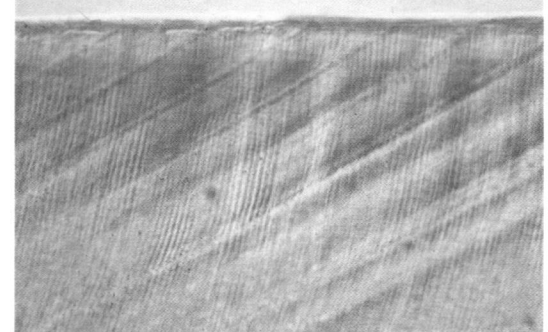 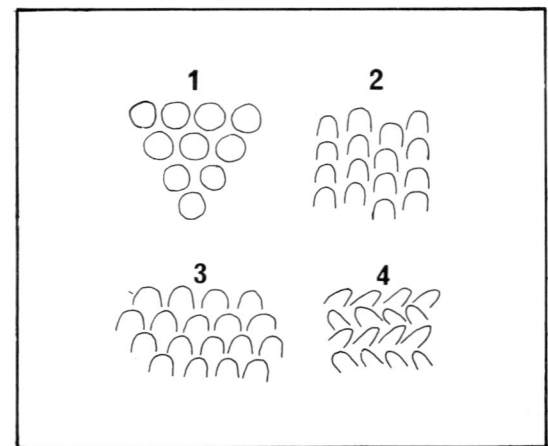

482 Ground longitudinal section through human enamel showing rods or prisms running approximately perpendicular to the enamel surface. As indicated previously, the prisms reflect the changing arrangements of crystallite orientation at the prism core and prism boundary. (×150)

483 Different types of prism patterns seen in mammalian enamel cut in cross-section.
Pattern 1 Complete cylindrical prism boundaries. This pattern predominates in the Sirenia, Chiroptera, Insectivora and Odontoceti.
Pattern 2 Longitudinal rows of prisms. This pattern predominates in Ungulates and the Macropodidae (Marsupialia).
Pattern 3 This arrangement is characteristic of human enamel though patterns 1 and 2 may also be found.
Pattern 4 This pattern is characterised by decussation of alternate transverse rows of prisms. It is seen in the inner enamel of Murine incisors.

Tubular enamel is a specialised form of prismatic enamel found in all marsupials (excepting the rodent-like teeth of the wombat *Phascolomis*) and in many placental mammals, including the hyrax and certain insectivores and lemurs.

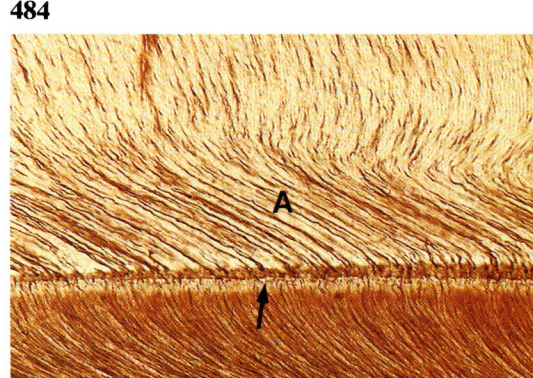

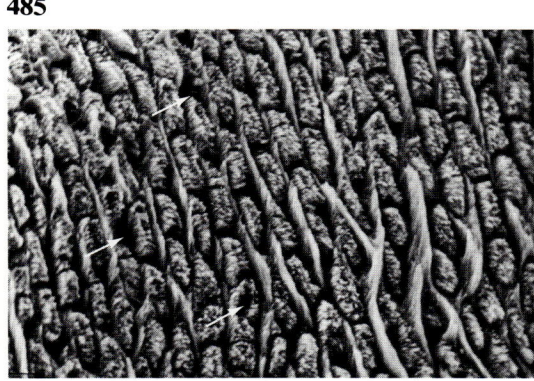

484 Longitudinal, ground section through tubular enamel (A) of a kangaroo (*Macropus rufus*). As the name suggests, tubular enamel is characterised by the presence of tubules running through the prismatic enamel. The tubules may be located both intraprismatically and interprismatically and appear to be continuous with the underlying dentinal tubules. The amelodentinal junction is arrowed. It has been suggested that, during development, the enamel tubules contain cell processes which are extensions of the ameloblast. An alternative explanation attempts to homologise the enamel tubule with the human enamel spindle. Thus, according to this theory, the enamel tubules are thought to develop around odontoblast processes. (×100)

485 Transverse section through the tubular prismatic enamel of a kangaroo (*Macropus rufus*). The enamel tubules are arrowed. The surface has been acid-etched to display the prisms which are of the pattern 2 type (see figure **483**). (*Scanning electron micrograph,* ×1,000)

Dentine

Two basic types of dentine may be recognised in living vertebrates; vasodentine and orthodentine. Orthodentine is characterised by the presence of tubules within the tissue, while, in the main, vasodentine is devoid of tubules, having vascular channels within it.

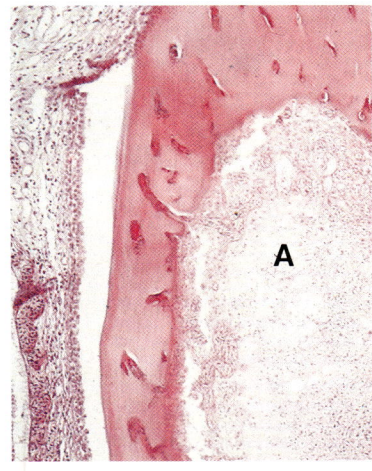

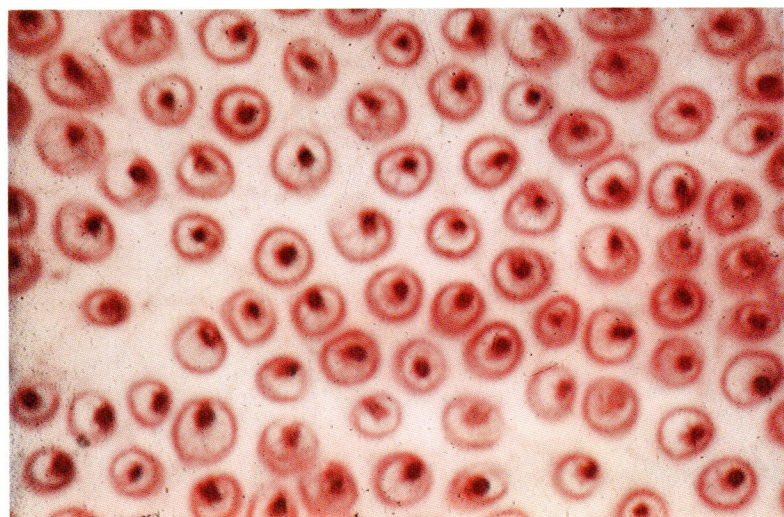

486 Decalcified, longitudinal section of a hake tooth (*Merluccius merluccius*) showing vasodentine. In the forming dentine of some fish, blood capillaries become entrapped. Tubules may be scarce or absent within the vasodentine. The significance of the capillaries within the vasodentine is not known. A, pulp. (*H&E,* ×90)

487 Ground, transverse section through the tubules of human orthodentine viewed in red light. (×1,500)

Unlike human orthodentine which is arranged around a single pulp chamber, the orthodentine of crossopterygian fishes, many fossil amphibians (especially the so-called 'labyrinthodonts') and a few lizards is arranged as a series of complicated folds of the pulp. Such dentine is referred to as plicidentine.

488 Ground, transverse section showing plicidentine at the base of a tooth of a monitor lizard (*Veranus sp.*). Note the folds of dentine, each with a central core of pulp tissue. (×8)

489 High power view of plicidentine of a monitor lizard (*Veranus sp.*) showing tubular nature of the dentine. (×30)

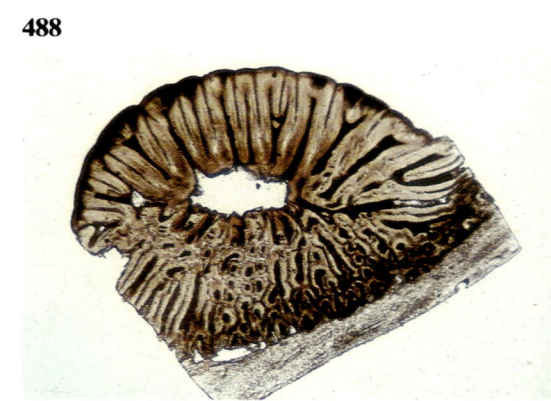
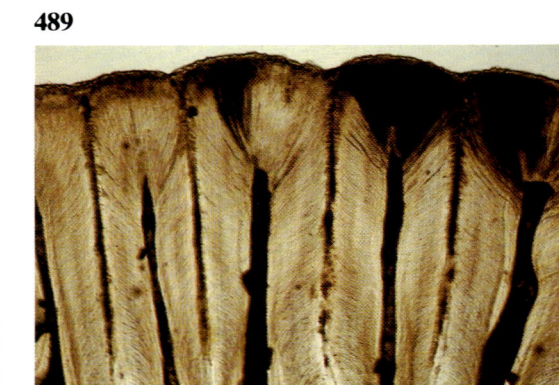

In some fish there is no clearly defined pulp cavity. Instead, the pulp cavity becomes divided by dentinal trabeculae. Because this tissue has a resemblance to bone, it has been termed osteodentine.

490 Longitudinal, ground section through a tooth of an eagle ray (*Myliobatis aquilla*) showing osteodentine. The osteodentine (A) shown here is regularly arranged in the form of parallel trabeculae. B, covering enameloid. C, pulp spaces. (*Basic fuchsin*, ×80)

491 Decalcified cross-section through osteodentine in a tooth of an eagle ray (*Myliobatis aquilla*). In cross-section, the osteodentine is seen to be traversed by vascular pulp canals (A) which are surrounded by concentric laminae of dentine termed denteons (B). Unlike bone, however, these laminae do not contain cells but house the processes of odontoblasts whose cell bodies line the vascular spaces. Between the denteons lies calcified interstitial tissue (C) which is generally devoid of cells. (*Mallory*, ×65)

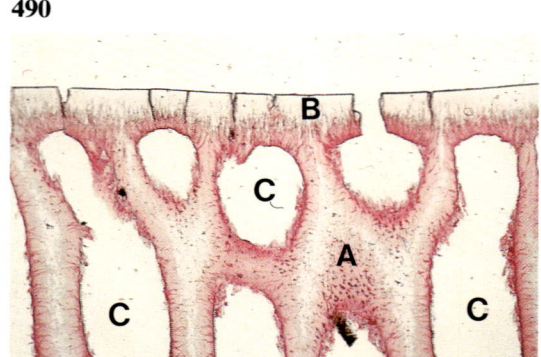
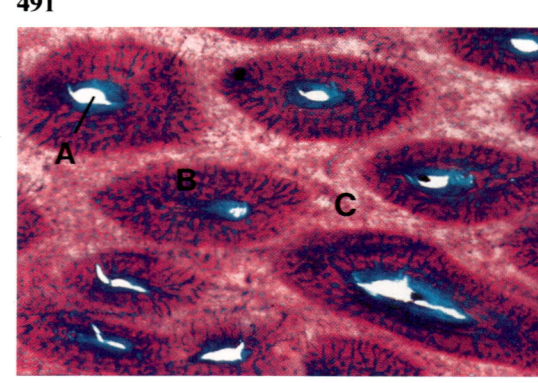

492 Decalcified, transverse section through part of the jaw of a blue shark (*Prionace glauca*) showing stages in the development of osteodentine. The section shows two teeth from the same tooth family, the lower tooth being the younger. Beneath the orthodentine (A), at the base of the younger tooth, osteodentine (B) in the form of dentinal trabeculae is being formed within the pulp chamber. In the older tooth, osteodentine formation is well advanced. Note that the osteodentine is more irregularly arranged compared with that of the eagle ray (figure **490**). (*Gomori-reticulum and van Gieson*, ×16)

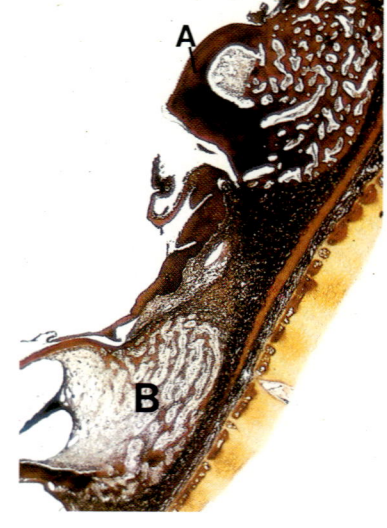

Types of tooth attachment

The attachment of teeth to the jaws may be accomplished either by means of a fibrous ligament or by direct union or ankylosis of the tooth to bone.

A variety of *fibrous tooth attachments* have been described, and these may be conveniently classified according to whether or not the teeth are socketed.

1 *Teeth without sockets* (a) Continuous fibrous attachment
　　　　　　　　　　　　(b) Local fibrous attachment
　　　　　　　　　　　　(c) Hinged attachment

2 *Teeth with sockets*　　(a) Thecodont gomphosis
　　　　　　　　　　　　(b) Gomphosis

493 Ground, transverse section through the jaw of a thornback ray (*Raia clavata*) demonstrating the continuous fibrous attachment of the teeth typical of elasmobranch fish. The bases of the teeth are attached to a sheet of connective tissue (*arrowed*) which overlies the jaw cartilages (D). The teeth are continuously replaced, being generated from a persistent dental lamina low down on the inner aspect of the jaw (immediately below position A). From this site they migrate around the jaw to become functional at or about position B. The teeth are shed at the front of the jaw (position C). ($\times 16$)

494 Decalcified, longitudinal section through the tooth of a piranha (*Serrasalmus rhombeus*) showing a local fibrous attachment. In this bony fish, each tooth is connected separately to the bone of the jaws by a narrow ring of fibrous tissue (*arrowed*) which here stains a darker green than either the dentine (A) or bone (B). The tip of a replacing tooth (C) is seen below the functional tooth. (*Masson's trichrome, $\times 80$*)

495 Decalcified, longitudinal section through a tooth in an eel (*Anguilla anguilla*). In this bony fish, instead of the fibrous attachment (A) of the tooth being inserted directly into the bone of the jaw, there is an intervening cell-free pedicel (B) composed of calcified collagen whose matrix is secreted by the odontoblasts. C, dentine. D, bone of jaw. (*Berenbaum's Sudan black, $\times 80$*)

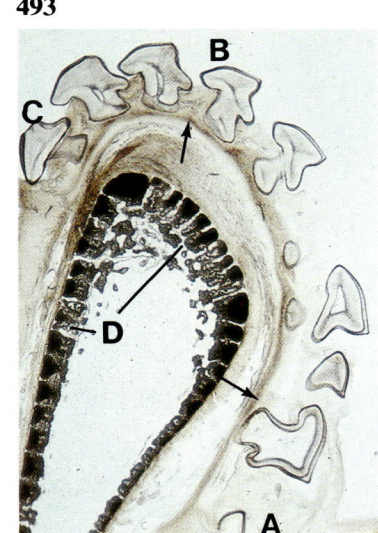

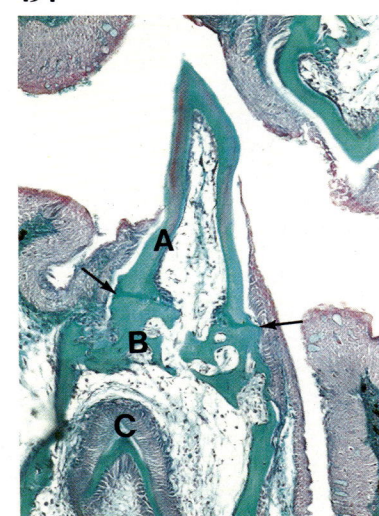

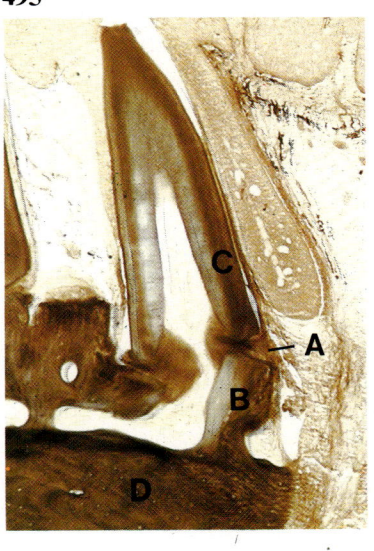

The degree of movement during feeding associated with fibrous attachments of teeth will depend, in part, on the length, distribution and elasticity of the fibres. In the above examples, there is relatively little movement of the teeth. However, in a number of carnivorous fishes, modification of the fibrous attachment may produce a hinged attachment which allows a greater range of movement.

496 Longitudinal decalcified section of a hake's tooth (*Merluccius merluccius*) showing an example of a hinged attachment. Prey entering the mouth will depress and pass over the hinged teeth which will subsequently spring upright should the prey try to leave the mouth to make its escape. The base of the outer part of the tooth (A) lies above the base of the inner part. The fibrous attachment between the base of the outer surface of the tooth and the jaw prevents lateral displacement. As shown in this section, there is a small, midline region (*arrowed*) which lacks such a fibrous attachment. The attachment between the base of the inner surface of the tooth and the jaw is in two parts, an outer, stiffened portion (B), apparently of unmineralised dentine which is elastic, and an inner fibrous portion (C). When the tooth is pushed back the outer band buckles, its subsequent recoil returning the tooth to the upright position when the load is removed from the tooth. (*Picro-indigo-carmine*, × 32)

497 Radiograph of a crocodile (*Crocodilus niloticus*) lower jaw showing a thecodont attachment. The Crocodilia are unique amongst the non-mammalian vertebrates in having roots situated in deep sockets to which they are attached by a periodontal ligament. In the radiograph, a radiolucent, periodontal space can be seen surrounding the teeth. The root surfaces of the teeth are covered with a layer of cementum. The socket in this thecodont condition differs from the gomphosis associated with mammalian teeth in that it is permanent and does not undergo significant remodelling, successive replacing teeth (*arrowed*) occupying the same socket.

498 Mammalian gomphosis is characterised by the independent development of successional teeth within their own sockets. A, deciduous tooth. B, permanent successor. (*H&E*, × 3)

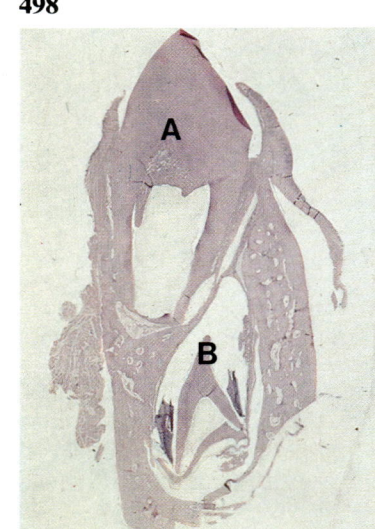

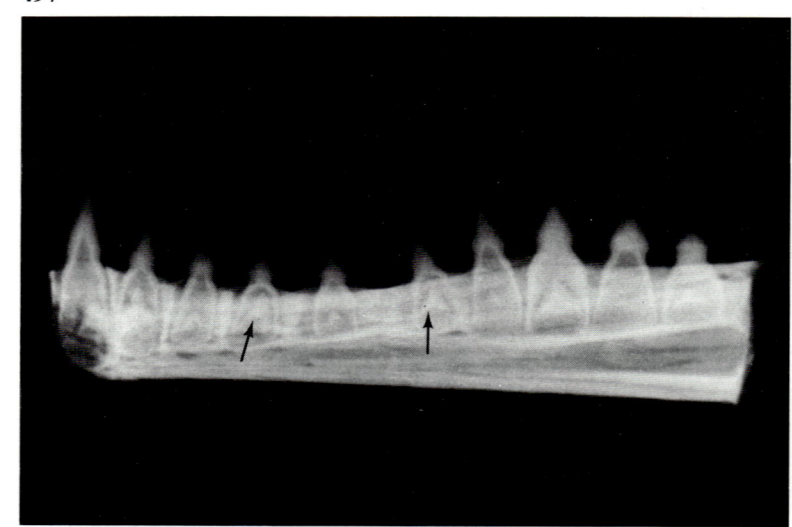

Bony attachment or *ankylosis* occurs commonly throughout the non-mammalian vertebrates.

499 Longitudinal decalcified section of a trout tooth (*Salmo gairdneri*) illustrating attachment by ankylosis. Note the attachment of dentine (A) directly to the bone of the jaw (B), without the intervention of fibrous tissue. (*Masson's trichrome, × 32*)

500 In reptiles, two basic types of ankylosis may be recognised. Pleurodont ankylosis (A) refers to the attachment of a tooth to the inner margin of the bone of the jaw. Acrodont ankylosis (B) refers to an attachment to the crest of the bone. Acrodont teeth are not replaced, pleurodont teeth are replaced.

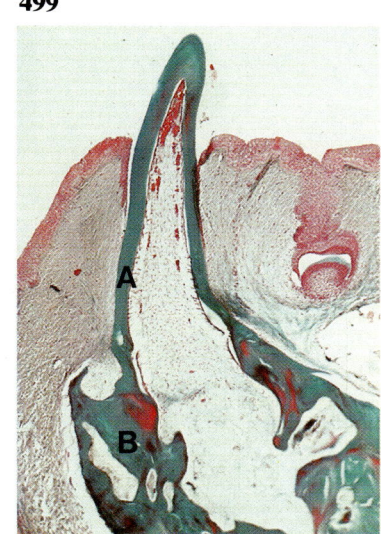

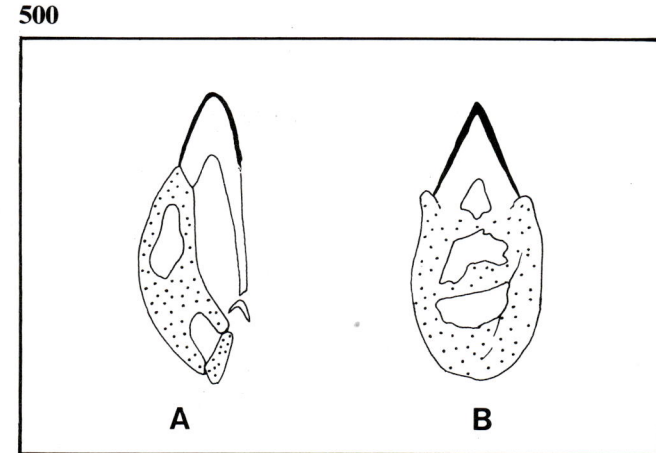

Tooth replacement

The teeth of most non-mammalian vertebrates are replaced throughout life (polyphyodonty), though in some animals – for example the chamaeleon (*Chamaeleo*) – the teeth are not replaced (monophyodonty). In polyphyodont dentitions, the speed of tooth replacement slows down with age, successive replacing teeth remaining functional for progressively longer periods. During growth of the animal, increase in jaw size is associated with an increase in tooth size. In some animals, for example the trout (*Salmo gairdneri*) and the green lizard (*Lacerta viridis*), the tooth number increases with growth of the animal, though in other species, for example the piranha (*Serrasalmus*), the tooth number remains constant. The rate of tooth replacement varies considerably. Teeth of young lemon sharks (*Negaprion brevirostris*) are replaced on average every nine days but may be functional for as little as two days. In young rainbow trout (*Salmo gairdneri*), teeth may be replaced every 10 to 18 weeks, and similar values have been obtained in lizards (see page 194).

From measurements of a series of jaws and teeth of crocodiles (*Crocodilus niloticus*), it has been calculated that during its lifespan there are about 50 replacements at each tooth position. The time interval between tooth loss and succession varies in different animals.

Teeth appear to have relatively fixed lifespans and are replaced whether or not they are worn. Tooth replacement generally occurs throughout the year but in the mud-puppy (*Necturus maculatus*), for example, replacement appears to be seasonal.

Should several adjacent teeth in a jaw be shed simultaneously, then extensive regions along the jaw might remain edentulous for a considerable period. Clearly, this situation would be disadvantageous. However, in those animals which have been studied, waves of tooth replacement pass through *alternate* tooth positions, thus generally ensuring that at any one time at least every alternate tooth is functional.

501 Lower jaw of the green lizard (*Lacerta viridis*) viewed medially (reconstructed model). The model shows both functional and replacing teeth at different stages of development. The arrangement of the teeth may appear random, especially when comparing adjacent teeth. However, if alternate teeth are compared a recognisable pattern emerges. Thus, starting for instance at tooth position 16 (*arrowed*), this tooth has recently erupted and, as yet, no successor is evident. As one progresses anteriorly through tooth positions 14, 12, 10, 8 and 6 the replacing teeth are at progressively younger stages of development. Thus, it can be assumed that these teeth will successively erupt in an alternate sequence from back to front.

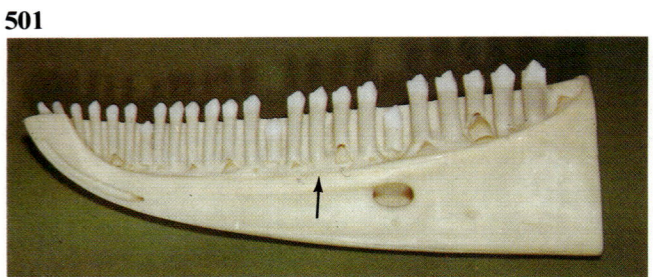

502 The same model as **501** with the waves of tooth replacement passing through alternate tooth positions being indicated by coloured wire.

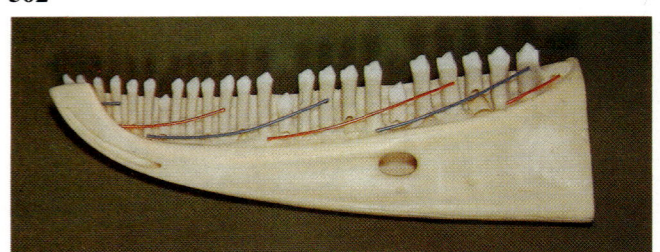

Though the sequence of tooth succession can be predicted from observations on the stages of development of the teeth in skeletal material, the precise pattern and timing of the sequence of eruption can only be adequately demonstrated by studies on living animals involving observations of the teeth at frequent, discrete intervals. Such studies have been undertaken in fish and reptiles either by taking dental impressions or radiographs.

503 A dental chart constructed from a series of dental impressions of teeth in an upper jaw quadrant of a lizard (*Lacerta bedriagae sardoa*) over a period of 7 months. The lizard was an adult female with a length from snout to vent of 7.5cm. The open circles show the period over which a tooth was functional. Small, closed circles indicate when teeth were emerging into the mouth. Blank spaces show unoccupied tooth positions. In the quadrant 23 teeth were present, the most anterior tooth being represented on the right side of the chart. The solid oblique lines are replacement waves which slope from the back forwards, passing through alternate tooth positions.

From the chart it can be seen that at no time are adjacent tooth positions simultaneously unoccupied. The posterior teeth have a longer life-cycle than the anterior teeth. Though the replacement waves here slope forwards, in other reptiles the waves may slope backwards. Perfect alternation (seen in the slow worm (*Anguis fragilis*)) would be indicated by a horizontal replacement wave.

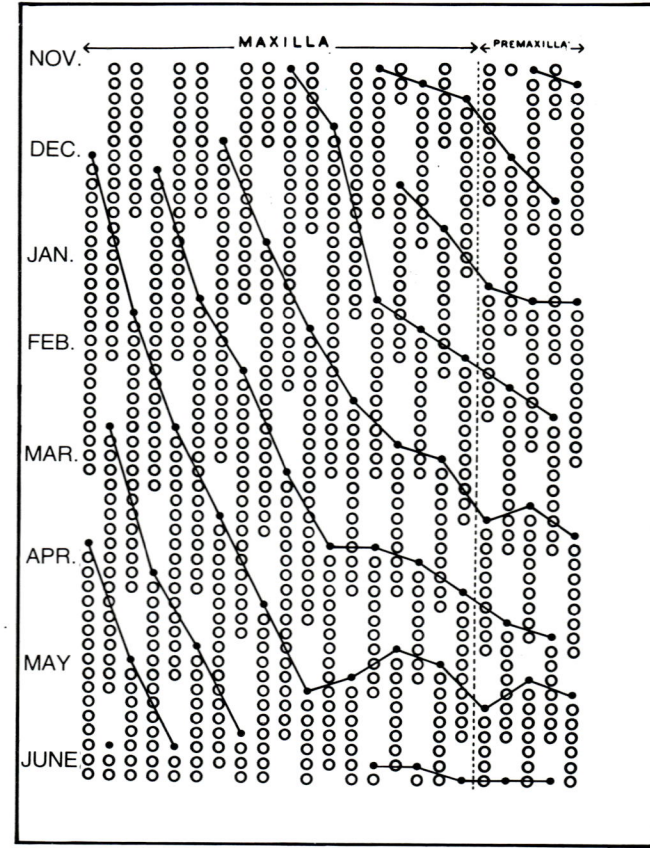

The underlying control mechanisms responsible for organising replacement patterns are not known. One view interprets these patterns as resulting from stimuli which initiate tooth production at individual loci, passing along the dental lamina from tooth position to tooth position. Alternatively, it has been suggested that control of replacement is a local mechanism involving the inhibition of growth of a tooth germ by adjacent teeth. According to this view, development of a tooth germ will only proceed when the inhibition is removed by migration of the adjacent maturing teeth towards the functional position.

504 An exception to the rule concerning alternate tooth replacement in non-mammalian vertebrates is the piranha (*Serrasalmus*). In each jaw quadrant the teeth are interlocked (see figure **514**), functioning as a single unit. Therefore, teeth in each quadrant develop and are replaced almost simultaneously. Also, each half of the jaw is generally out of phase with the other half. Thus, the radiographs illustrated show all the replacing teeth in one half of the lower jaw at the same advanced stage of development while in the opposite half of the lower jaw none of the replacing teeth has yet begun to calcify.

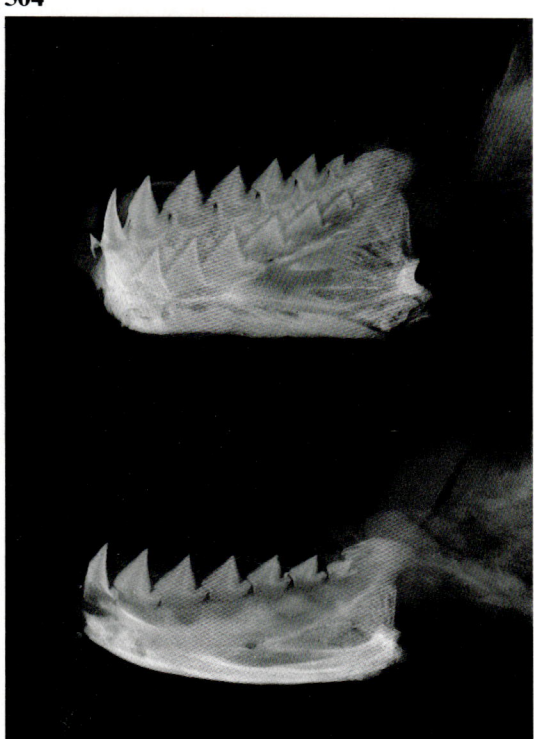

In mammals there is usually evidence of two dentitions (diphyodonty), though there are many examples (e.g. cetaceans, certain rodents and edentates) where only a single dentition develops. In such cases it is difficult to homologise this dentition with either a deciduous or a permanent series.

Features of vertebrate dentitions

Dentition of fishes

Agnatha

505 Mouth of a sea lamprey (*Petromyzon marinus*). The living agnathans, as represented by the lampreys and hagfishes, do not possess true calcified teeth. They attach themselves to other fish by means of a sucker-like mouth and rasp off flesh by means of horny teeth. In the sea lamprey, these horny teeth are arranged circumferentially and are of different shapes and sizes. Horny teeth can also be seen on the tongue in the centre of the mouth.

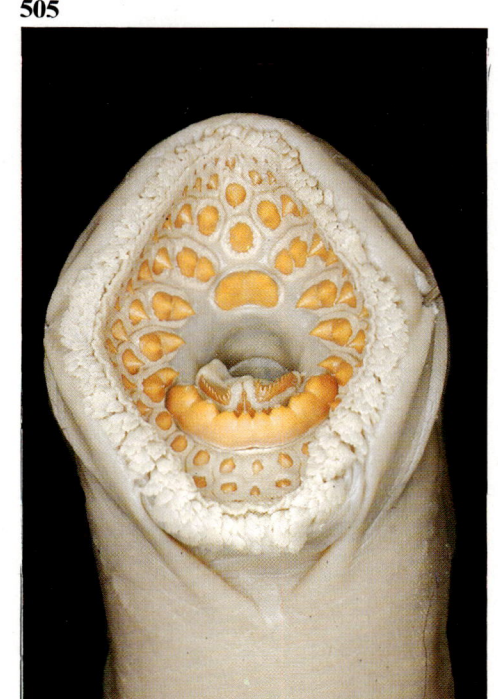

Chondrichthyes

In the cartilaginous fishes (and also bony fishes), all types of dental specialisations may be seen. The dentition is generally homodont and polyphyodont and the teeth are covered by enameloid. Large numbers of teeth are usually present.

506 Lower jaw of a Porbeagle shark (*Lemna nasus*). The teeth of sharks are triangular with sharp, serrated, cutting edges. In addition to the main cusp, subsidiary cusps may be present near the base. The teeth are arranged in rows. As well as the functional tooth row, a number of rows of replacing teeth at varying stages of development lie against the inner surface of the jaw. The rate of tooth replacement is rapid.

507 Lower jaw of a monk fish (*Squatina squatina*). In some carnivorous elasmobranchs, the teeth become erect when the jaw is opened. Photograph **507A** shows some teeth in the lower jaw which is only partly opened. In photograph **507B** the jaw is fully opened and the teeth become erect with more of the underlying replacement teeth being seen. This uprighting of the teeth is brought about by means of fibres which run out from the bases of the teeth and become interwoven with a band of fibrous tissue which surrounds the jaw cartilages.

508 Cross-section of the lower jaw of a blue shark (*Prionace glauca*). This shows a functional tooth (A) beneath which can be seen three successional teeth (S_1, S_2, and S_3) at progressively younger stages of development. B, continuous fibrous band. C, Meckel's cartilage. (*Gomori-reticulin and van Gieson, ×8*)

509 Dentition of a thornback ray (*Raia clavata*) viewed anteriorly. Unlike the sharks whose teeth specialise in cutting, the dentition of rays (and skates) is adapted for crushing molluscs and other shelled creatures. The teeth are blunt and crowded together forming a 'mosaic pavement' pattern. Teeth are continuously generated posteriorly and carried anteriorly into function where they are eventually exfoliated (see figure **493**).

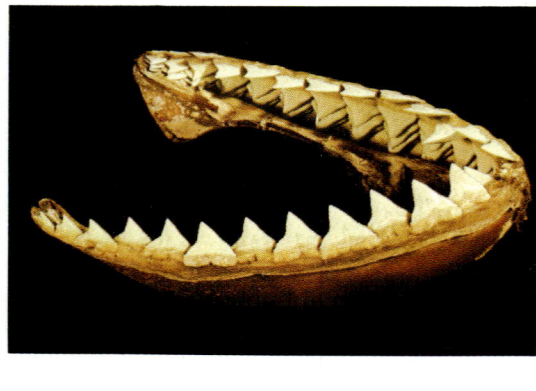

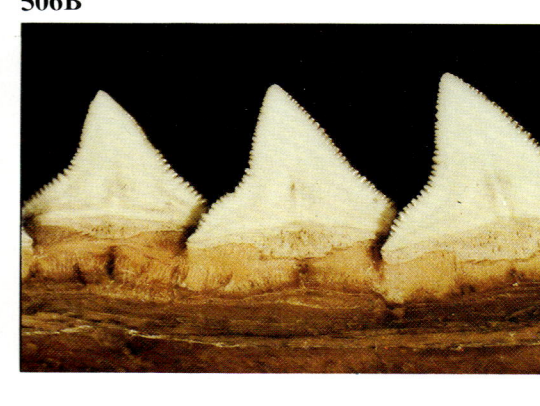

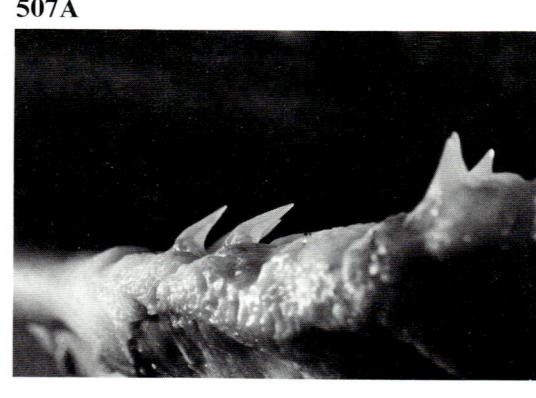

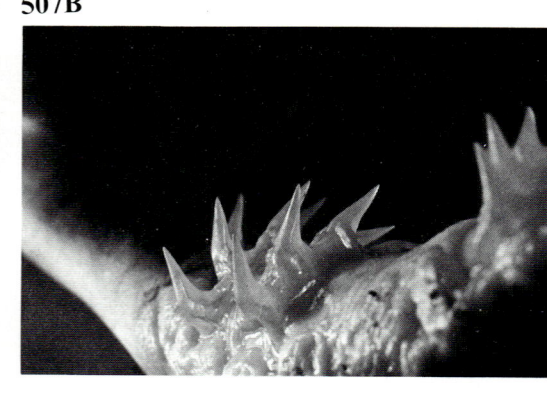

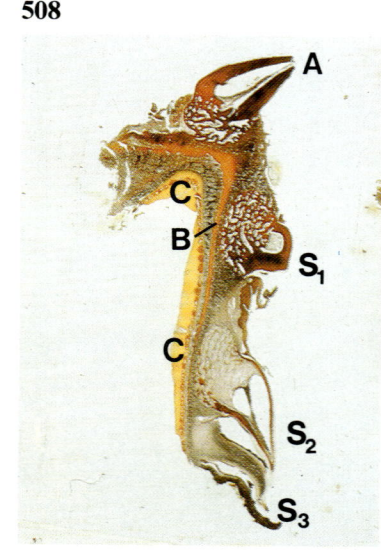

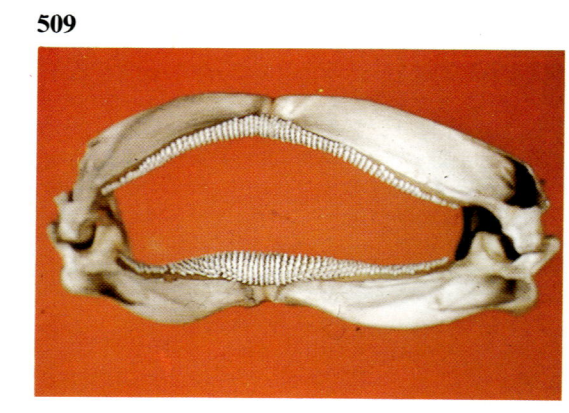

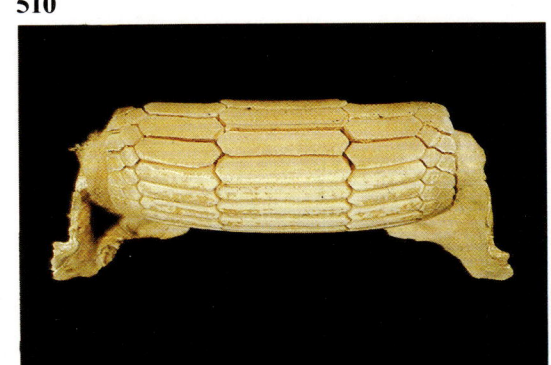

510 Occlusal view of the teeth of an eagle ray (*Myliobatis aquilla*). The teeth are arranged in the form of a mosaic pavement. The central teeth are elongated transversely and interdigitate laterally with hexagonally-shaped teeth.

Osteichthyes

Though a number of bony fish lack teeth (e.g. sturgeon (*Acipenser*)), the teeth of bony fish tend to be conical in shape (i.e. haplodont) and are primarily used for prehension. The dentition is polyphyodont.

511 Trout (*Salmo gairdneri*). A large number of small, conical teeth are ankylosed to the marginal bones of the jaws. However, teeth in bony fish are not necessarily restricted to the marginal jaw bones but may be found on a number of other bones lining the mouth and also within the pharynx. In the trout, for example, teeth are also present in the roof of the mouth, on the vomer and palatine bones, and on the tongue.

512 The lower jaw of an angler fish (*Lophius piscatorius*). The buccal surface shows two main rows of recurved, conical teeth. The outer row of smaller teeth is ankylosed to the jaw. The teeth of the inner row have a hinged-type of tooth attachment. **512B** shows one of the hinged teeth (*arrowed*) bent inwards.

513 Heterodonty in fish. Though the teeth of fish are generally homodont, examples of heterodonty can be found. This illustration shows the lower right jaw quadrant of a sheepshead fish (*Sargus ovis*) from the medial side. The anterior teeth are incisiform in shape and are used to prise shellfish from rocks. The rounded and elongated posterior teeth are used for crushing.

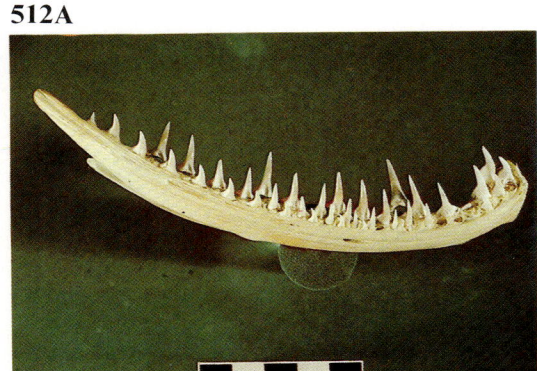

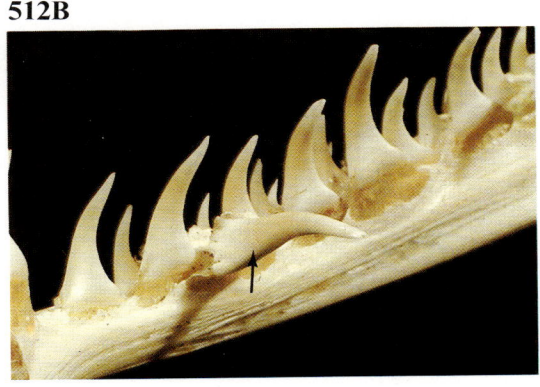

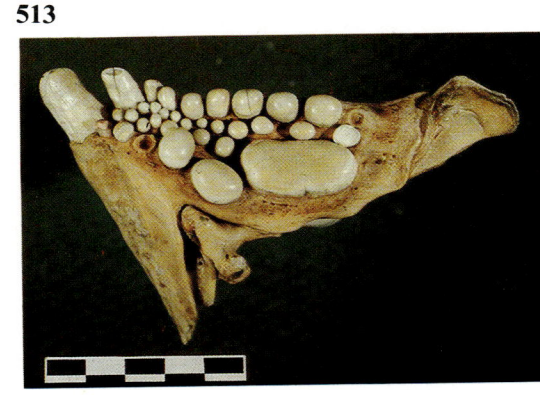

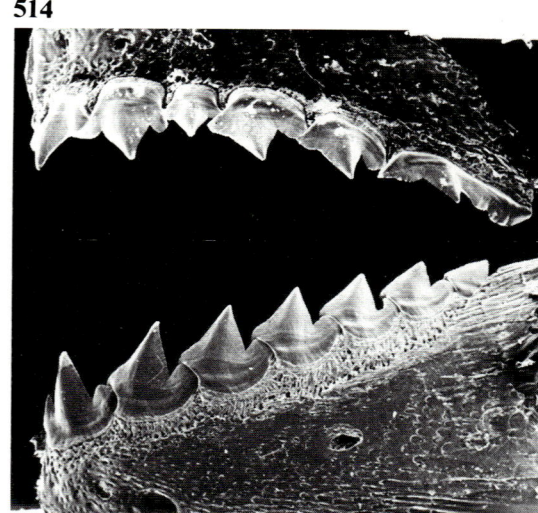

514 The dentition of a piranha (*Serrasalmus rhombeus*). The dentition of this fish is highly specialised for a carnivorous diet. There are six upper and seven lower, narrow, blade-like teeth. The sixth upper tooth is considerably elongated and is the main slicing component of the upper jaw. The lower teeth, especially, show a remarkable degree of interlocking which produces an almost continuous cutting unit. On jaw closure, the lower four posterior teeth pass upwards and inwards against the elongated upper posterior tooth. The close interlocking of the teeth necessitates that eruption occurs almost simultaneously in any jaw quadrant (see figure **504**). (*Scanning electron micrograph*)

Dentitions of amphibia

Where present, the teeth are small, homodont and polyphyodont and are used primarily for prehension.

515 Frog (*Rana temporaria*). Small teeth are present on the upper jaw. The teeth are homodont, haplodont (cone-shaped), ankylosed and polyphyodont. No teeth are present on the lower jaw.

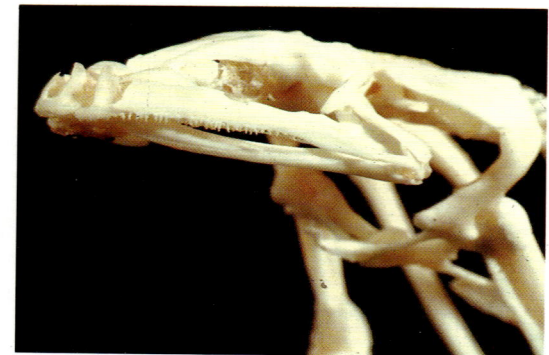

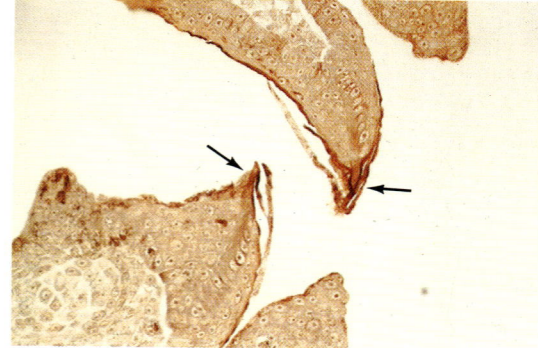

516 Transverse section through the jaws of a tadpole (*Rana temporaria*) showing horny teeth (*arrowed*). The horny teeth are in the form of columns of proliferating epithelial cells which keratinize as they approach the surface. (*Haematoxylin and van Gieson, × 100*)

517 Mud-puppy (*Necturus maculatus*). A double row of teeth is present in the upper jaw, the anterior and outer row being on the premaxilla, the posterior and inner row being on the maxilla. On each dentary there is a single row of teeth. Tooth replacement is not continuous throughout the year but is apparently seasonal.

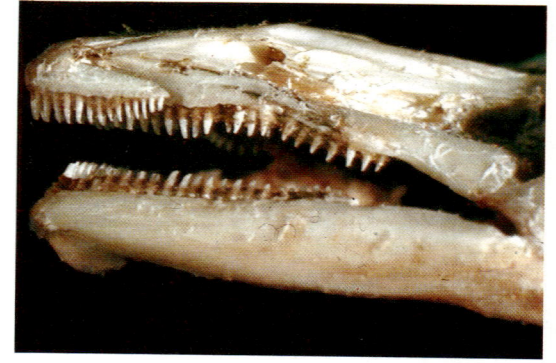

Dentition of reptiles

In general, the teeth are homodont and polyphyodont. In shape, the teeth tend to be tricuspid or haplodont. Except for the Crocodilia, the teeth are ankylosed. The enamel is ectodermal and non-prismatic (except for *Uromastyx*, see page 188).

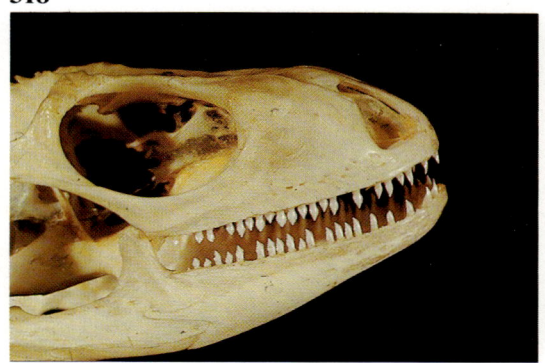

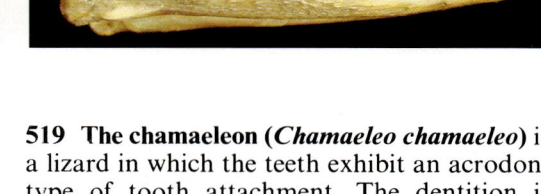

518 The iguana (*Iguana iguana*). A number of small, conical teeth having a pleurodont ankylosis are present. Along the margins of the jaws of this lizard, gaps in the dentition indicate sites where a tooth has been exfoliated and not yet been replaced.

519 The chamaeleon (*Chamaeleo chamaeleo*) is a lizard in which the teeth exhibit an acrodont type of tooth attachment. The dentition is monophyodont.

There is usually considerable movement (kinesis) between the upper jaw and the cranium of lizards. This allows for a wider gape and more complex prey-grasping and swallowing mechanisms than would be possible if all the gapes were achieved by movement of the mandible alone. In snakes, the degree of mobility of the mouthparts is even greater.

The dentition of the bearded lizard (*Amphibolurus barbartus*, figure **468**) is unusual in that the extreme anterior teeth are pleurodont while the remaining teeth are acrodont. Though there is some replacement of the anterior pleurodont teeth, there is no replacement of the posterior acrodont teeth. The number of teeth in the dentition increases with age by addition of teeth at the posterior end of the row, this being somewhat analogous to the replacement pattern in mammals.

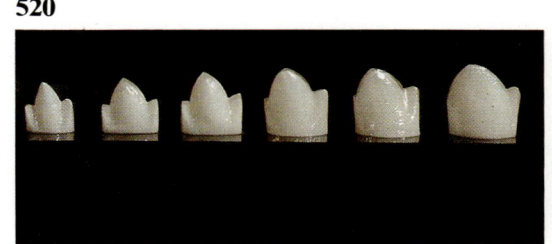

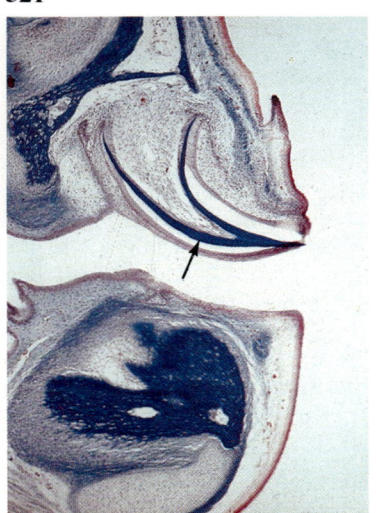

520 Comparing the teeth of young and old reptiles, a change in crown morphology may be seen. The models show the changing tooth morphology in the green lizard (*Lacerta viridis*). The 'young' tooth form on the left is tricuspid, the 'old' tooth form on the right bicuspid. ($\times 10$)

521 Egg teeth. In the embryos of lizards and snakes an egg tooth, generally a single, median tooth, develops on the premaxilla. The egg tooth is used by the embryo to break out of its shell and is shed soon afterwards. The section illustrated is a median longitudinal section through the head of a developing rainbow lizard (*Agama agama*). The egg tooth (*arrowed*) is a true tooth, being composed primarily of dentine. Whether or not there is a thin covering of enamel has yet to be fully investigated. (*Masson's blue trichrome*, $\times 40$)

522 Egg tooth of the rainbow lizard (*Agama agama*) – model. A, lateral view. B, view from above showing pulp chamber. (× 50)

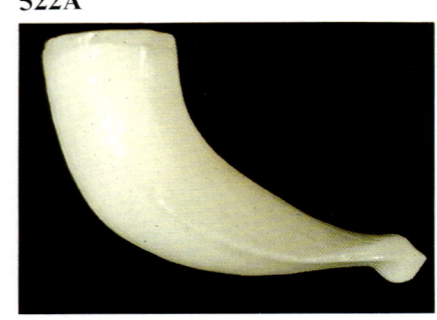
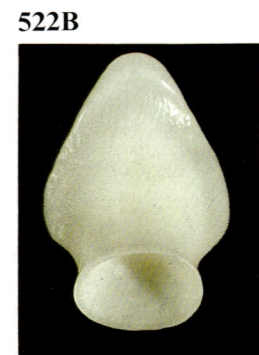

522A   522B

Some lizard embryos possess teeth which are resorbed without becoming functional.

523 Alligator (*Alligator mississippiensis*). The dentition is homodont and the teeth are conical. The upper and lower teeth interdigitate and are used for prehension. There is variation in the size of some of the teeth along the jaw (the first, fourth and eleventh in the lower, and the fourth and tenth teeth in the upper jaw being enlarged). The enlarged lower teeth pass inside the upper teeth (unlike the situation in the crocodile, *Crocodilus*, where the enlarged lower teeth fit into deep notches on the outer side of the upper jaw). The teeth are socketed and the successional teeth erupt into the same sockets as their predecessors (thecodont gomphosis). The roots of the teeth have a covering of cementum and show wide-open apices. The skull is non-kinetic, the bones of the upper jaw being fixed rigidly to the braincase.

524 Python (*Python sp.*) is a non-poisonous snake which kills its prey by crushing. The teeth are conical, recurved and used for prehension. Two rows of ankylosed teeth are present in the upper jaw, an outer row on the premaxilla and maxilla and an inner row on the palatine and pterygoid bones. A single row of teeth is present on the dentary.

The successional teeth move vertically upwards until, near the surface, they assume a horizontal position, though they finally erupt vertically. This horizontal positioning may prevent injury to the mucous membrane from the unerupted teeth during distension of the jaws which occurs when swallowing prey.

525 Adder (*Vipera berus*). This snake poisons its prey. The venom is produced by the parotid gland from which it passes into a canal lying within the dentine of the fangs. This enlarged tooth (A) alone occupies the short maxilla and only one is usually functional at any one time. The fang is erected for use. Ankylosed, recurved teeth are also present in both jaws.

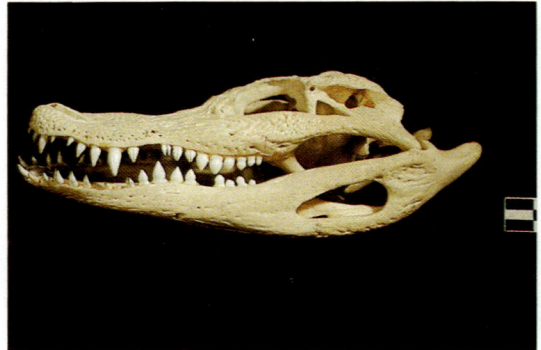

523

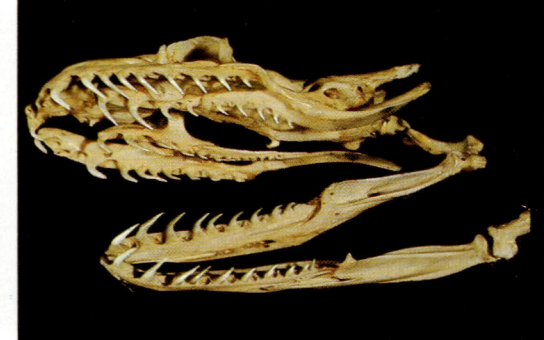

524

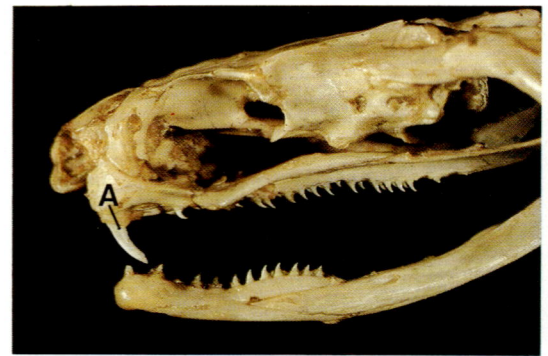

525

526 Ground, transverse section of a poison fang of a puff-adder (*Bitis arietans*). In some poisonous snakes, such as the sea snake (*Hydrophis*), the poison from the parotid gland runs along a groove on the surface of the fang. In other snakes, the poison runs along a poison canal. In the puff-adder, the poison canal (A) lies completely within the dentine (B) of the tooth, the pulp chamber (C) occupying only a thin crescent-shaped space. ($\times 40$)

Dentitions of mammals

Unlike reptiles, the dentitions of mammals are generally heterodont and diphyodont. The mammalian dentition is composed of four different morphological types – incisors, canines, premolars and molars, the premolars and molars having a more complicated form associated with the ability to masticate food. The teeth are restricted to two rows, one in the mandible, the other in the maxilla. In adult placental mammals, there is generally a maximum of 11 teeth in each jaw quadrant ($I_3^3 \, C_1^1 \, P_4^4 \, M_3^3$).

In amphibians and reptiles, the teeth are used mainly for prehension, the prey being seized head first and swallowed whole. Jaw activity is associated with relatively simple up and down movements with little lateral displacement. In mammals, the shape of the molar teeth become broadened so that, with forceful jaw closure, food can be squashed between opposing occlusal surfaces and partly divided by the penetration of cusps. The ability to masticate and break down food in the mouth produces an enormous gain in digestive efficiency which is considered necessary for the high rate of metabolism associated with homothermy.

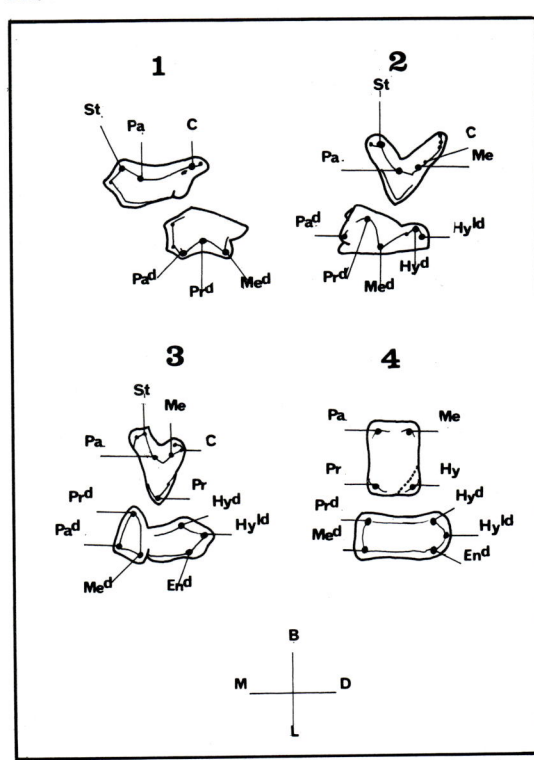

527 The evolution of the mammalian molar.
Upper teeth: Pa, paracone. Me, metacone. Pr, protocone. Hy, hypocone. C, C cusp. St, stylocone.
Lower teeth: Ra^d, paraconid. Me^d, metaconid. Pr^d, protoconid. Hy^d, hypoconid. Hy^{ld}, hypoconulid. En^d, entoconid.
The cross at the bottom of the figure gives the orientation of the mesial (M), distal (D), buccal (B) and lingual (L) surfaces.

1 *Kuehneotherium*. The cheek teeth of this early mammal (found in the late Triassic period) had, as those of reptiles, three cusps. However, the cusps were no longer in alignment, in the upper teeth the prominent paracone being situated more lingually, in the lower teeth the large protoconid being placed more buccally. The upper teeth interdigitate with the lower teeth, producing a scissor-like action without direct tooth contact.

2 *Peramus*. Compared to *Kuehneotherium*, the molars of this mammal (found in the late Jurassic period) showed the following additional cusps; a metacone in the upper molars and a hypocorid and hypoconulid in the lower molars. In the upper molars, there was also the beginnings of a new palatal cusp, the future protocone. The lower molars can be subdivided into an anterior triangular element, the trigonid, and a low posterior heel, the talonid. Like the molars of *Kuehneotherium*, there was no contact between upper and lower molars.

3 The molars of *Pappotherium* (a mid-cretaceous mammal) differ from *Peramus* in the following respects. The lower molars show an expanded talonid basin with an additional cusp, the entoconid. The upper molars show a well developed protocone which occludes into the talonid of the lower molars. This arrangement is consistent with masticatory activity. At this stage in its evolution, the upper molar with its triangular shape and its three main cusps (paracone, metacone and protocone) is termed a trigone. The stylocone and C-cusp are now considerably reduced in size.

4 The form of primate molars can be derived from the primitive tritubercular molar pattern typified by *Pappotherium*. In the upper molars, this is achieved by the addition of a further cusp, the hypocone, at the disto-palatal corner of the primitive trigone. In the lower molars, the cusps of the talonid are raised to the level of those on the trigonid. The paraconid in the first molar and the hypoconid in the second and third molars are lost.

Other features associated with mastication which are peculiar to mammals include:
A   A temporomandibular jaw articulation.
B   Salivary glands.
C   Prismatic enamel.
D   Diphyodonty.
E   Secondary palate.
F   Significant muscle development associated with lips, cheeks, tongue and muscles of mastication.
G   Gomphosis type of tooth attachment.

The development of a temporomandibular articulation and the muscles of mastication allow the force of the bite and the range of movement for chewing to be increased. Saliva moistens and lubricates the food during mastication. Its enzyme content allows digestion to commence at an early stage in the mouth. The prismatic arrangement of enamel and its greater thickness in mammals is said to be more efficient in resisting masticatory loads and attrition than non-prismatic enamel. The development of a secondary palate is thought to be related to the necessity of maintaining ventilation during prolonged masticatory periods. The development of muscles within the lips, cheeks and tongue is associated with manipulation of the bolus within the mouth. The change from polyphyodonty to diphyodonty has been related to a 'grinding-in' period necessary to produce an efficient cutting or grinding tooth surface, it seeming inefficient to replace such teeth too frequently. The gomphosis type of attachment may be associated with the increased stresses and strains brought to bear on the tooth during mastication.

The chewing cycle of mammals

Mammals generally chew on one side at a time. Two methods of chewing have been distinguished depending upon the texture of the food:

1 *Puncture-crushing*. The food is crushed and pierced between the teeth without direct tooth contact. This method of chewing results in abrasion of the teeth especially at the tips of the cusps.

2 *Shearing (power) stroke*. This method involves tooth contacts which only takes place after the food has been sufficiently reduced. This type of movement produces attrition facets with characteristic directional scratch lines.

The chewing cycle involves three basic movements of the lower jaw in relation to the upper. From a situation in which the jaws are open, the mandible is lifted upwards and outwards, bringing the buccal parts of the lower teeth into contact with those of the uppers – the preparatory stroke. The lower teeth then move upwards and inwards against the upper teeth – the power stroke. The jaw is then opened – the recovery stroke. Though the chewing cycle is common to all mammals, the direction and dimensions of the individual phases of the masticatory cycle vary considerably. In carnivores, the main movement of the jaws is in the vertical plane and the lateral component of the power stroke is minimal; in herbivores, the lateral component of the power stroke is greatly exaggerated.

The class Mammalia may be subdivided into Prototheria or egg-laying mammals, Metatheria or marsupials and Eutheria or placental mammals.

Dentitions of Prototheria

The spiny ant-eater (*Echidna*) is edentulous. The duck-billed platypus (*Ornithorhyncus*) has three functional posterior teeth in each jaw quadrant which, however, soon drop out leaving horny plates. A number of additional teeth develop but do not erupt and are rapidly resorbed.

Dentitions of Metatheria

Marsupials have a number of dental features which distinguish them from placental mammals. With the exception of the wombat (*Phascolomis*), the upper incisors outnumber the lower. The dental formula for the cheek teeth is $P\frac{3}{3} M\frac{4}{4}$. Apart from the wombat, the enamel is tubular (see figure **484**). An unusual feature of the marsupial dentition is the manner of tooth replacement, only the last tooth in the premolar series having a successor (see figure **536**). This has led to some difficulty in homologising the teeth with the deciduous and permanent series in placental mammals. The situation is further complicated by a variable number of small teeth which develop anteriorly but which do not become functional, being rapidly resorbed. Apart from these distinguishing features, the overall morphology of the teeth of marsupials is similar to that of placental mammals with corresponding diets. It is possible, therefore, to distinguish insectivorous, rodent-type, carnivorous and herbivorous marsupial dentitions.

528 & 529 Virginian opossum (*Didelphis virginianis*). $I\frac{5}{4} C\frac{1}{1} P\frac{3}{3} M\frac{4}{4}$. The diet of this South American marsupial is small mammals and insects. Its incisors exceed in number those of the eutheria. It has large canines and its molar teeth resemble those of placental insectivores (see figures **537 & 538**). The posterior part of the hard palate is characteristically fenestrated.

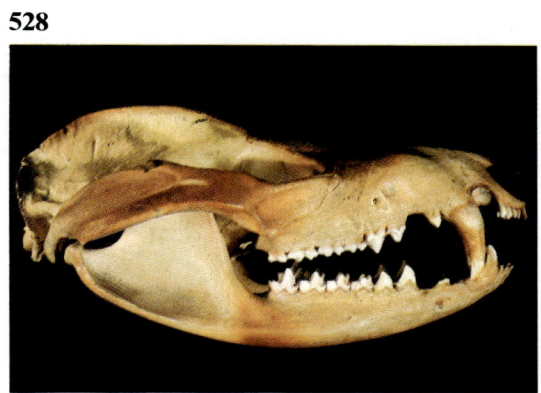
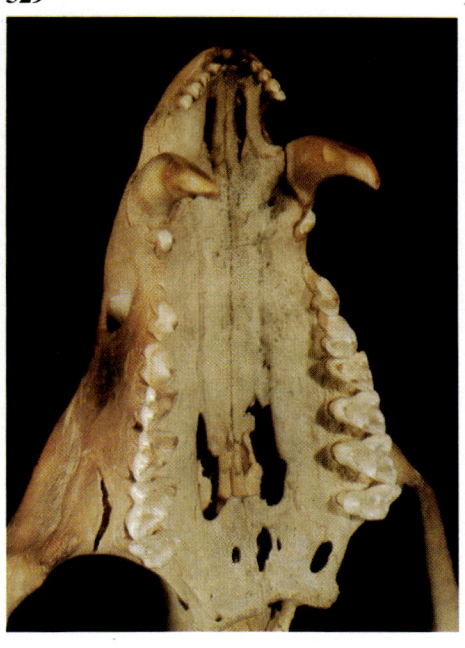

530 & 531 Wombat (*Phascolomis ursinus*). $I\frac{1}{1} C\frac{0}{0} P\frac{1}{1} M\frac{4}{4}$. This animal feeds on grass and roots and shows many features characteristic of the rodent dentition (see figure **542**). All of its teeth are of continuous growth. A prominent gap or diastema is found between the incisor and cheek teeth.

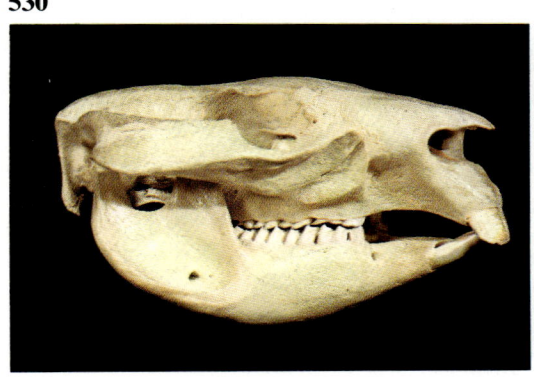
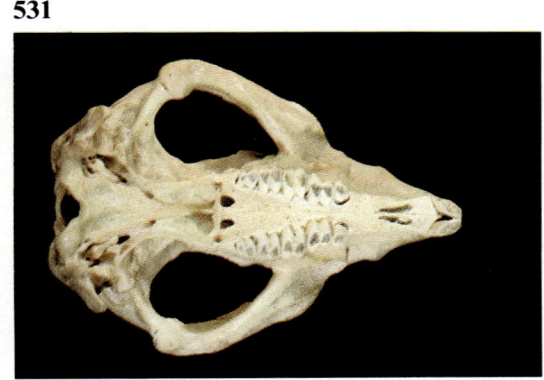

532 & 533 Thylacine wolf (*Thylacinus cynocephalus*). $I\frac{4}{3}$ $C\frac{1}{1}$ $P\frac{3}{3}$ $M\frac{4}{4}$. These rare creatures are the largest carnivorous marsupials. They possess prominent canines and though there are no specialised carnassial teeth corresponding to those of some placental carnivores (see figure **548**), some of the cheek teeth do allow for a slicing action.

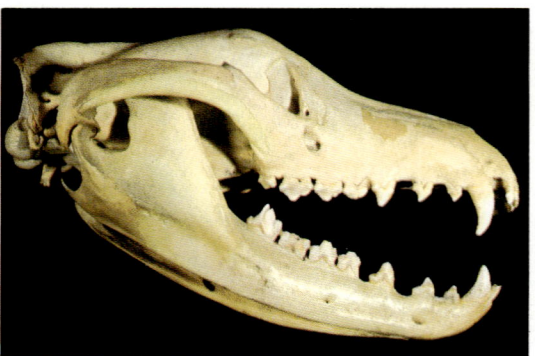

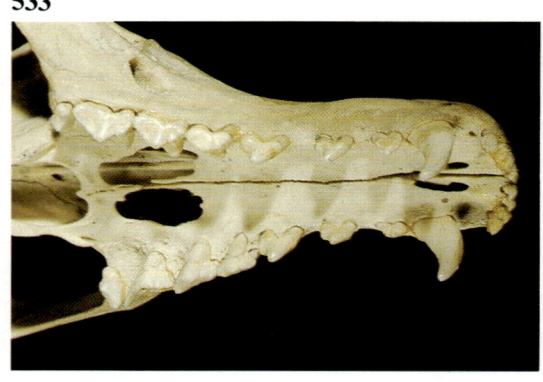

534 & 535 Red kangaroo (*Macropus rufus*). $I\frac{3}{1}$ $C\frac{0}{0}$ $P\frac{1}{1}$ $M\frac{4}{4}$. Kangaroos feed on various types of plant material. The lower incisor is procumbent and, acting against the upper incisors, allows the food to be firmly grasped; cropping is then accomplished by an upward jerk of the head. Of the upper incisors, the third is the largest. A diastema separates the incisors from the cheek teeth. The mesial and distal cusps of the molars are joined together to form transverse ridges or lophs. In this specimen, the anterior cheek tooth has yet to be replaced and the last molar tooth is just erupting. With age, the cheek teeth may gradually be lost from before backwards. The angle of the mandible is inflected, a characteristic of marsupials.

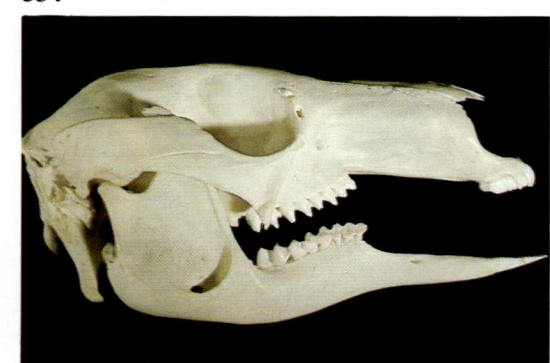

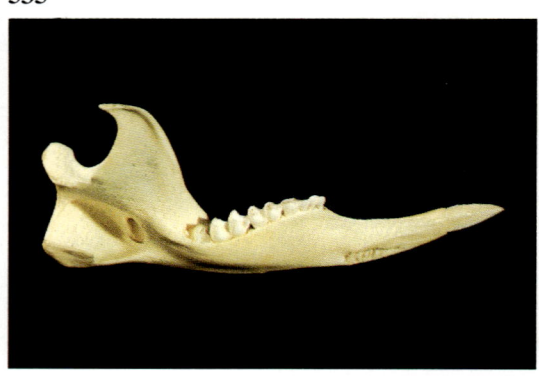

536 Lower jaw of a red kangaroo illustrating the distinctive pattern of tooth replacement of marsupials. Note that only a single tooth is replaced, the last of the premolar series (*arrowed*). However, there is no tooth replacement in the wombat (*Phascolomis*), and in thylacines (*Thylacinus*), the 'deciduous' tooth being resorbed or shed before any other teeth erupt. In some herbivorous marsupials (e.g. *Hypsiprymnodon*) the successional tooth may be a specialised, elongated sectorial tooth which displaces two teeth. (*Radiograph*)

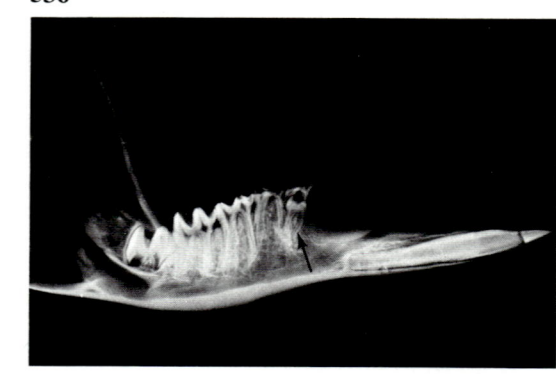

Dentitions of Eutheria

A Insectivora

The insectivores are an ancient Order, though recent forms still have high tooth numbers with sharp cusps for piercing insects. The precise homologies of the teeth are not known because of reduction of the deciduous dentition.

537 Hedgehog (*Erinaceus europaeus*). $I\frac{3}{2}$ $C\frac{1}{1}$ $P\frac{3}{2}$ $M\frac{3}{3}$. The upper first incisors are enlarged, procumbent and separated by a small space. Into this space, the procumbent lower first incisors fit, thus providing a forceps-like mechanism for picking up its prey. The canines are small. The molars have a primitive tritubercular form with sharp, high cusps which interdigitate with those of the opposite jaw, an adaptation suitable for crushing the chitinous shells of insects.

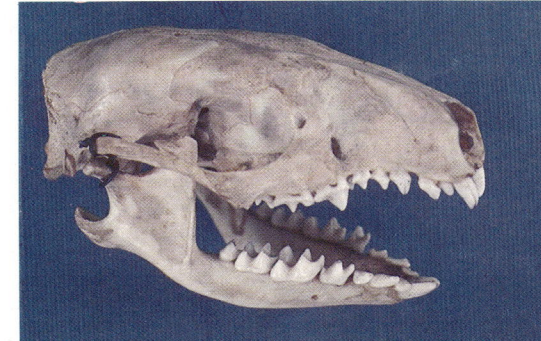

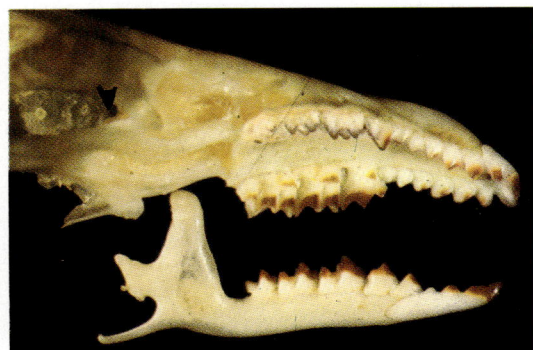

538 Long-tailed shrew (*Sorex araneus*). $I\frac{3}{2}$ $C\frac{1}{0}$ $P\frac{3}{1}$ $M\frac{3}{3}$. The upper first incisors are comparatively large, hook-shaped teeth. The lower incisors are large, procumbent and have a notched upper border. The molars have the primitive tritubercular form. The enamel is tubular. The tips of the teeth contain an iron pigment which gives them a reddish appearance. A number of non-functional deciduous teeth develop but are soon resorbed. Indeed, the deciduous dentition is so reduced that some of these teeth are said to appear *after* the respective permanent teeth.

B Chiroptera

Bats are the only flying mammals. Their dentitions provide examples of adaptive radiation, being suited to diets of insects, fruit or blood. However, whatever the diet, the canines of all groups are relatively large.

539 South American spear-nosed bat (*Phyllostomus hastatus*). $I\frac{2}{3}$ $C\frac{1}{1}$ $P\frac{2}{2}$ $M\frac{3}{3}$. This insectivorous bat shows features reminiscent of the dentition of the Insectivora, the most obvious feature being sharp-cusped cheek teeth.

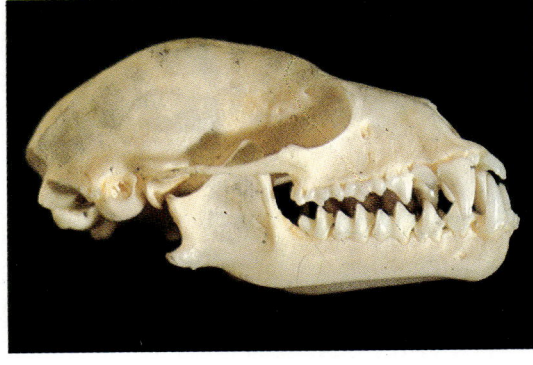

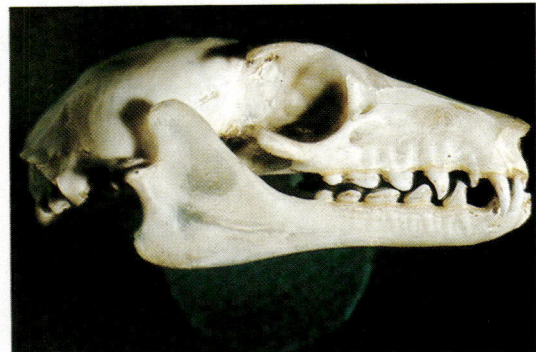

540 Fruit bat (*Pteropus sp.*). $I\frac{2}{2}$ $C\frac{1}{1}$ $P\frac{2}{3}$ $M\frac{3}{3}$. In this bat, the molar teeth are laterally compressed, lack cusps and are spaced. The fruit tends to be crushed by the tongue against the palate.

541 Common vampire bat (*Desmodus rotundus*). $I\frac{1}{2} \ C\frac{1}{1} \ P + M\frac{2}{3}$. The most conspicuous teeth are the upper incisors and canines which the animal uses for puncturing the skin of its prey. Apart from the lower canines, the remaining teeth are greatly reduced. The saliva of this bat contains an anticoagulant.

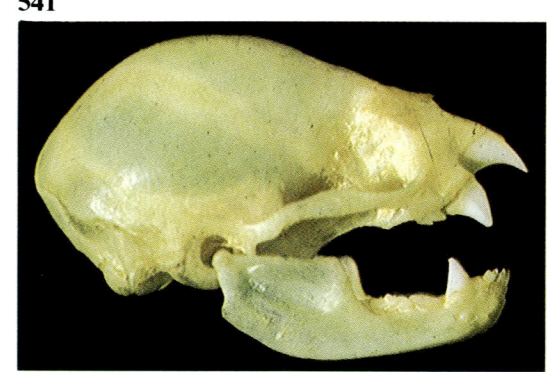

C Rodentia

Rodents are a heterogeneous group whose dentition is reduced in number compared with the archetypal mammalian dentition and whose most conspicuous feature is the possession of continuously growing incisors. Many rodents are monophyodont. The rat and mouse have been widely used as experimental animals in dental science.

542 & 543 Laboratory rat (*Rattus norvegicus*). $I\frac{1}{1} \ C\frac{0}{0} \ P\frac{0}{0} \ M\frac{3}{3}$. The dentition of the rat is monophyodont. Note the conspicuous, continuously growing (and erupting) incisors which are constantly worn to a chisel-shaped edge. The upper incisors are more curved than the lower. The surface enamel contains an iron pigment which imparts a yellow-orange colouration to the enamel surface. The incisors are separated from the cheek teeth by a diastema. Intrusion of the cheeks into the diastema separates the dentition into an anterior gnawing compartment and a posterior grinding compartment. Enamel is not formed on the tips of the molar cusps. The molar cusps are joined by transverse ridges. When these ridges become worn, gradually widening areas of dentine are exposed surrounded by rings of enamel. This arrangement of tissues is said to increase masticatory efficiency. The upper incisors overhang the lowers which are brought forward in gnawing. This movement is reflected in the elongation of the condyles in the anteroposterior plane.

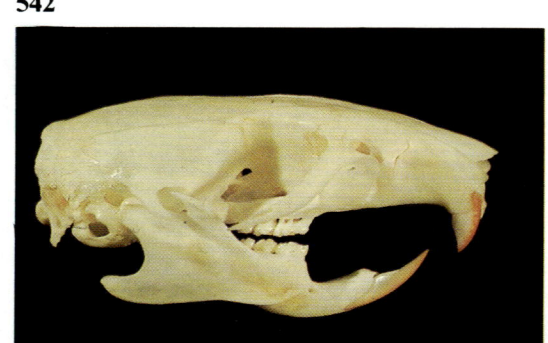
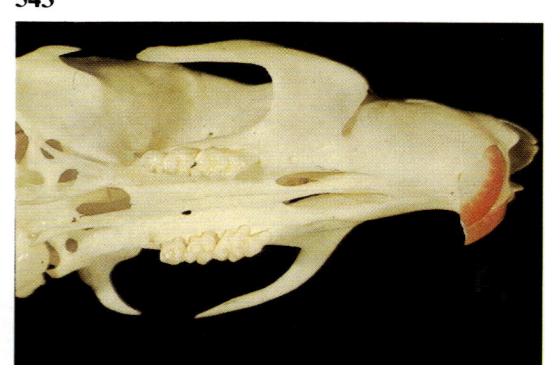

544 Continuously growing rat incisor drawn to show the distribution of tissues. In essence, this tooth presents root tissue (i.e. dentine and cementum) on its lingual side and crown tissue (i.e. dentine and enamel) on its labial side. A, enamel. B, dentine. C, cementum. D, pulp. On the lingual side of the tooth, a true periodontal ligament (E) passes from the cementum to the alveolar bone while labially connective tissue intervenes between, though it is not attached to, the enamel surface and the alveolar bone. In the region of the proliferative 'root' apex, structures homologus with an epithelial root sheath (F) and an enamel organ (G) continually produce new dental tissues to compensate for attritional loss. In the laboratory rat, incisor teeth in occlusion erupt at a rate of about 400um/day (impeded eruption rate). If the teeth are cut out of occlusion, their eruption rate attains levels of about 1mm/day (unimpeded eruption rate). To prevent pulp exposure during gnawing, secondary dentine (H) is continually deposited beneath the incisal edge.

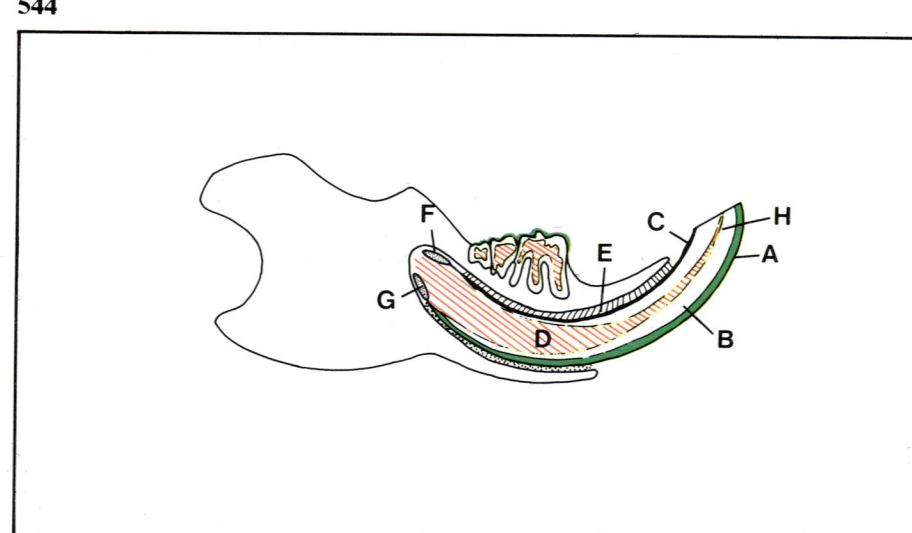

The dentition of the mouse (*Mus musculus*) is similar to, but smaller than, that of the rat. The mouse has deciduous incisors as has the squirrel (*Sciuridae*). The guinea pig (*Cavia*) and the squirrel possess an additional functional anterior cheek tooth or premolar in each quadrant. The incisors of the guinea pig are unpigmented. The molars of the guinea pig, as the incisors, are of continuous growth. The guinea pig is born at a relatively advanced stage of development with all teeth erupted, some of which may even be worn. The anterior cheek tooth has a deciduous predecessor which is shed *in utero*. This deciduous tooth exhibits wear facets, showing that attrition can occur *in utero*.

D Lagomorpha

Despite the apparent resemblance of their dentitions to those of rodents, the pikas, hares and rabbits are placed in a separate Order since other features show that they are but remotely related.

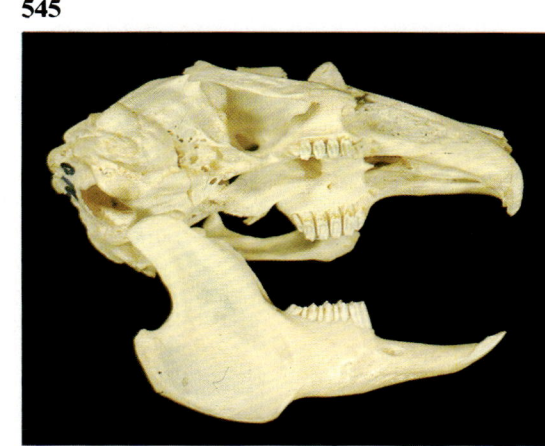

545 Rabbit (*Oryctolagus cuniculus*). $I_1^2 \ C_0^0 \ P_2^3 \ M_3^3$. Unlike rodents, the rabbit possesses a small pair of additional incisors lying behind the large continuously growing upper incisors. The incisors are unpigmented. All the cheek teeth are of continuous growth.

The deciduous dentition has the formula $DI_2^2 \ DC_0^0 \ DM_3^3$ but the teeth are lost early.

546 Jaws of a rat (A) and rabbit (B). Note that only the incisors of the rat are of continuous growth, while this is true for all the teeth of the rabbit. (*Radiographs*)

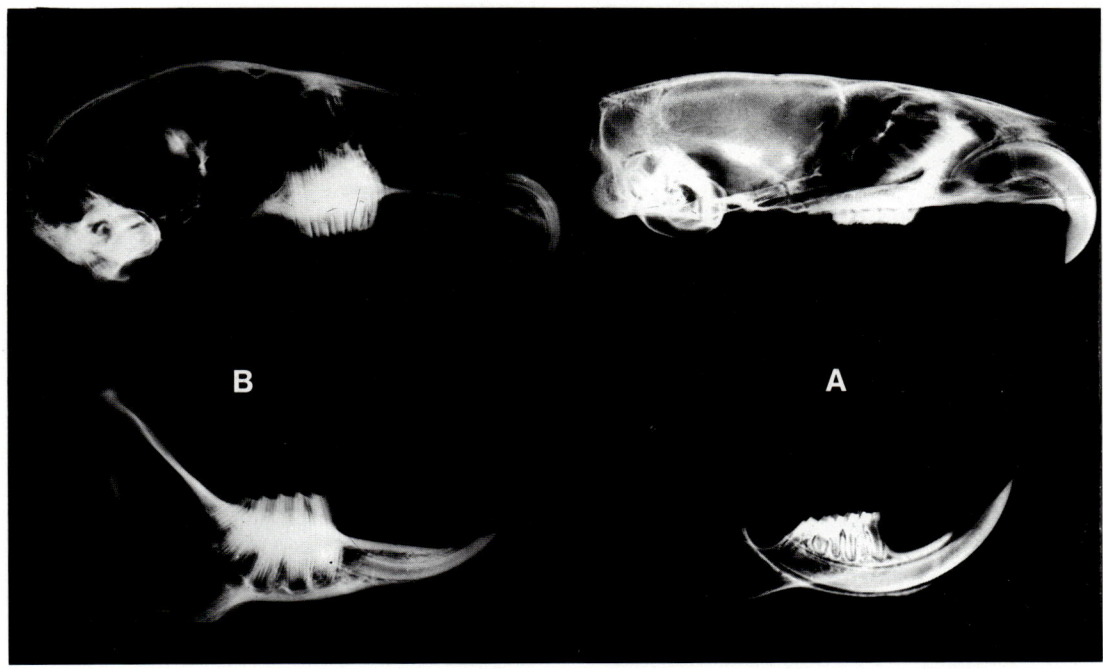

E Carnivora

Carnivores, as their name suggests, are predominantly meat eaters and show a number of dental specialisations, particularly enlarged canines and the presence of carnassial teeth. A great variety of animals are found in the Order Carnivora, including Felidae (cats), Canidae (dogs), Ursidae (bears), Mustelidae (ferrets), Hyaenidae (hyaenas), and Viverridae (mongooses) and some marine carnivores. Carnivorous dental specialisations are most pronounced in the cat family (Felidae).

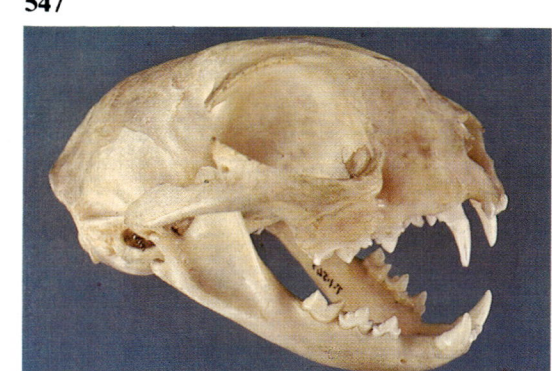

547 Domestic cat (*Felis catus*). $I\frac{3}{3}$ $C\frac{1}{1}$ $P\frac{3}{2}$ $M\frac{1}{1}$. The incisors are small and arranged more or less in a straight line. The canines, often used as offensive weapons, are very large, pointed teeth, the lower fitting into a distema in front of the upper. Both the canines and incisors are used for tearing flesh. The cheek teeth are reduced in number. The last upper premolar and the lower first molar are specialised to form elongated, blade-like, carnassial teeth. These teeth are used for cutting up the prey by a scissor-like action. The teeth immediately anterior to the carnassials, though smaller, have a carnassial-type function. The upper molar tooth is a small, rotated, instanding tooth which by contacting the posterior element of the lower carnassial appears to act as a stop. Jaw movement is primarily of the hinge-type, though a small degree of lateral movement can occur. To stabilise the temporomandibular joint, the articular condyles of the mandible are transversely elongated and fit into a deep, close fitting glenoid fossa with flanges both in front and behind.

The deciduous dentition has the formula $DI\frac{3}{3}$ $DC\frac{1}{1}$ $DM\frac{3}{2}$. In this dentition, the upper carnassial tooth is the middle of the three deciduous molars and the lower carnassial the second deciduous molar. Thus, the permanent carnassial teeth erupt one tooth position behind the deciduous carnassial teeth.

The dentition of the dog (family *Canidae*) reflects a more omnivorous diet than that of the cat.

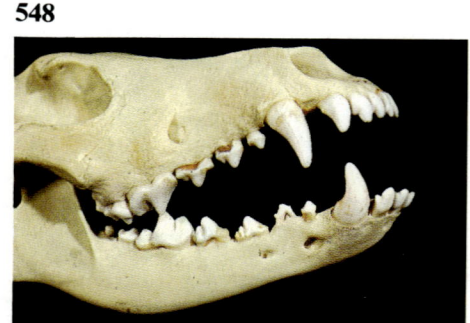

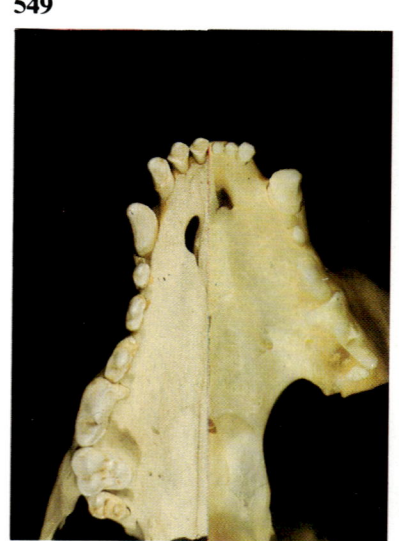

548 Dog (*Canis familiaris*). $I\frac{3}{3}$ $C\frac{1}{1}$ $P\frac{4}{4}$ $M\frac{2}{3}$. Compared with the cat, the number of teeth present in the dog is greater. The anterior teeth are similar to those of the cat. Opposing premolars do not occlude. The carnassial teeth are less sectorial than those of the cat. The presence of extra molar teeth, especially the broad upper first molar, provides an additional grinding surface.

The formula of the deciduous dentition is $DI\frac{3}{3}$ $DC\frac{1}{1}$ $DM\frac{3}{3}$. The first permanent premolar, as in other placentals with four premolars, has no deciduous predecessor.

549 Comparison of the upper jaw of a dog (left) and a cat (right) viewed occlusally.

550 Bear (*Ursus sp.*). $I\frac{3}{3} C\frac{1}{1} P\frac{4}{4} M\frac{3}{3}$. Bears (family Ursidae) are omnivorous and may subsist on a vegetable diet. The anterior teeth resemble those of other carnivores, the canines being conspicuous. The premolars are usually considerably reduced in size and sometimes number. The carnassial teeth do not show sectorial specialisation and the molar teeth have broad flat crowns with blunt cusps. The right half of the figure shows maxillary teeth, the left half mandibular teeth.

The dental formulae for some other land carnivores are:

Viverridae $I\frac{3}{3} C\frac{1}{1} P\frac{4}{4} M\frac{2}{2}$
Hyaenidae $I\frac{3}{3} C\frac{1}{1} P\frac{4}{4} M\frac{1}{1}$
Mustelidae $I\frac{3}{3} C\frac{1}{1} P\frac{4}{4} M\frac{1}{2}$

551 Californian seal (*Zalophus californianus*). $I\frac{3}{3} C\frac{1}{1} P\frac{4}{4} M\frac{1}{1}$. The dentition of this aquatic carnivore reflects its piscivorous diet, the simple, cone-shaped, interdigitating cheek teeth being well suited to hold the slippery prey. The carnassial elements have been lost but enlarged canines are retained. The deciduous dentition is much reduced in size and function.

Another aquatic carnivore is the walrus (*Odobenus rosmarus*), with a dental formula of $I\frac{1}{1} C\frac{1}{1} P\frac{3}{3} M\frac{0}{0}$. Its deciduous dentition has been reported as $DI\frac{3}{3} DC\frac{1}{1} DM\frac{5}{4}$. It lives primarily on shellfish. Its cheek teeth are low and blunt and the most outstanding dental feature is the pair of tusks which are continuously growing upper canines.

F Arteriodactyla

This group of even-toed ungulates has dentitions suited mainly for an herbivorous diet, though some (e.g. the pig) are omnivorous. Where the diet is herbivorous, there is a tendency towards a reduction in number of upper anterior teeth and a broadening of the cheek teeth to produce an efficient grinding surface.

552 & 553 Domestic pig (*Sus scrofa*). $I\frac{3}{3} C\frac{1}{1} P\frac{4}{4} M\frac{3}{3}$. The upper central incisors are the largest incisors. Their roots are separated but because they are inclined mesially, their crowns meet in the midline. The third incisors are the smallest. The lower incisors are deeply implanted and are almost horizontal. They are used for rooting up the ground in search of food. The canine teeth or tusks are of continuous growth. In the male they are well-developed and project out of the mouth in an upward and outward direction. In the female, the tusks are considerably reduced. The convex surface of the canine is covered with enamel, the concave surface with cementum. Except for the upper fourth premolar which is molariform, the premolars are somewhat narrow, cutting teeth which increase in size from before backwards. The molar crowns increase in size from before backwards and have cone-shaped cusps (bunodont). Four main cusps may be distinguished in each molar, though each cusp has numerous accessory cusps. The dental formula for the deciduous dentition is $DI\frac{3}{3} DC\frac{1}{1} DM\frac{3}{3}$.

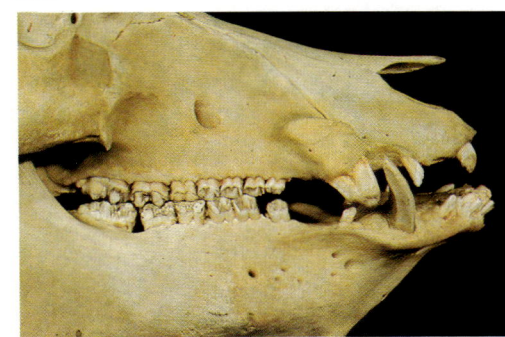

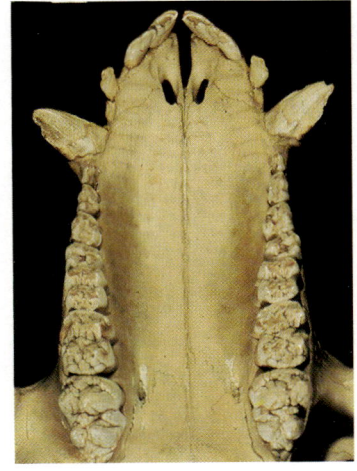

554 & 555 Domestic cattle (*Bos taurus*). $I\frac{0}{3} C\frac{0}{1} P\frac{3}{3} M\frac{3}{3}$. Incisors and canines are absent from the upper jaw, this region being covered by a dense pad of mucous membrane. The lower canines are incisiform and with the lower incisors form a row of shovel-shaped teeth with sharp edges. Grass is held against the upper gum pad by the lower anterior teeth and cropped by abrupt movement of the head. A diastema separates the incisor group of teeth from the cheek teeth. The cheek teeth are described as being hypsodont having long crowns and short roots. The hypsodonty allows the teeth to slowly erupt over long periods thus compensating for wear incurred during grinding of the teeth. The cusps of the cheek teeth are crescent-shaped (selenodont) and the enamel is thrown into multiple folds. Coronal cementum fills the clefts between the enamel folds. Because of the differing hardnesses of enamel, dentine and cementum, with wear a roughened occlusal table suitable for grinding is maintained, the enamel standing proud.

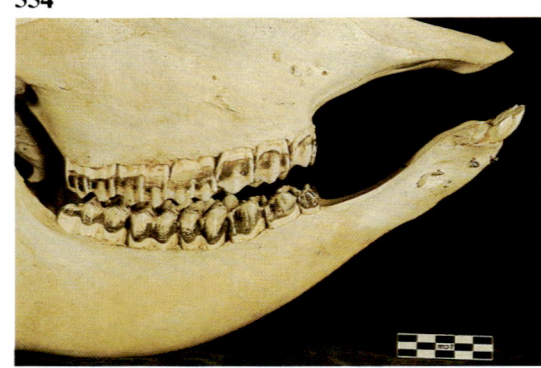

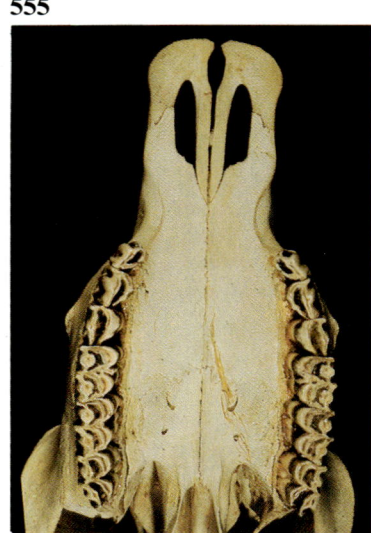

The deciduous dentition has the formula $DI\frac{0}{3} DC\frac{0}{1} DM\frac{3}{3}$.

556 Molar teeth of the hippopotamus (*Hippopotamus amphibius*). The hippopotamus has four premolars and three molars in each jaw quadrant. The molars when first erupted (A) are bunodont, this shape being unsuited for an herbivorous diet. However, with subsequent wear, (B), a ridged surface of enamel and dentine highly suitable for grinding vegetable matter is formed. The incisors and canines ($I\frac{2}{2} C\frac{1}{1}$) of the hippopotamus are of continuous growth, the lower canines being large and tusk-like.

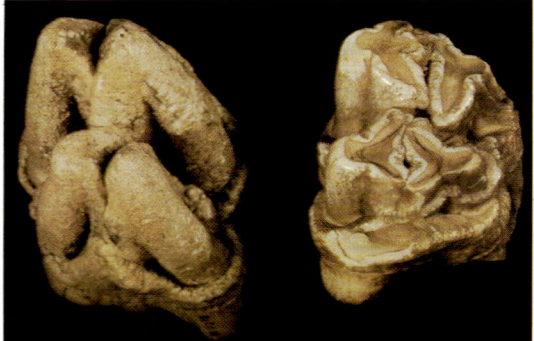

G Perissodactyla

Like the arteriodactyla, the perissodactyla or odd-toed ungulates are mainly herbivorous.

557 & 558 Horse (*Equus caballus*). $I\frac{3}{3} C\frac{1}{1} P\frac{4}{4} M\frac{3}{3}$. The columnar crowns of the incisors are covered by a thin layer of cementum and the incisal edges initially show a central pit (the 'mark') which, depending upon the degree of wear, is used in ageing. The relatively small canine tooth (which may be absent in mares) is separated from both the incisors and the cheek teeth by a diastema. The first premolar is much reduced in size. It is rarely seen in the functioning dentition, however, being either unerupted or shed. The remaining cheek teeth are similar in form, the premolars being difficult to distinguish from the molars (molarisation). Like the cow, the cheek teeth are adapted for grinding, being hypsodont and having a complicated series of enamel folds covered by coronal cementum. The darker-staining material in the central areas of the occlusal table is secondary dentine.

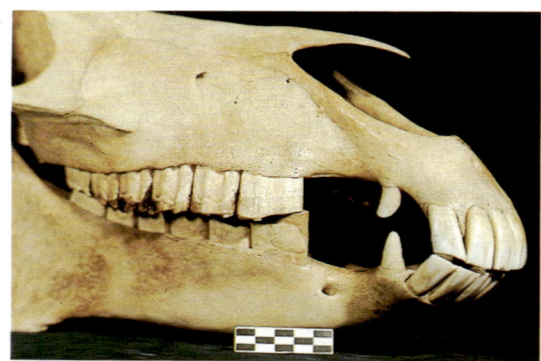

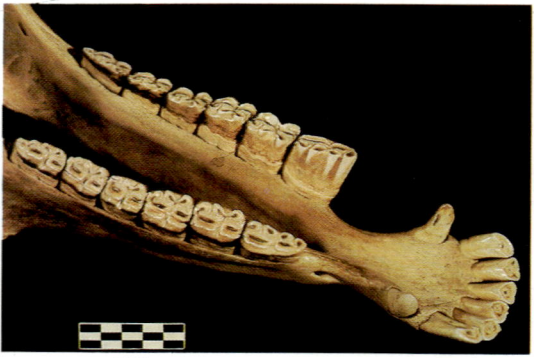

559 Section of a horse's mandible demonstrating the hypsodont nature of the cheek teeth. (*Radiograph*)

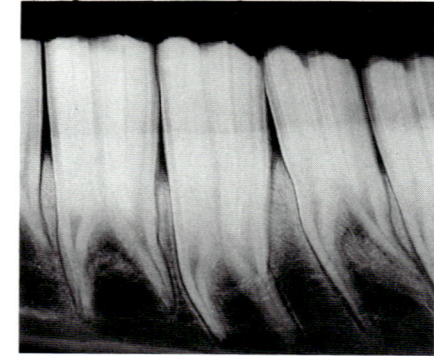

H Proboscidea

The elephant is the only existing genus in this group. The dental formula for the elephant is $I_0^1 C_0^0 P + M_0^6$. The precise homology of the cheek teeth is uncertain. The upper incisor has a deciduous predecessor. The upper incisors form tusks which erupt continuously throughout life. The tusk is composed primarily of dentine which has a thin covering of cementum. When the tusk first erupts it is surmounted by a cap of enamel. The dentine of the elephant's incisor is known as ivory. The arrangement of the dentinal tubules in ivory is unique. The tubules pass in regular sinuous curves across the whole thickness of the tooth in distinct groups. Within each group, the curvatures are all in phase but are in the reverse phase from those of the adjacent groups. The pulp in the adult tusk is limited to the base of the tooth.

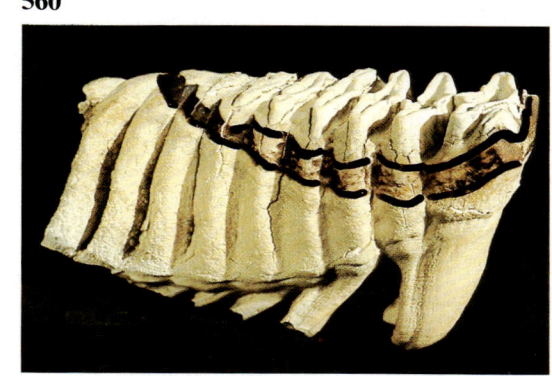

560 The third permanent molar of an African elephant (*Loscodonta africana*). The molars of the elephant increase in size from before backwards. Only one whole tooth in each quadrant (or portions of two when the anterior molar is extremely worn) is in function at any one time. Each new molar erupts obliquely from behind and moves forwards to replace the preceding worn tooth. This type of replacement is referred to as horizontal tooth succession. The molar illustrated had partly erupted, being worn only on its anterior part. The site of the gingival margin at the time this tooth was removed from the jaws has been drawn in. The cheek teeth are composed of plates of dentine covered by enamel which are united by cementum. Differential wear, therefore, maintains a roughened occlusal surface. When worn, the plates appear 'lozenge-shaped'. In the Indian elephant (*Elephas maximus*) the cheek teeth have more plates and their outline is slot-shaped and wrinkled.

J Cetacea

The Order Cetacea comprises two main groups of mammals, the toothed whales (Odontoceti) and the whalebone whales (Mystacoceti). The toothed whales feed primarily upon squids and fish while the whalebone whales are plankton feeders. The dentition of toothed whales is homodont and monophyodont. The teeth of whalebone whales are resorbed *in utero*.

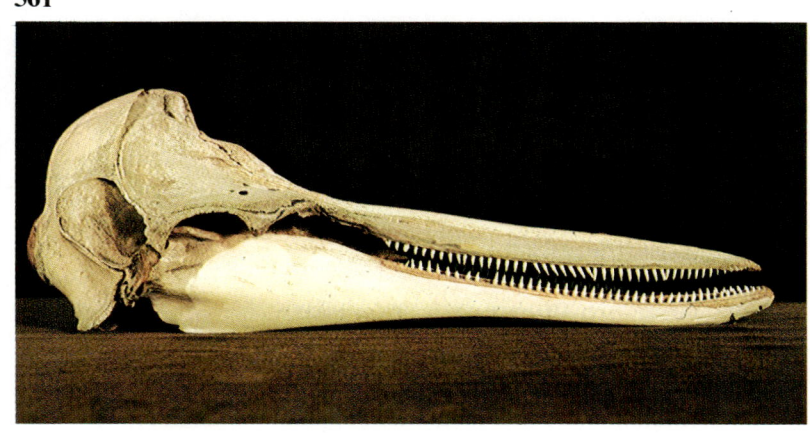

561 Dolphin (*Delphinus delphis*) is a toothed whale. The number of teeth in its dentition far exceeds the typical mammalian tooth number, being approximately 200. Each tooth is conical, sharply pointed and interdigitates with teeth in the opposing jaw. The teeth in the middle of the tooth row tend to be the largest.

The sperm whale (*Physeter catodon*) has about 54 large conical teeth in the lower jaw. In the upper jaw, there are no functional teeth: those that do develop there remain unerupted or are lost.

A most unusual dental specialisation is seen in the narwal (*Monodon monoceros*) where only two teeth develop in the anterior region of the upper jaw. As a rule, those of the female and one (usually the right) of the male remain unerupted. In the male, the remaining tooth grows continuously to form a straight tusk 10–12 feet long with a spiral winding from right to left. Its functional significance is not understood.

K Edentata

This group comprises the sloths (*Bradypodidae*), armadillos (*Dasypodidae*), and anteaters (*Myrmecophagidae*). The term Edentata may be misleading for it is only the anteaters that are toothless. The other forms have well-developed, functional cheek teeth, only the incisors and canines being absent. The dentitions are generally homodont and monophyodont and the teeth lack enamel. They are vegetable and/or insect eaters.

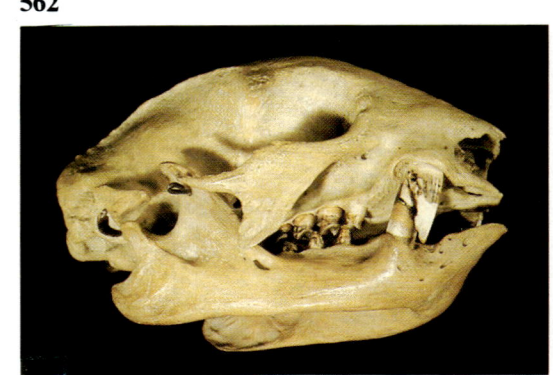

562 Two-toed sloth (*Choloepus didactylus*). Five cheek teeth are present in each upper jaw quadrant and four in each lower quadrant. The most anterior tooth is separated from the remainder by a diastema and is caniniform. The teeth are cylindrical in shape and of continuous growth.

L Sirenia

This Order comprises the herbivorous dugongs (*Dugong dugon*) and manatees (*Trichechus manatus*). Manatees have two incisors in each jaw quadrant, which lie beneath horny plates and are lost before maturity. The cheek teeth are bilophodont and number up to ten in each jaw quadrant. Only six cheek teeth are present in each quadrant at a time and exhibit horizontal succession.

M Hyracoidea

The animals in this Order have a diet of vegetables and/or insects. The dental formula has been given as $I\frac{1}{2} C\frac{0}{0} P\frac{4}{4} M\frac{3}{3}$. The upper incisor is of continuous growth, the lower incisors of non-continuous growth. The premolars are molariform; the cheek teeth are selenodont and bear some resemblance to those of horses.

N Tubulidentata

The dentition of the aardvark (*Orycteropus afer*) usually contains no more than five, continuously growing, cylindrical cheek teeth at any time. The deciduous dentition is represented by a number of functionless rudiments.

O Pholidota

Pangolins (*Maris*) are insectivorous and have no teeth.

P Primates

The Order Primates is one of the most ancient of the mammalian Orders. The diet of Primates is mainly fruit and vegetables. However, in some, the diet may be insectivorous or omnivorous. For purposes of classification, the Primates are divided into two suborders, the Prosimii or lemur-type primates and the Anthropoidea, containing monkeys, apes and man. Each suborder is eventually subdivided into six distinct families.

Classification of living primates		
Order	*Suborder*	*Family*
		Tupaiidae
		Lemuridae
	Prosimii	Indriidae
		Daubentonidae
		Lorisidae
		Tarsiidae
Primates		
		Cebidae
		Callitricidae
	Anthropoidea	Cercopithecidae
		Hylobatidae
		Pongidae
		Hominidae

Prosimii

Tupaiidae

The precise classification of this group is still a matter of some controversy, for while the animals in this group have features considered to be characteristic of Primates, they also bear a distinct resemblance to some of the Insectivores. The dental formula for the permanent dentition of the Tupaiidae is $I\frac{2}{3} \ C\frac{1}{1} \ P\frac{3}{3} \ M\frac{3}{3}$.

563, 564A & 564B Tree-shrew (*Tupaia glis*). $I\frac{2}{3}$ $C\frac{1}{1} \ P\frac{3}{3} \ M\frac{3}{3}$. The lower incisors are procumbent and form a dental 'comb'. The lower third incisor is the smallest and may be functionless or lost. The upper incisors are caniniform. The upper canine is relatively small and is well-spaced from the first premolar which it resembles. The lower canine is well developed but is not procumbent and, unlike the lemurs and lorises, is not involved in the dental comb. The cheek teeth in both jaws are primitive in form and have sharply pointed cusps. The first premolars in both jaws are small and functionless. The premolars increase in size from before backwards. The molars decrease in size from before backwards and tend to be tritubercular in form.

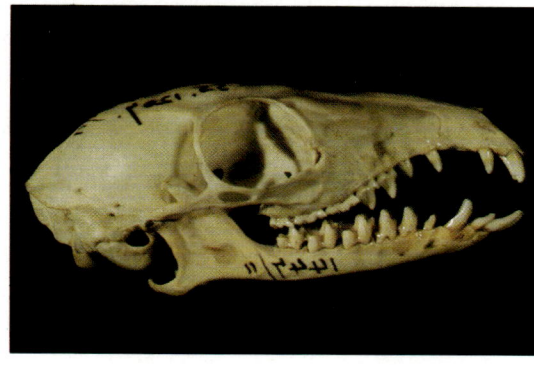

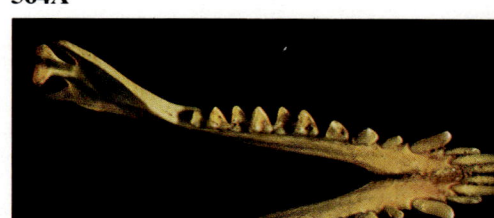

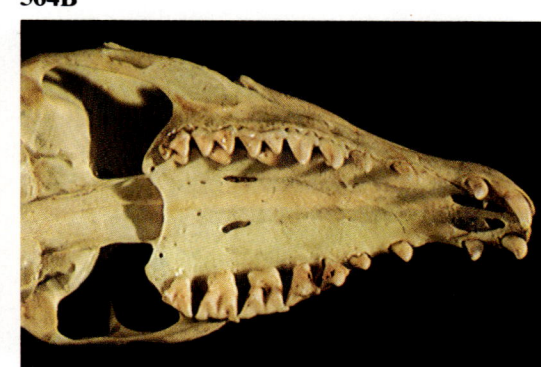

Lemuridae

The lemurs are generally vegetable feeders though the diet may also be insectivorous.

565 & 566 Ring-tailed lemur (*Lemur calta*). $I\frac{2}{3}$ $C\frac{1}{1} \ P\frac{3}{3} \ M\frac{3}{3}$. Both the lower incisors and canines are procumbent and form the dental comb. The canines are the largest teeth in the comb. The upper incisors are small and there is a midline diastema. The upper canines are blade-like and are large and prominent. The premolars increase in size from front to back though the lower first premolar is caniniform and is the largest of the premolars. The upper third premolar has an additional palatal cusp. The upper molars are tritubercular though sometimes additional palatal cusps may be seen. The upper molars decrease in size from before backwards. The lower first and second molars each have four cusps and transverse ridges. The lower third molar is reduced in size. The cusp pattern of the molars of the lemur are said to show greater variability in form than those of any other Primates. The dental formula for the deciduous dentition is $DI\frac{2}{2} \ DC\frac{1}{1} \ DM\frac{3}{3}$.

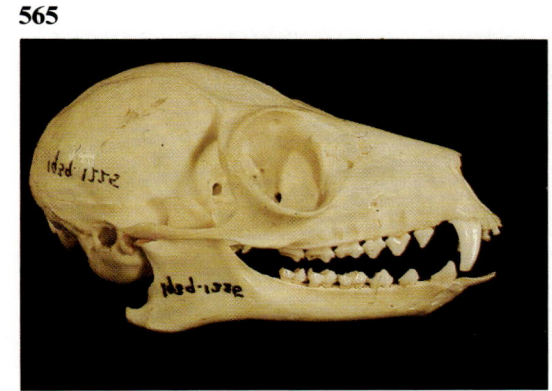

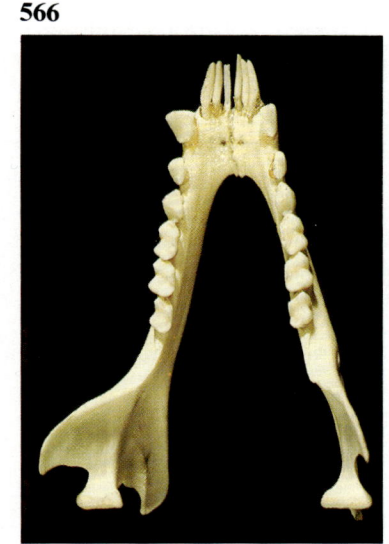

Indriidae

The members of this Order are lemur-like, the dentition varying from the Lemuridae in terms of the numbers of teeth (dental formula $I_1^2 C_1^1 P_2^2 M_3^3$) and the quadritubercular form of the upper molars. The dental formula for the deciduous dentition is said to be $DI_2^2 DC_1^1 DM_3^3$.

Daubentoniidae

567A & 567B Lower jaw of the aye-aye (*Daubentonia madagascariensis*). $I_1^1 C_0^0 P_0^1 M_3^3$. The dentition is unique among the primates, being 'rodent-like'. Note from the radiograph that the incisors are of continuous growth. There is a diastema between the incisors and the cheek teeth. The cheek teeth are small and have flat occlusal surfaces. The diet is chiefly insectivorous. Deciduous dentition is $DI_2^2 DC_1^1 DM_2^2$.

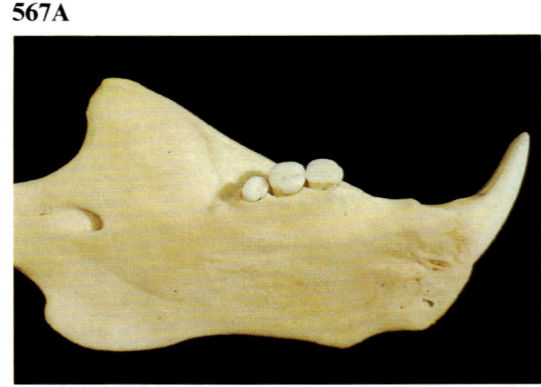

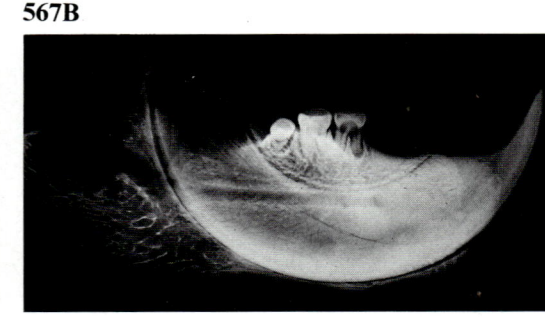

Lorisidae

The dentitions of this group do not differ significantly from those of the Lemuridae though the teeth forming the dental comb are less procumbent and the upper molars are less primitive in form. The diet of the lorises is insectivorous though vegetables, fruits and animal matter may be ingested.

568 & 569 African slow loris (*Perodicticus potto*). $I_2^2 C_1^1 P_3^3 M_3^3$. Note that the upper first and second molars each have four cusps with oblique ridges on the occlusal surfaces. The upper third molar is small and has two main cusps.

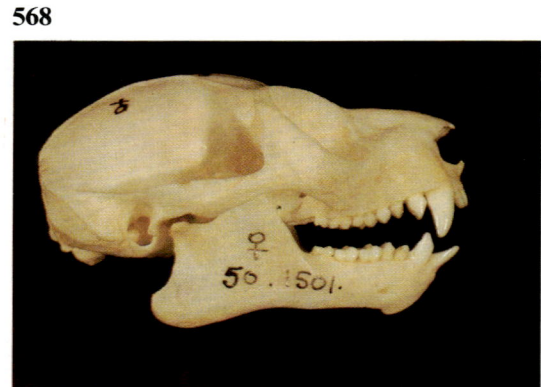

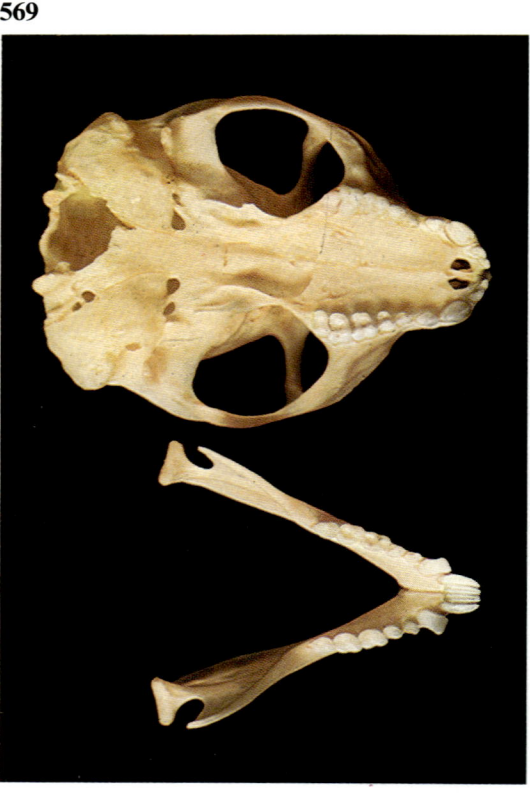

Tarsiidae

The Tarsiidae are the closest link between the Prosimii and Anthropoidea. The diet of the Tarsiidae is insectivorous. The dentition of this group differs markedly from that of other Prosimii particularly in the mandibular anterior region.

570 & 571 Tarsius (*Tarsius banconus*). $I\frac{2}{1} C\frac{1}{1} P\frac{3}{3} M\frac{3}{3}$. Unlike the lemurs and lorises, the mandibular incisors and canines are not procumbent and do not form a dental comb. The upper central incisors are large and pointed. The upper lateral incisors are small. Compared to the loris, the upper canine is much reduced. The premolars increase in size from front to back, though unlike the loris, the lower first premolar is not caniniform. The upper second and third premolars have a palatal cingulum. The molar teeth of Tarsius are more primitive in form than those of other living primates. The first and second upper molars are of equal size, the third molar being smaller. The upper molars are primarily trituberular in shape, with an incipient hypocone. The lower molars are about equal in size, the first and second molars having five 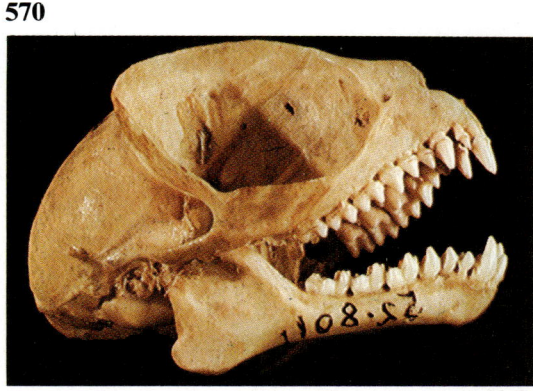 cusps, the third molars six. Only three of the permanent dentition have deciduous predecessors, the canine and the two distal premolars. The deciduous formula is therefore $DI\frac{0}{0} DC\frac{1}{1} DM\frac{2}{2}$.

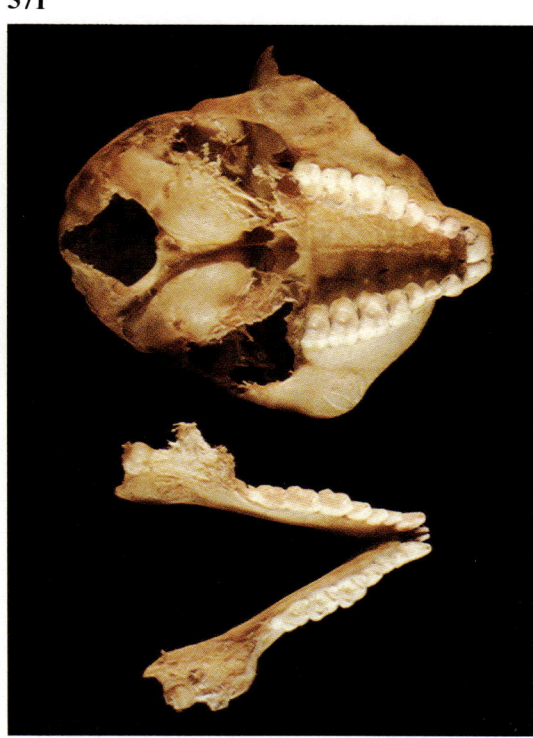

Anthropoidea

The New World Monkeys are classified into two families, the Cebidae and Callitricidae. The Old World Monkeys comprise but a single family, the Ceropithecidae. The anthropoid apes (including man) are classified into three families, the Hylobatidae, Pongidae and Hominidae.

Cebidae

572 & 573 Squirrel monkey (*Saimiri sciureus*). $I\frac{2}{2} C\frac{1}{1} P\frac{3}{3} M\frac{3}{3}$. The diet of the squirrel monkey, as of all New World monkeys, consists mainly of fruit and insects. The incisors are spatulate, the canines are large and tusk-like. The upper canine is separated from the lateral incisor by a diastema which accommodates the lower canine. The premolars are bicuspid, the buccal cusp being the most prominent. The lower first premolar, however, is unicuspid. The buccal and lingual cusps of both the second and third lower premolars are united by a transverse crest. Typically, the lower premolars have two roots, the upper premolars three roots. The molars decrease in size from before backwards and have four sharp cusps. The reduced upper third molar, however, tends to have three cusps. The mesiopalatal cusp (protocone) of each upper molar is joined to the distobuccal cusp 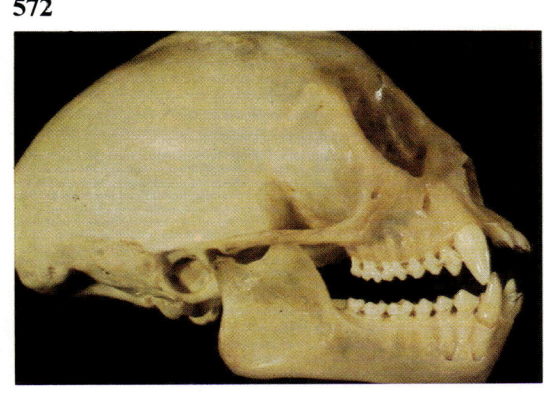 (metacone) by an oblique ridge. The upper molars have three roots, the lowers two. The deciduous dentition has the formula $DI\frac{2}{2} DC\frac{1}{1} DM\frac{3}{3}$.

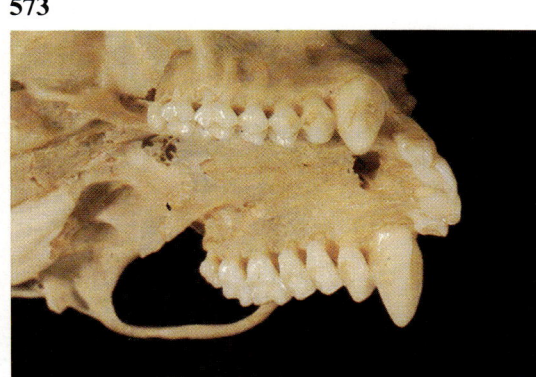

Callitrichidae

This family comprises the marmosets and tamarins. The dentition is similar to the Cebidae, except for the absence of third molars in the Callitrichidae and the triangular appearance of their upper molars, which lack a well defined hypocone.

Cercopithecidae

The dentition of Old World monkeys differs from that of New World monkeys in a number of respects. In Old World monkeys only two premolars are present in each jaw quadrant. The lower first premolar of Old World monkeys is a sectorial tooth. Unlike those of New World monkeys, the cusps of the molars of Old World monkeys are connected by distinct transverse ridges or lophs and the third molars are well developed.

574 & 575 Stump-tailed macaque (*Macaca arctoides*). $I\frac{2}{2} \ C\frac{1}{1} \ P\frac{2}{2} \ M\frac{3}{3}$. The incisors are spatulate. The canines are long, dagger-like teeth, being especially prominent in the male. The upper canine is separated from the incisors by a diastema. The well-marked groove on the anterior surface of the upper canine is said to help guide the lower canines into occlusion. The upper premolars and lower second premolar are bicuspid. The lower first premolar is a highly specialised sectorial tooth. Its crown slopes sharply backwards to leave a wedge-shaped space between it and the crown of the lower canine into which the upper canine occludes. It has been suggested that the posterior edge of the upper canine may be sharpened against the sloping surface of the lower sectorial premolar. The upper molars have four cusps, the anterior and posterior pairs each being linked by a transverse ridge. Viewed occlusally, the crowns show distinct

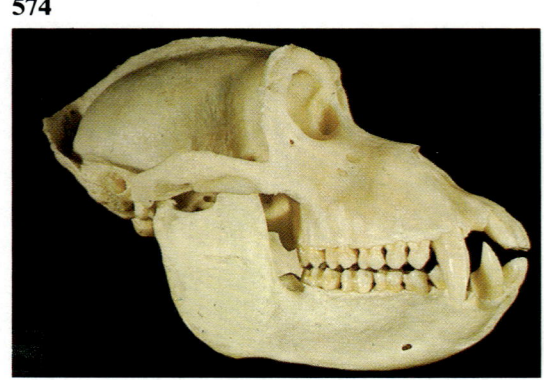

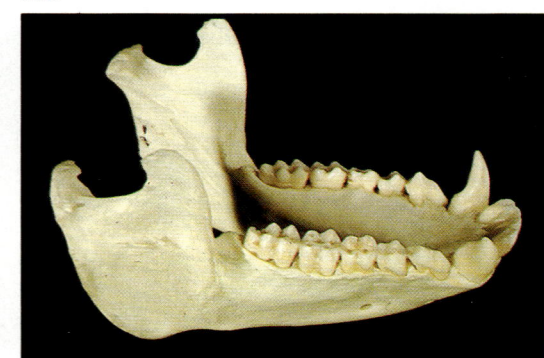

mesial and distal constrictions in the midline, giving the teeth a characteristic bilophodont appearance. The upper first molar is the smallest, the second and third molars being approximately equal in size. The lower molars are also bilophodont and increase in size from before backwards. The lower third molar has an additional posterior cusp (hypoconulid). The upper molars and premolars have three roots, the corresponding lower teeth two roots. The dental formula for the deciduous dentition is $DI\frac{2}{2} \ DC\frac{1}{1} \ DM\frac{2}{2}$.

The dental formula for the anthropoid apes is the same as the Old World monkeys, namely, $I\frac{2}{2} \ C\frac{1}{1} \ P\frac{2}{2} \ M\frac{3}{3}$.

Hylobatidae

The gibbons and siamangs in this family differ from the other anthropoid apes in terms of the size of incisors and canines and the shape of the arches; the incisors being small, the canines large and the arches converging posteriorly. They have a sectorial type of lower first premolar similar to that of Old World monkeys.

Pongidae

There are three genera within this family, the chimpanzee (*Pan*), the orang-utan (*Pongo*) and the gorilla (*Gorilla*).

Principal differences between the dentitions of the great apes and man.

Apes	*Man*	*Apes*	*Man*
The dental arches are U-shaped.	The dental arches are parabolic.	The upper premolars have three roots, the lower premolars two.	The premolars usually have one root except for the upper first which has two.
The incisors are large, procumbent and meet edge-to-edge.	The incisors are smaller and are more vertically inclined. The maxillary incisors usually overlap the mandibular incisors anteriorly.	The lower first premolar is predominantly unicuspid; the second premolar is bicuspid with a well-developed talonid.	The lower premolars are similar in shape and are bicuspid.
The canines are large in males (sexual dimorphism). They erupt late, sometimes after the third molar.	The canines are smaller and there is no sexual dimorphism. They erupt relatively early.	The lower molars all have five cusps.	The second and third lower molars usually have four cusps.
		Cusps more pointed.	Cusps more rounded.
The maxillary canine and lateral incisor are separated by a diastema.	There is no diastema.		

---

576 & 577 Chimpanzee (*Pan troglodytes*). Of the great apes, the permanent teeth of the chimpanzee most closely resemble the permanent teeth of man. However, the incisors are procumbent and the canines in the male are powerful, pointed teeth. The upper molars decrease in size from before backwards. The lower molars have five cusps. The lower second molar tends to be the largest of the lower molars. The arrow indicates the simian shelf. This shelf is a ridge of bone lying in the midline on the inferior aspect of the medial surface of the mandible. It is a site for muscle attachments and corresponds in the human to the genial tubercles. It has been suggested that the simian shelf strengthens the front of the mandibular arch in order to support the large canines.

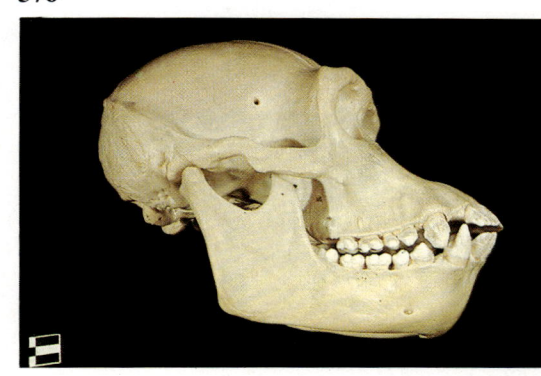

576

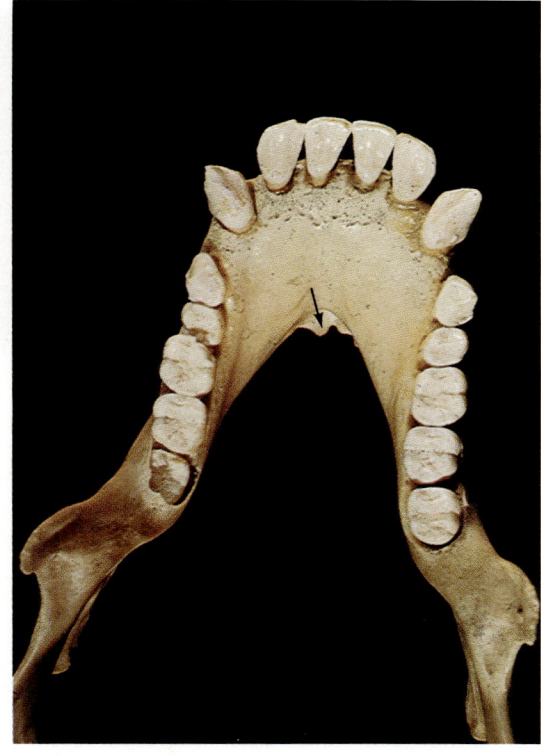

577

578 & 579 Deciduous dentition of Chimpanzee. DI$\frac{2}{2}$ DC$\frac{1}{1}$ DM$\frac{2}{2}$. The deciduous incisors are similar in shape to those of man, though they are disproportionately smaller compared to the permanent incisors. The canines remain proportionately large. There is no sexual dimorphism. The diastema between the maxillary incisors and canine is still a conspicuous feature in the deciduous dentition. The morphology of the deciduous lower first molar differs from that of man in that there is a greater disproportion between the anterior trigonid element which is high and the posterior talonid element which is low and without cusps. Compared with the corresponding human tooth, the upper first deciduous molar of apes has a more pointed buccal cusp and a reduced palatal cusp. As in the human, the second deciduous molars closely resemble the first permanent molars. Note the gubernacular canals leading down to the underlying permanent teeth.

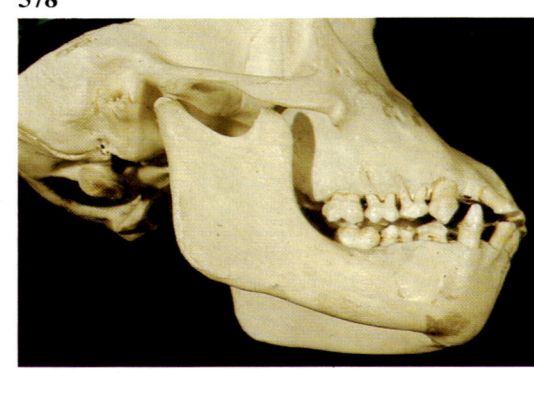
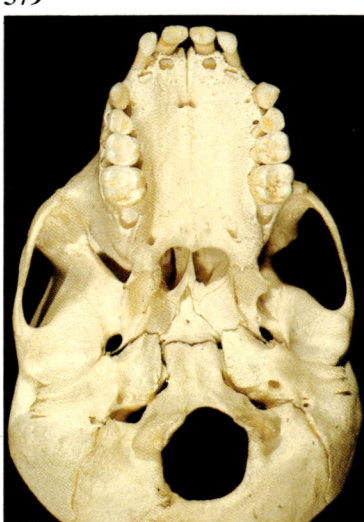

580 & 581 Orang-utan (*Pongo pygmaeus*). The teeth and jaws are large. There is considerable wrinkling of the enamel on the molar teeth. The simian shelf is arrowed.

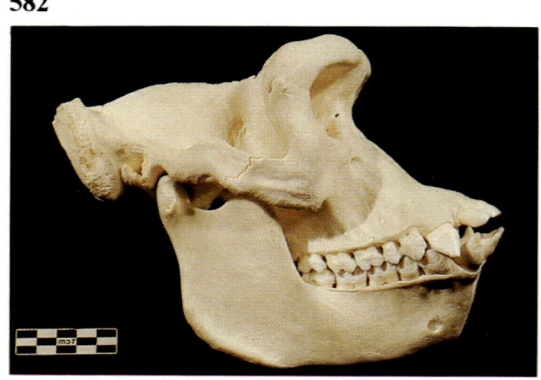
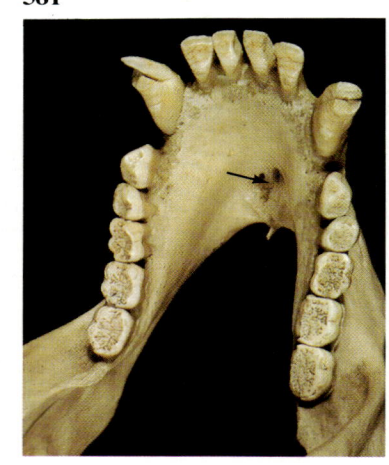

582 & 583 Lowland gorilla (*Gorilla gorilla*). In this specimen the upper left central incisor is absent. Note the characteristic crenated folds of enamel at the bases of the cusps of the molars.

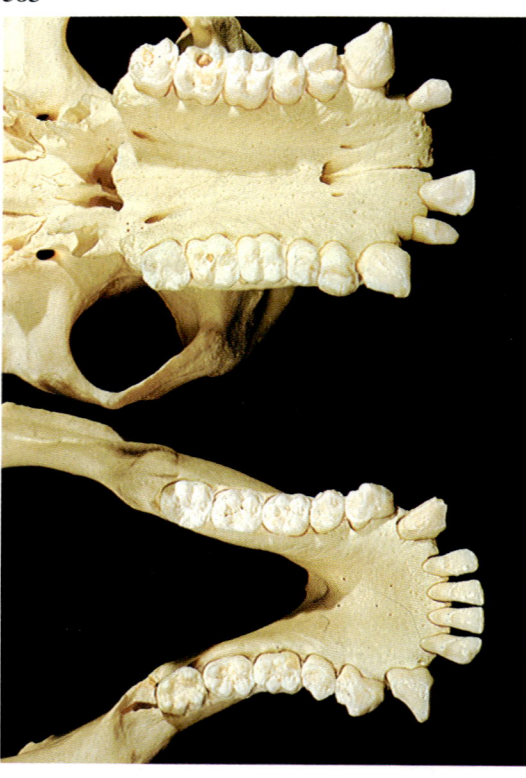

Hominidae

Modern man (*Homo sapiens*) is the only living species in this family, though fossil remains of other species and genera have been discovered. In order to relate the remains to either ape or man, great emphasis has been placed upon distinguishing features of the teeth and jaws. The principal differences between the teeth of apes and man have already been described. The following features help distinguish the skulls of apes and man. The ape mandible is square and massive, lacks a chin and has a shallow mandibular notch. The simian shelf of apes corresponds to the genial tubercles of the human mandible. In the ape skull, the front of the face slopes markedly forward and downwards. Large supraorbital ridges and a sagittal crest reflect the great development of the masticatory apparatus of apes. The cranial capacity of the great apes is relatively small (chimpanzee 400cc, gorilla 500cc) compared to man (1300cc).

The oldest fossil remains regarded as ancestral to the great apes and *Homo sapiens* belong to two primate genera, *Propliopithecus haeckeli* and *Aegyptopithecus zeuxis*, which lived about 30 million years ago in the Fayum region of Egypt. It has been postulated that *Propliopithecus* was ancestral to *Aegyptopithecus*.

584 & 585 *Aegyptopithecus zeuxis*. In several features, *Aegyptopithecus* bears a strong resemblance to the ancestors of living great apes, the dryopithecines. It had large canines, a sectorial lower first premolar, molars that increased in size from before backwards and a dryopithecine Y-5 cusp pattern on the lower molars. *Aegyptopithecus* was probably an herbivorous and/or frugivorous, tree-living quadruped.

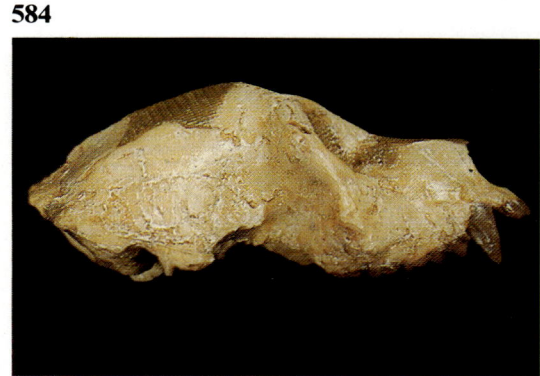

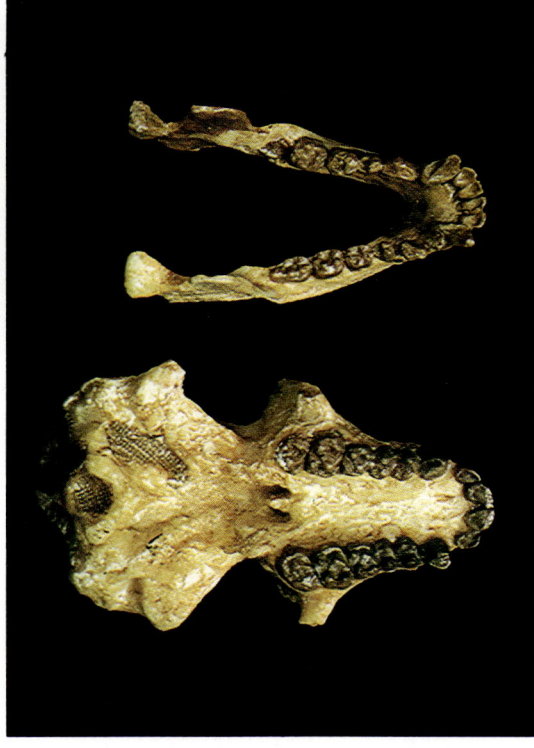

Nothing is known about the evolution of man from about 27 to 14 million years ago. Considerably more is known about the evolution of the great apes during this period. The genus *Dryopithecus* with its 3 subgenera colonised the Old World at this time: *D. dryopithecus* in Europe; *D. proconsul* in Africa and *D. sivapithecus* in Asia. Among these forms can be recognised the ancestors of modern apes.

586 *Ramapithecus wickeri*. **586A**, occlusal view. **586B**, buccal view. At least two species are recognised, *Ramapithecus wickeri* and *Ramapithecus punjabicus*. It existed from over 14 million years to at least 9 million years ago. Jaw fragments of this animal have been discovered in north-west India, Kenya, Hungary, Pakistan, Turkey and Greece. Among the features distinguishing *Ramapithecus* from other fossil apes were the anterior position of the canines and the reduced size of the anterior teeth. The cheek teeth have flat, broad chewing surfaces suggesting that the diet was coarse. The gradient of tooth wear along the molars was very marked. This pattern of wear indicates that, unlike apes, there was a considerable interval of time between the eruption of successive molars. The dental arcade had slightly diverging straight tooth rows. Among its more ape-like features were the facts that the canines projected slightly beyond the adjacent teeth and there may even have been a diastema present. The crown of the lower first premolar was unicuspid. Although some of the features which differentiate *Ramapithecus* from other fossil apes do not particularly resemble those of *Homo sapiens*, nevertheless they do anticipate characteristics of *australopithecines*. Thus, *Ramapithecus* is the most likely candidate representing the earliest ancestral hominid.

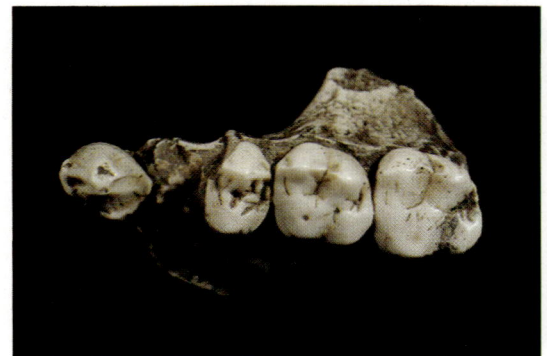

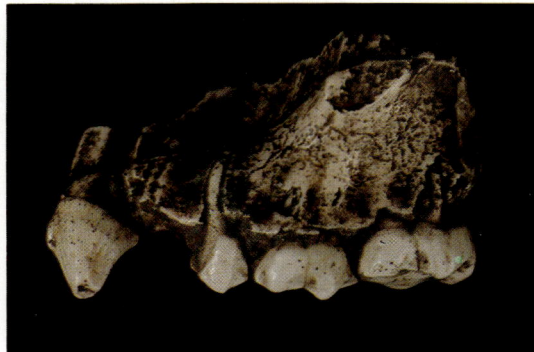

If *Ramapithecus* was a hominid, then man's early ancestors differentiated within and at the edge of the forests where they lived on vegetable foods, in particular seeds and nuts which were gathered on the ground in the open areas around rivers and lakes. The locomotory behaviour of this animal is not known.

About five million years ago there appeared a more advanced hominid genus, *Australopithecus*, which survived until as recently as one million years ago. Three species of *Australopithecus* have been described: *A. africanus*, *A. robustus* and *A. boisei*. The best known specimens have been found in South and East Africa but the genus may also have inhabited Asia. Their environment was probably grassland and open woodland. The evidence available suggests that the early australopithecines were bipedal though they were relatively inefficient at this form of locomotion. The use of and ability to make tools was established by these creatures, the oldest known stone tools being over 2 million years old.

587 & 588 *Australopithecus africanus*. This hominid was small (122cm to 137cm) and had a cranial capacity of about 450cc. The teeth had features typical of hominids. The incisors were spatulate and vertically-implanted in the jaws. The canines were short and hardly projected above the other teeth. There was no diastema between incisors and canines. The dental arcade was parabolic. The molars were larger than in later hominids but morphologically were very similar to those of *Homo*. The third molars erupted relatively late. Moderate brow ridges surmounted a projecting face.

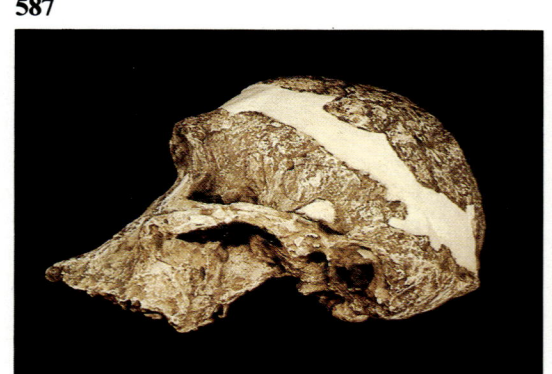

Australopithecus robustus was a more robust form than *A. africanus* and possessed an increased cheek-tooth size. Associated with the increased tooth size was evidence of more powerful masticatory musculature.

589 & 590 *Australopithecus boisei*. This probably represents a later form of *A. robustus*. This almost complete cranium, 1.75 million years old, was found in Olduvai Gorge, Tanzania. Its molars and premolars were enormous relative to the incisors and canines and were broad compared with those of other *Australopithecus* species, hence his familiar name 'Nutcracker man'. The sagittal crest indicates well-developed temporal muscles.

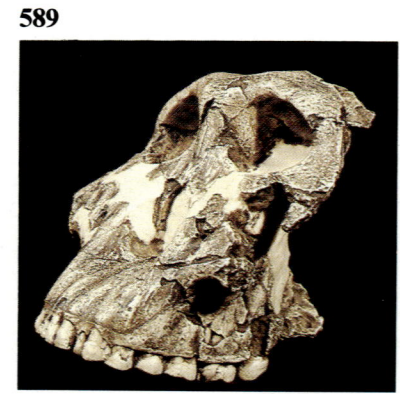
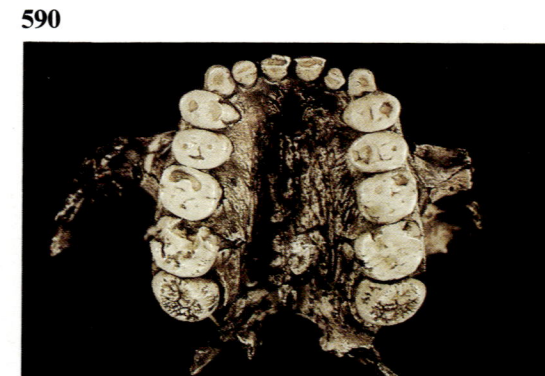

The remains of a gracile hominid type (*Homo habilis*) having some characteristics of *Australopithecus* and others of *Homo* have been found in Olduvai Gorge. This creature was thought to inhabit the Gorge approximately 1.75–0.75 million years ago.

591 *Homo habilis*. Some of the features which distinguish *Homo habilis* from *Australopithecus* are:
1 Its greater cranial capacity (600–650cc).
2 Its larger incisors and canines relative to the size of the cheek teeth.
3 A tendency towards buccolingual narrowing and mesiodistal elongation of all the teeth, especially the cheek teeth.
4 Unlike the early australopithecines, *Homo habilis* may have been a better biped.

Despite these differences, however, some authorities regard *Homo habilis* as an advanced australopithecine.

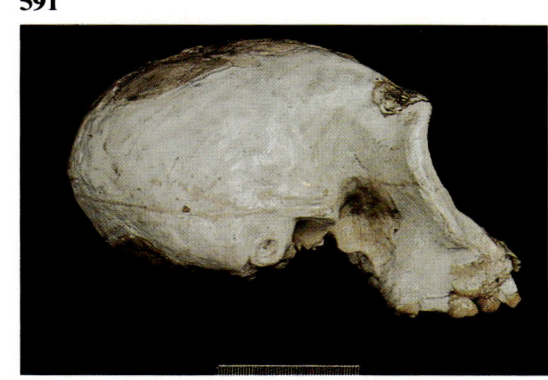

591

Recent fossil finds suggest that the genera *Homo* and *Australopithecus* diverged some time between 2 and 5 million years ago, the date being somewhat controversial. However, the problem of deciding which hominid fossils should be regarded as the earliest members of the genus *Homo* is not an easy one to solve, mainly because of the difficulty in defining the characteristics distinctive of *Homo*.

592 Cranium KNM-ER 1470. This skull collected from Kenya has yet to be fully analysed, but is probably about 2 million years old. The supraorbital tori were weakly developed. There was no indication of a nuchal crest or other powerful muscle attachments. Its cranial capacity has been given as approximately 775cc. No teeth from this fossil have been found, though teeth attributed to the same type of hominid have recently been discovered e.g. KN-ER 1590 and 1802.

593 *Homo erectus*. This hominid was apparently widely distributed throughout the Old World (e.g. Indonesia, China, Africa and Europe) about 1.5–0.5 million years ago. This species shows a number of significant advances compared with *Australopithecus*. It was taller, had a greater cranial capacity and had a relatively smaller face and teeth. It was completely adapted to bipedal locomotion. Illustrated here is *Homo erectus* from Java. The oldest specimens possessed thick cranial bones and a marked flattening of the profile of the cranial vault. They had huge brow ridges, pronounced post-orbital constrictions, a sloping forehead and a cranial capacity of about 850cc. The crania of the later specimens of *H. erectus* were rounder and higher, had smaller brow ridges and a cranial capacity of approximately 1050cc.

A number of fossils intermediate in position between *H. habilis* and *H. erectus* have been found.

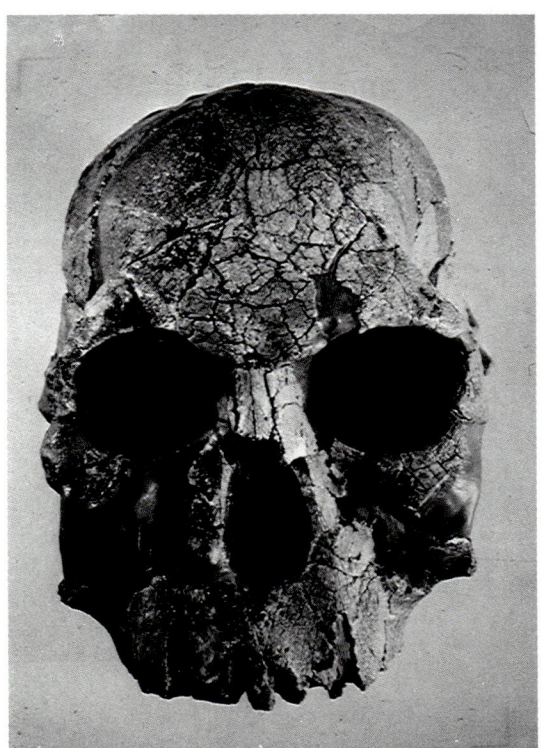

592

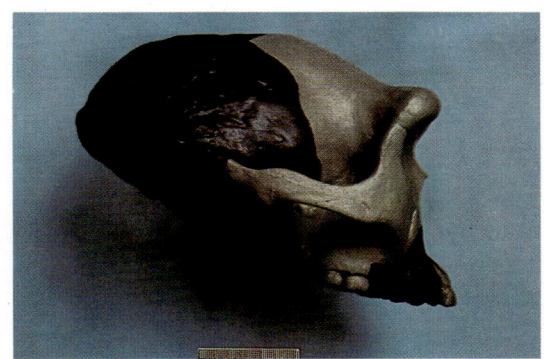

593

594 Occlusal view of jaws of *Homo erectus*. The upper jaw is from a specimen unearthed in Java, the lower jaw from Algeria. Although the teeth had an appearance similar to that of modern man, they were larger. The canines were more robust. The molars were more equal in size and the lower second and third molars tended to possess five rather than four cusps.

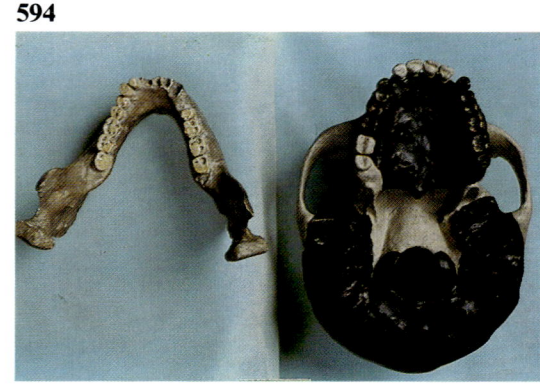

The major evolutionary changes from *H. erectus* to *H. sapiens* were restricted almost entirely to the head. The brain capacity increased to about 1300cc, the jaws became less robust and the teeth slightly smaller. The skull became rather shorter and higher. Though some fossils exist of 'archaic' man whose position lies between *H. erectus* and modern *H. sapiens* (e.g. Heidelberg and Swanscombe) considerable gaps exist in our knowledge concerning the affinities of the various fossils.

595 & 596 *Homo sapiens neanderthalensis*. The picture of the final emergence of modern *Homo sapiens* is further complicated by the appearance of 'Neanderthal' man in Europe about 100,000 years ago. The Neanderthals had long, low, robust skulls with prominent occiputs and well-developed brow ridges. They had a cranial capacity of 1450+cc and possessed taurodont molars (i.e. the pulp chamber extends well into roots). They became extinct about 35,000 years ago. Recent evidence suggests that they were not direct ancestors of modern *H. sapiens* but may have been a cold-adapted sub-species of *H. sapiens*.

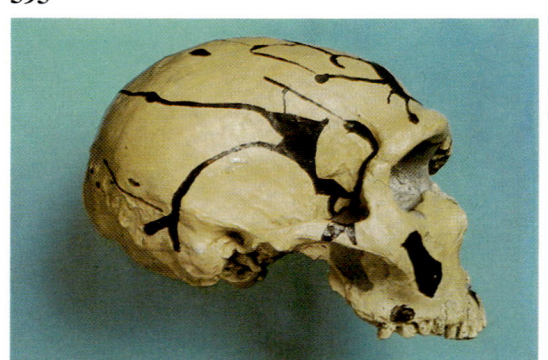
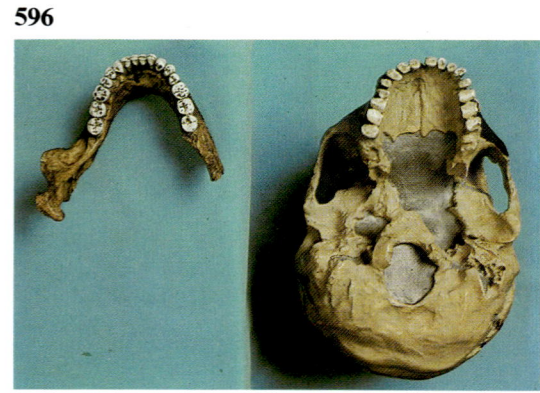

597 & 598 The first appearance of modern *Homo sapiens* in Europe was about 35,000 years ago (Cro-magnon man), though isolated finds suggest that modern man may have existed 100,000 years ago. This Cro-magnon specimen is dated about 22,000 years ago.

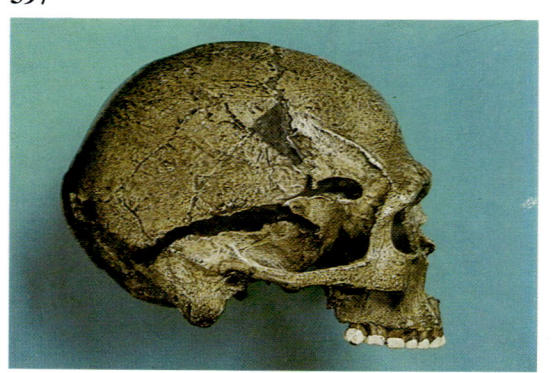
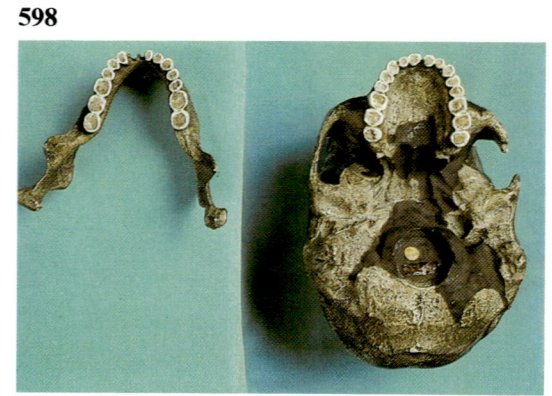

Suggested family tree for the evolution of *Homo sapiens*

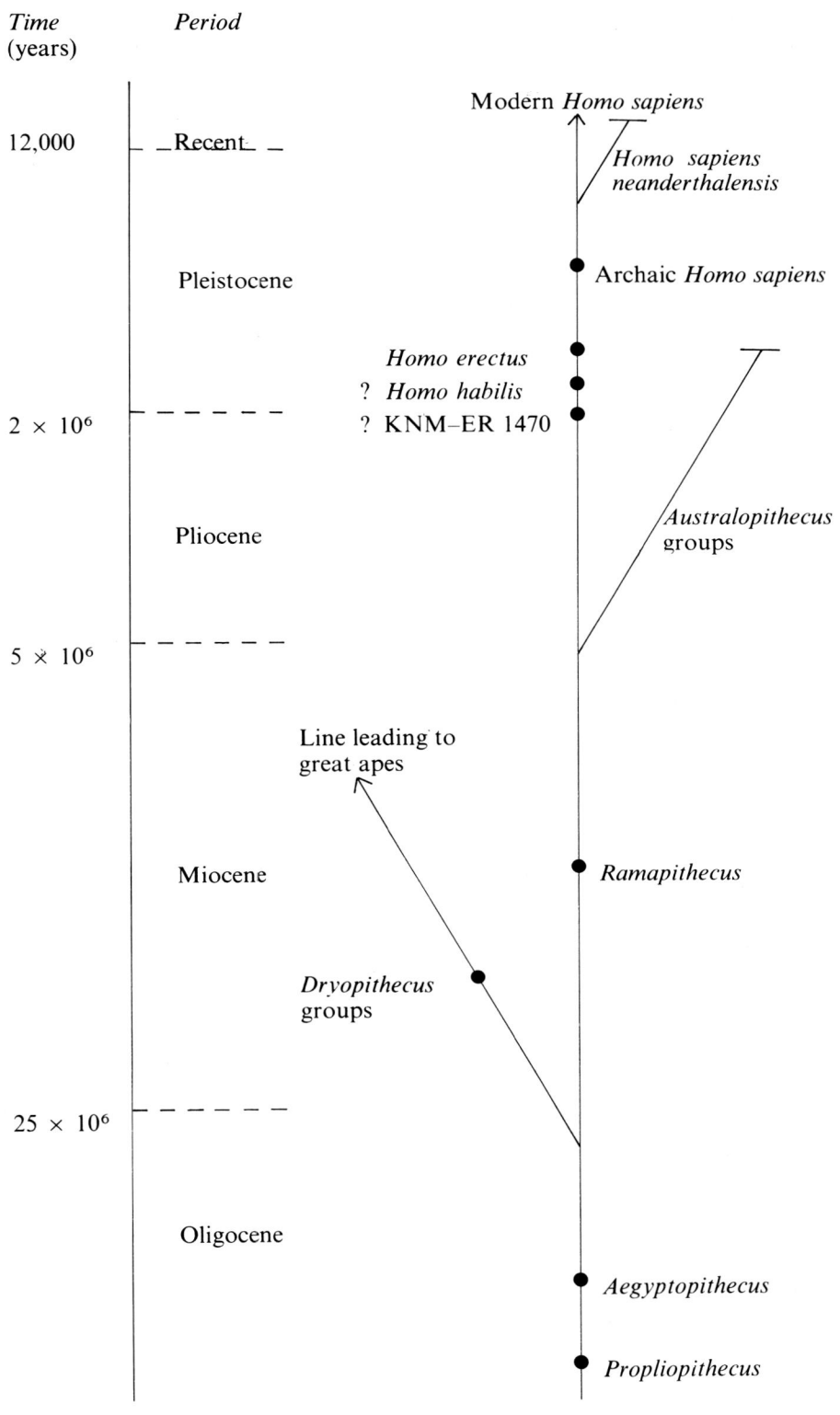

Suggestions for further reading

Macroscopic appearance of the oral cavity and environs

Tooth morphology
Downer, G. C. (1975). *Dental morphology*. Wright, Bristol.
Harty, F. J. (1976). *Endodontics in clinical practice*. Wright, Bristol.
Kraus, B. S., Jordan, R. E. and Abrams, L. (1969). *Dental anatomy and occlusion*. Williams and Wilkins, Baltimore.
Wheeler, R. C (1974). *A textbook of dental anatomy and physiology*. 5th ed. Saunders, Philadelphia.

Occlusion
Anderson, D. J. and Matthews, B. (eds.). (1976). *Mastication*. Wright, Bristol.
Graber, T. M. (1972). *Orthodontics*. 3rd ed. Saunders, Philadelphia.
Houston, W. J. B. (1976). *Walther's orthodontic notes*. 3rd ed. Wright, Bristol.
Ramfjord, S. P. and Ash, M. M. Jr. (1971). *Occlusion*. 2nd ed. Saunders, Philadelphia.
Thomson, H. (1975). *Occlusion*. Wright, Bristol.

Oro-facial soft tissues
Anderson, D. J. and Matthews, B. (eds.). (1976). *Mastication*. Wright, Bristol.
Berry, D. C. and Yemm, R. (1976). Muscle function and the occlusion of the teeth. In – *Scientific foundations of dentistry*. B. Cohen and I. R. H. Kramer (eds.). Heinemann, London. P. 583.
Carter, R. B. and Keen, E. N. (1971). The intramandibular course of the inferior alveolar nerve. *J. Anat.*, 108: 433.
Hollingshead, W. H. (1968). *Anatomy for surgeons*. Vol. 1. Head and neck. 2nd ed. Harper and Row, Maryland.
Jones, F. W. (1939). The anterior superior alveolar nerve and vessels. *J. Anat.*, 73: 583.
Killey, H. C., Seward, G. R. and Kay, L. W. (1975). Anatomical factors influencing the mode of spread of infection in the soft tissues around the jaw. In – *An outline of oral surgery*. Part 1. Wright, Bristol. P. 76.
Potter, G. D. (1971). *Sectional anatomy and tomography of the head*. Heinemann, London.
Sessle, B. J. and Hannam, A. J. (eds.). (1976). *Mastication and swallowing*. University of Toronto, Toronto.
Sicher, H. and Du Bruel, E. L. (1975). *Oral anatomy*. 6th ed. Mosby, St. Louis.
Warwick, R. and Williams, P. L. (eds.). (1973). *Gray's anatomy*. 35th ed. Longman, Edinburgh.

Radiographic appearance of jaws and teeth
Clarke, K. C. (1974). *Positioning in radiography*. Vols. 1 and 2. 9th ed. Heinemann, London.
Graber, T. M. (1972). Cephalometric radiographs. In – *Orthodontics*. 3rd ed. Saunders, Philadelphia. P. 431.
Potter, G. D. (1971). *Sectional anatomy and tomography of the head*. Heinemann, London.
Wuehrmann, A. H. and Manson-Hing, L. R. (1977). *Dental radiography*. 4th ed. Mosby, St. Louis.

Microscopic appearance of dental tissues

Enamel
Boyde, A. (1975). Scanning electron microscopy of enamel surfaces. *Brit. med. Bull.*, 31: 120.
Boyde, A. (1976). Amelogenesis and the structure of enamel. In – *Scientific foundations of dentistry*. B. Cohen and I. R. H. Kramer (eds.). Heinemann, London. P. 335.
Braden, M. (1976). Biophysics of the tooth. *Front. oral Physiol.*, 2: 1.
Brudevold, F. and Söremark, R. (1967). Chemistry of the mineral phase of enamel. In – *Structural and chemical organisation of teeth*. Vol. II. A. E. W. Miles (ed.). Academic Press, London. P. 247.
Fearnhead, R. W. and Stack, M. V. (eds.). (1971). *Tooth enamel. II*. Wright, Bristol.
Gustafson, G. and Gustafson, A.-G. (1967). Microanatomy and histochemistry of enamel. In – *Structural and chemical organisation of teeth*. Vol. II. A. E. W. Miles (ed.). Academic Press, London. P. 76.
Gwinnett, A. J. (1967). The ultrastructure of the prismless enamel of permanent human teeth. *Archs oral Biol.*, 12: 381.
Helmcke, J.-G. (1967). Ultrastructure of enamel. In – *Structural and chemical organisation of teeth*. Vol. II. A. E. W. Miles (ed.). Academic Press. P. 135.
Lavelle, C. L. B., Shellis, R. P. and Poole, D. F. G. (1977). *Evolutionary changes to the primate skull and dentition*. Thomas, Illinois. P. 197.
Newman, H. N. and Poole, D. F. G. (1974). Observations with scanning and transmission electron microscopy on the structure of human surface enamel. *Archs oral Biol.*, 19: 1135.
Orams, H. J., Phakey, P. P., Rachinger, W. A. and Zybert, J. J. (1974). Visualisation of micropore structure in human dental enamel. *Nature*, 252: 584.
Osborn, J. W. (1973). Variations in structure and development of enamel. In – *Dental enamel*. Oral Science Reviews, Vol. 3. Munksgaard, Copenhagen. P. 3.
Robinson, C., Weatherell, J. A. and Hallsworth, S. A. (1971). Variation in composition of dental enamel within thin ground tooth sections. *Caries Res.*, 5: 44.
Schmidt, W. J. and Keil, A. (1971). *Polarising microscopy of dental tissues*. Pergamon Press, Oxford.
Silverstone, L. M., Saxton, C. A., Dogon, I. L. and Fejerskov, O. (1975). Variation in the pattern of acid etching of human dental enamel examined by scanning electron microscopy. *Caries Res.*, 9: 373.
Stack, M. V. (1967). Chemical organisation of the organic matrix of enamel. In – *Structural and chemical organisation of teeth*. Vol. II. A. E. W. Miles (ed.). Academic Press, London. P. 317.
Stack, M. V. and Fearnhead, R. W. (eds.). (1965). *Tooth enamel I*. Wright, Bristol.
Weatherell, J. A. (1975). Composition of dental enamel. *Brit. med. Bull.*, 31: 115.
Zimmerman, S. (1976). Physicochemical properties of enamel and dentine. In – *Dental biochemistry*. 2nd ed. E. P. Lazzari (ed.). Lea and Febiger, Philadelphia. P. 112.

Investing organic layers on enamel surfaces
Armstrong, W. G. (1968). Origin and nature of the acquired pellicle. *Proc. R. Soc. Med.*, 61: 923.
Dawes, C., Jenkins, G. N., and Tonge, C. H. (1963). The nomenclature of the integuments of the enamel surface of teeth. *Brit. dent. J.*, 115: 65.
Hodson, J. J. (1966). The distribution, structure, origin and nature of the dental cuticle of Gottlieb. Parts I and II. *J. Am. Soc. Periodont.*, 5: 235, 295.
McHugh, W. D. (ed.). (1970). *Dental plaque*. Livingstone, Edinburgh.
Newman, H. N. (1973). The organic films on enamel surfaces. Parts 1 and 2. *Brit. dent. J.*, 135: 106, 164.
Newman, H. N. and Poole, D. F. G. (1974). Structural and ecological aspects of dental plaque. In – *Normal microbial flora of man*. F. A. Skinner and J. D. Carr (eds.). Academic Press, London. P. 111.
Provenza, D. V. and Sisca, R. F. (1970). Fine structure features of monkey (*Macaca mulatta*) reduced enamel epithelium. *J. Periodont.*, 4: 313.
Schroeder, H. E. and Listgarten, M. A. (1971). *Fine structure of the developing epithelial attachment in human teeth*. Monographs in developmental biology. Vol. 2. A. Wolskey (ed.). Karger, Basel.
Stallard, R. E., Diab, M. A. and Zander, H. A. (1965). The attaching substance between enamel and epithelium. A product of the epithelial cells. *J. Periodont.*, 36: 130.

Dentine
Anderson, D. J. (1975). Pain from dentine and pulp. *Brit. med. Bull.*, 31: 111.
Boyde, A. (1974). Transmission electron microscopy of ion-beam thinned dentine. *Cell Tiss. Res.*, 152: 543.
Braden, M. (1976). Biophysics of the tooth. *Front. oral Physiol.*, 2: 1.
Bradford, E. W. (1967). Microanatomy and histochemistry of dentine. In – *Structural and chemical organisation of teeth*. Vol. II. A. E. W. Miles (ed.). Academic Press, London. P. 3.
Brannstrom, M. and Astrom, A. (1972). The hydrodynamics of the dentine; its possible relationship to dentinal pain. *Int. dent. J.*, 22: 219.
Byers, M. R. and Kish, S. J. (1976). Delineation of somatic nerve endings in rat teeth by radioautography of axon-transported protein. *J. dent. Res.*, 55: 419.
Eastoe, J. E. (1967). Chemical organisation of the organic matrix of dentine. In – *Structural and chemical organisation of teeth*. Vol. II. A. E. W. Miles (ed.). Academic Press, London. P. 279.
Frank, R. M. (1968). Ultrastructural relationship between the odontoblast, its process and the nerve fibre. In – *Dentine and pulp*. N. B. B. Symons (ed.). Livingstone, Edinburgh. P. 115.
Garberoglio, R. and Brannstrom, M. (1976). Scanning electron microscopic investigations of human dentinal tubules. *Archs oral Biol.*, 21: 355.
Holland, G. R. (1975). The dentinal tubule and odontoblast process in the cat. *J. Anat.*, 120: 169.

Holland, G. R. (1976). An ultrastructural survey of cat dentinal tubules. *J. Anat.*, 122: 1.
Johansen, E. (1967). Ultrastructure of dentine. In – *Structural and chemical organisation of teeth*. Vol. II. A. E. W. Miles (ed.). Academic Press, London. P. 35.
Kawasaki, K. and Fearnhead, R. W. (1975). On the relationship between tetracycline and the incremental lines in dentine. *J. Anat.*, 119: 49.
Lester, K. S. and Boyde, A. (1968). Morphology of some crystalline components of dentine. In – *Dentine and pulp*. N. B. B. Symons (ed.). Livingstone, Edinburgh. P. 197.
Mjör, I. A. (1972). Human coronal dentine: Structure and reactions. *Oral Surg.*, 33: 810.
Rowles, S. L. (1967). Chemistry of the mineral phase of dentine. In – *Structural and chemical organisation of teeth*. Vol. II. A. E. W. Miles (ed.). Academic Press, London. P. 201.
Schmidt, W. T. and Keil, A. (1971). *Polarising microscopy of dental tissues*. Pergamon Press, Oxford.
Ten Cate, A. R. (1972). An analysis of Tomes' granular layer. *Anat. Rec.*, 172: 137.

Dental pulp

Anderson, D. J., Hannam, A. G. and Matthews, B. (1970). Sensory mechanisms in mammalian teeth and their supportive structures. *Physiol. Rev.*, 50: 171.
Arwill, T. (1968). The ultrastructure of the pulpo-dentinal border zone. In – *Dentine and pulp*. N. B. B. Symons (ed.). Livingstone, Edinburgh. P. 147.
Beerstecher, E. Jr. (1976). Biochemistry of the dental pulp. In – *Dental biochemistry*. 2nd ed. E. P. Lazzari (ed.). Lea and Febiger, Philadelphia. P. 178.
Brown, A. C., Barrow, B. L., Gadd, G. N. and Van Hassell, H. J. (1969). Tooth pulp transcapillary osmotic pressure in dog. *Archs oral Biol.*, 14: 491.
Corpron, R. C., Avery, J. K. and Lee, S. D. (1973). Ultrastructure of terminal pulpal blood vessels in mouse molars. *Anat. Rec.*, 179: 527.
Dahl, E. and Mjör, I. A. (1973). The fine structure of the vessels in the human dental pulp. *Acta odont. scand.*, 31: 223.
Fearnhead, R. W. (1967). Innervation of dental tissues. In – *Structural and chemical organisation of teeth*. Vol. I. A. E. W. Miles (ed.). Academic Press, London. P. 247.
Finn, S. B. (ed.). (1968). *Biology of the dental pulp organ*. University of Alabama Press, Alabama.
Garant, P. R., Szabo, G. and Nalbandian, J. (1968). The fine structure of the mouse odontoblast. *Archs oral Biol.*, 13: 857.
Gotjamanos, T. (1969). Cellular organization in the subodontoblastic zone of the dental pulp. 1. A study of cell-free and cell-rich layers in pulps of adult rat and deciduous monkey teeth. *Archs oral Biol.*, 14: 1007.
Holland, G. R. (1975). Membrane junctions on cat odontoblasts. *Archs oral Biol.*, 20: 551.
Jessen, H. (1967). The ultrastructure of odontoblasts in perfusion fixed, demineralised incisors of adult rats. *Acta odont. scand.*, 25: 491.
Kramer, I. R. H. (1960). The vascular architecture of the human dental pulp. *Archs oral Biol.*, 2: 177.
Matthieson, M. E. and von Bülow, F. A. (1970). The ultrastructure of human foetal odontoblasts. *Z. Zellforsch.*, 105: 569.
Saunders, R. L. De C. H. and Röckert, H. Ö. E. (1967). Vascular supply of dental tissues, including lymphatics. In – *Structural and chemical organisation of teeth*. Vol. I. A. E. W. Miles (ed.). Academic Press, London. P. 199.
Setzer, S. and Bender, I. B. (1975). *The dental pulp*. 2nd ed. Lippincott, Philadelphia.
Stanley, H. R. and Rainey, R. R. (1962). Age changes in the human dental pulp. *Oral Surg.*, 15: 1396.
Zerlotti, E. (1964). Histochemical study of the connective tissue of the dental pulp. *Archs oral Biol.*, 9: 149.

Cementum

Boyde, A. and Jones, S. T. (1968). Scanning electron microscopy of cementum and Sharpey fibre bone. *Z. Zellforsch.*, 92: 536.
El Mostehy, M. R. and Stallard, R. E. (1968). Intermediate cementum. *J. periodont. Res.*, 3: 24.
Furseth, R. (1967). A microradiographic and electron microscopic study of the cementum of human deciduous teeth. *Acta odontol. scand.*, 25: 613.
Furseth, R. (1969). The fine structure of the cellular cementum of young human teeth. *Archs oral Biol.*, 14: 1147.
Furseth, R. and Mjör, I. A. (1973). Cementum. In – *Histology of the human tooth*. I. A. Mjör and J. J. Pindborg (eds.). Munksgaard, Copenhagen. P. 97.
Jones, S. J. and Boyde, A. (1972). A study of human root cementum surfaces as prepared for and examined in the scanning electron microscope. *Z. Zellforsch.*, 130: 318.

Linden, L-Å. (1968). Microscopic observations of fluid flow through cementum and dentine. An *in vitro* study on human teeth. *Odontol. Revy*, 19: 367.
Lorber, M. (1951). A study of the histochemical reactions of the dental cementum and alveolar bone. *Anat. Rec.*, 111: 129.
Paynter, K. J. and Pudy, C. (1958). A study of the structure, chemical nature and development of cementum in the rat. *Anat. Rec.*, 131: 233.
Rodriguez, M. S. and Wilderman, M. N. (1972). Amino acid composition of the cementum matrix from human molar teeth. *J. Periodont.*, 43: 438.
Selvig, K. A. (1965). The fine structure of human cementum. *Acta odontol. scand.*, 23: 423.
Zander, H. A. and Hürzler, B. (1958). Continuous cementum apposition. *J. dent. Res.*, 37: 1035.

Periodontal ligament

Anderson, D. J., Eastoe, J. E., Melcher, A. H. and Picton, D. C. S. (eds.). (1967). *Mechanisms of tooth support*. Wright, Bristol.
Anderson, D. J., Hannam, A. G. and Matthews, B. (1970). Sensory mechanisms in mammalian teeth and their supportive structures. *Physiol. Rev.*, 50: 171.
Beertsen, W., Everts, V. and Van den Hooff, A. (1974). Fine structure of fibroblasts in the periodontal ligament of the rat incisor and their possible role in tooth eruption. *Archs oral Biol.*, 19: 1087.
Castelli, W. A. and Dempster, W. T. (1965). The periodontal vasculature and its response to experimental pressures. *J. Am. dent. Ass.*, 70: 890.
Eastoe, J. E. (1976). Collagen chemistry and tissue organisation. In – *The eruption and occlusion of teeth*. Colston Papers No. 27. D. F. G. Poole and M. V. Stack (eds.). Butterworths, London. P. 229.
Fullmer, H. M. (1967). Connective tissue components of the periodontium. In – *Structural and chemical organisation of teeth*. Vol. II. A. E. W. Miles (ed.). Academic Press, London. P. 349.
Fullmer, H. M., Sheetz, J. H. and Narkates, A. J. (1974). Oxytalan connective tissue fibres: A review. *J. oral Path.*, 3: 291.
Gianelly, A. A. and Goldman, H. M. (1971). *Biological basis of orthodontics*. Lea and Febiger, Philadelphia.
Griffin, C. J. and Harris, R. (1967). The fine structure of the developing human periodontium. *Archs oral Biol.*, 12: 971.
Hannam, A. G. (1976). Periodontal mechanoreceptors. In – *Mastication*. D. J. Anderson and B. Matthews (eds.). Wright, Bristol. P. 43.
Kindlová, M. and Matěna, V. (1962). Blood vessels of the rat molar. *J. dent. Res.*, 41: 650.
Melcher, A. H. and Bowen, W. A. (eds.). (1969). *Biology of the periodontium*. Academic Press, London.
Melcher, A. H. and Walker, T. W. (1976). The periodontal ligament in attachment and as a shock absorber. In – *The eruption and occlusion of teeth*. Colston Papers No. 27. D. F. G. Poole and M. V. Stack (eds.). Butterworths, London. P. 183.
Pearson, C. H., Wohlleble, M., Carmichael, D. J. and Chovelon, A. (1975). Bovine periodontal ligament: an investigation of the collagen, glycosaminoglycan and insoluble glycoprotein components at different stages of tissue development. *Connect. tissue Res.*, 3: 195.
Rippin, J. W. (1975). The metabolism and functions of the soft connective tissues of the mouth. In – *Applied physiology of the mouth*. C. L. B. Lavelle (ed.). Wright, Bristol. P. 1.
Sloan, P., Shellis, R. P. and Berkovitz, B. K. B. (1976). Effect of specimen preparation on the appearance of the rat periodontal ligament in the scanning electron microscope. *Archs oral Biol.*, 21: 633.
Ten Cate, A. R. (1974). The role of the fibroblast in collagen turnover in the functioning periodontal ligament of the mouse. *Archs oral Biol.*, 19: 339.
Valderhaug, J. P. and Nylen, M. V. (1966). Function of epithelial rests as suggested by their ultrastructure. *J. periodont., Res.*, 1: 69.

Alveolar bone

Atkinson, P. J. (1976). Patterns of bone growth. In – *The eruption and occlusion of teeth*. Colston Papers No. 27. D. F. G. Poole and M. V. Stack (eds.). Butterworths, London. P. 5.
Birn, H. (1966). The vascular supply of the periodontal ligament. *J. periodont. Res.*, 1: 51.
Bourne, G. H. (ed.). *The biochemistry and physiology of bone*. 2nd ed. Vols. I and II (1972), Vol. III (1971), Vol. IV (1976). Academic Press, London.
Boyde, A. and Hobdell, M. H. (1969). Scanning electron microscopy of lamellar bone. *Z. Zellforsch.*, 93: 213.
Boyde, A. and Jones, S. J. (1968). Scanning electron microscopy of cementum and Sharpey fibre bone. *Z. Zellforsch.*, 92: 536.
Cohn, S. A. (1972). A re-examination of Sharpey's fibres in alveolar bone of the mouse. *Archs oral Biol.*, 17: 255.
Cohn, S. A. (1972). A re-examination of Sharpey's fibres in alveolar bone of the marmoset (*Saguinus fuscicollis*). *Archs oral Biol.*, 17: 261.
McLean, F. C. and Urist, M. R. (1968). *Bone: fundamentals of the physiology*

of skeletal tissue. 3rd ed. University of Chicago Press, Chicago.
Moore, W. J. (1975). Bone growth and remodelling. In – *Applied physiology of the mouth.* C. L. B. Lavelle (ed.). Wright, Bristol. P. 73.
Ranley, D. M. (1976). Bone apposition and resorption. In – *Dental biochemistry.* 2nd ed. E. P. Lazzari (ed.). Lea and Febiger, Philadelphia. P. 134.
Weinmann, J. P. and Sicher, H. (1955). *Bone and bones: fundamentals of bone biology.* 2nd ed. Mosby, St. Louis.

Oral mucosa
Ainamo, J. and Löe, H. (1966). Anatomical characteristics of gingiva. A clinical and microscopic study of the free and attached gingiva. *J. Periodont.,* 37: 5.
Ainamo, J. and Talari, A. (1976). Eruptive movements of teeth in human adults. In – *The eruption and occlusion of teeth.* Colston Papers No. 27. D. F. G. Poole and M. V. Stack (eds.). Butterworths, London. P. 97.
Cimasoni, G. (1974). *The crevicular fluid.* Monographs in oral science. Vol. 3. H. M. Myers (ed.). Karger, Basel.
Dolby, A. E. (ed.). (1975). *Oral mucosa in health and disease.* Blackwell Scientific, Oxford.
Egelberg, J. (1966). The blood vessels of the dento-gingival junction. *J. periodont. Res.,* 1: 163.
Kindlová, M. (1967). Glomerular vascular structures in the periodontium. In – *The mechanisms of tooth support.* D. J. Anderson, J. E. Eastoe, A. H. Melcher and D. C. A. Picton (eds.). Wright, Bristol. P. 76.
Listgarten, M. A. (1972). Normal development, structure, physiology and repair of gingival epithelium. In – *Gingival epithelium.* Oral science reviews. Vol. 1. Munksgaard, Copenhagen. P. 3.
Loë, H. (1967). The structure and physiology of the dento-gingival junction. In – *Structural and chemical organisation of teeth.* Vol. II. A. E. W. Miles (ed.). Academic Press, London. P. 415.
Nuki, K. and Hock, J. (1974). The organisation of the gingival vasculature. *J. periodont. Res.,* 9: 305.
Schroeder, H. E. (1976). Gingival tissue. In – *Scientific foundations of dentistry.* B. Cohen and I. R. H. Kramer (eds.). Heinemann, London. P. 426.
Schroeder, H. E. and Listgarten, M. A. (1971). *Fine structure of the developing epithelial attachment of human teeth.* Monographs in developmental biology. Vol. 2. E. Wolsky (ed.). Karger, Basel.
Smith, C. J. (1969). Gingival epithelium. In – *Biology of the periodontium.* A. H. Melcher and W. H. Bowen (eds.). Academic Press, London. P. 105.
Squier, C. A., Johnson, N. W. and Hopps, R. M. (1976). *Human oral mucosa: development, structure and function.* Blackwell Scientific Publications, Oxford.
Squier, C. A. and Meyer, J. (eds.). (1971). *Current concepts of the histology of oral mucosa.* Thomas, Illinois.

Temporomandibular joint
Blackwood, H. J. J. (1976). The mandibular joint: development, structure and function. In – *Scientific foundations of dentistry.* B. Cohen and I. R. H. Kramer (eds.). Heinemann, London. P. 590.
Carlsson, G. E. and Öberg, T. (1974). Remodelling of the temporomandibular joints. In – *Temporomandibular joint function and dysfunction.* II. Oral science reviews, 6. Munksgaard, Copenhagen. P. 53.
Choukas, N. C. and Sicher, H. (1960). The structure of the temporomandibular joint. *Oral Surg.,* 13: 1263.
Durkin, J., Heeley, J. and Irving, J. T. (1973). The cartilage of the mandibular condyle. In – *Temporomandibular joint function and dysfunction.* I. Oral science reviews, 2. Munksgaard, Copenhagen. P. 29.
Rees, L. A. (1954). The structure and function of the mandibular joint. *Brit. dent. J.,* 96: 125.
Sarnat, B. G. (1964). *The temporomandibular joint.* 2nd ed. Thomas, Illinois.
Shore, N. E. (1976). *Temporomandibular joint dysfunction and occlusal equilibration.* 2nd ed. Lippincott, Philadelphia.
Storey, A. (1976). Temporomandibular joint receptors. In – *Mastication.* D. J. Anderson and B. Matthews (eds.). Wright, Bristol. P. 50.

Salivary glands
Amsterdam, A., Ohad, I. and Schramm, M. (1969). Dynamic changes in the ultrastructure of the acinar cell of the rat parotid gland during the secretory cycle. *J. Cell Biol.,* 41: 753.
Castle, J. D., Jamieson, J. D. and Palade, G. E. (1972). Radioautographic analysis of the secretory process in the parotid acinar cell of the rabbit. *J. Cell Biol.,* 53: 290.
Ferguson, D. B. (1975). Salivary glands and saliva. In – *Applied physiology of the mouth.* C. L. B. Lavelle (ed.). Wright, Bristol. P. 145.
Garrett, J. R. (1976). Structure and innervation of salivary glands. In – *Scientific foundations of dentistry.* B. Cohen and I. R. H. Kramer. Heinemann, London. P. 499.
Harrop, T. J. and Garrett, J. R. (1974). Effects of preganglionic sympathectomy on secretory changes in parotid acinar cells of rats on eating. *Cell Tissue Res.,* 154: 135.
Harrop, T. J. and McKay, B. (1968). Electron microscopic observations on myoepithelial cells and secretory nerves in rat salivary glands. *J. Canad. dent. Ass.* 34: 480.
Kim, S. K., Nasjleti, C. E. and Han, S. S. (1972). The secretion processes in mucous and serous secretory cells of the rat's sublingual gland. *J. Ultrastruct. Res.,* 38: 371.
Riva, A., Motta, G. and Riva-Testa, F. (1974). Ultrastructural diversity in secretory granules of human major salivary glands. *Am. J. Anat.,* 139: 293.
Riva, A. and Riva-Testa, F. (1973). Fine structure of acinar cells of human parotid gland. *Anat. Rec.,* 176: 149.
Shackleford, J. C. and Schneyer, L. H. (1971). Ultrastructural aspects of the main excretory duct of rat submandibular gland. *Anat. Rec.,* 169: 679.
Tandler, B. and Erlandson, R. A. (1972). Ultrastructure of the human submaxillary gland. IV. Serous granules. *Am. J. Anat.,* 135: 419.

Development of oro-dental tissues

Development of the face, palate and jaws
Baume, L. J. (1962). Ontogenesis of the temporomandibular joint. *J. dent. Res.,* 41: 1327.
Enlow, D. H. (1976). Postnatal growth and development of the face and cranium. In – *Scientific foundations of dentistry.* B. Cohen and I. R. H. Kramer (eds.). Heinemann, London. P. 29.
Haywood, A. F. (1968). Ultrastructural changes in the epithelium during fusion of the palatal processes in rats. *Archs oral Biol.,* 14: 661.
Humphrey, T. (1969). The relation between human fetal mouth opening reflexes and closure of the palate. *Am. J. Anat.,* 125: 317.
Kraus, B. S., Kitamura, H. and Latham, R. A. (1966). *Atlas of the developmental anatomy of the face.* Harper and Row, New York.
Latham, R. A. (1970). Maxillary development and growth: the septopremaxillary ligament. *J. Anat.,* 107: 471.
Manson, J. D. (1968). *A comparative study of the postnatal growth of the mandible.* Kimpton, London.
Moore, W. J. and Lavelle, C. L. B. (1974). *Growth of the facial skeleton in the hominoidea.* Academic Press, London.
Moss, M. L. (1968). The primacy of functional matrices in oro-facial growth. *Trans. Brit. Soc. Orthodont.,* 54: 107.
Moyers, R. E. and Krogman, W. M. (eds.). (1971). *Cranio-facial growth in man.* Pergamon Press, Oxford.
Pourtois, M. (1972). Morphogenesis of the primary and secondary palate. In – *Developmental aspects of oral biology.* H. S. Slavkin and L. A. Bavetta (eds.). Academic Press, London. P. 81.
Pratt, R. M. and Martin, G. R. (1975). Epithelial cell death and elevated cyclic AMP during palatal development. *Proc. Nat. Acad. Sci. U.S.A.* 72: 814.
Sperber, G. H. (1976). *Cranio-facial embryology.* 2nd ed. Wright, Bristol.
Tonge, C. H. and Luke, D. A. (1976). Cleft palate. *Dent. Update,* 3: 138.

Early tooth development
Berkovitz, B. K. B. (1967). An account of the enamel cord in *Setonix brachyurus* (Marsupialia) and on the presence of an enamel knot in *Trichosurus vulpecula. Archs oral Biol.,* 12: 49.
Butler, P. M. (1956). The ontogeny of molar pattern. *Biol. Rev.,* 31: 30.
Dahlberg, A. A. (ed.). (1971). *Dental morphology and evolution.* University of Chicago Press, Chicago.
Decker, J. D. (1963). A light and electron microscope study of the rat molar enamel organ. *Archs oral Biol.,* 8: 301.
Decker, J. D. (1967). The development of a vascular supply to the rat molar enamel organ. *Archs oral Biol.,* 12: 453.
Gaunt, W. A. (1959). The vascular supply to the dental lamina during early development. *Acta anat.,* 37: 232.
Gaunt, W. A. (1963). An analysis of the growth of the cheek teeth of the mouse during ontogeny. *Acta anat.,* 54: 220.
Gaunt, W. A. and Miles, A. E. W. (1967). Fundamental aspects of tooth morphogenesis. In – *Structural and chemical organisation of teeth.* Vol. I. A. E. W. Miles (ed.). Academic Press, London. P. 151.
Kollar, E. (1972). Histogenetic aspects of dermal-epidermal interactions. In – *Developmental aspects of oral biology.* H. C. Slavkin and L. A. Bavetta (eds.). Academic Press, New York. P. 125.
Ooë, T. (1957). On the early development of human dental lamina. *Okajimas Folia anat. Jap.,* 30: 197.
Ooë, T. (1959). On the development of position of the tooth germs in the human deciduous molar teeth. *Okajimas Folia anat. Jap.,* 32: 97.
Pannese, E. (1960). Observations on the ultrastructure of the enamel organ. I. Stellate reticulum and stratum intermedium. *J. Ultrastruct. Res.,* 4: 372.

Pannese, E. (1961). Observations on the ultrastructure of the enamel organ. II. Involution of the stellate reticulum. *J. Ultrastruct. Res.,* 5: 328.
Pannese, E. (1962). Observations on the ultrastructure of the enamel organ. III. Internal and external enamel epithelia. *J. Ultrastruct. Res.,* 6: 186.
Paynter, K. J. and Hunt, A. M. (1964). Morphogenesis of the rat first molar. *Archs oral Biol.,* 9: 611.
Pourtois, M. (1961). Contribution à l'étude des bourgeons dentaires chez la Souris. I. Périodes d'induction et de morphodifférentiation. *Arch. Biol., Liege,* 72: 17.
Provenza, D. V. and Sisca, R. F. (1971). Electron microscopic study of human dental primordia. *Archs oral Biol.,* 16: 121.
Silva, D. and Kallis, D. (1972). Ultrastructural studies on the cervical loop and the development of the amelo-dentinal junction in the cat. *Archs oral Biol.,* 17: 279.
Slavkin, H. C. (1974). *Embryonic tooth formation.* Oral science reviews. Vol. 4. Munksgaard, Copenhagen.

Amelogenesis
Allen, J. H. (1967). Maturation of enamel. In – *Structural and chemical organisation of teeth.* Vol. I. A. E. W. Miles (ed.). Academic Press, London. P. 467.
Boyde, A. (1976). Amelogenesis and the structure of enamel. In – *Scientific foundations of dentistry.* B. M. Cohen and I. R. H. Kramer (eds.). Heinemann, London. P. 335.
Crabb, H. S. M. and Darling, A. I. (1962). *The pattern of progressive mineralisation in human dental enamel.* Pergamon Press, Oxford.
Eggert, F. M., Allen, G. A. and Burgess, R. C. (1973). Amelogenesis: purification and partial characterization of proteins from developing bovine dental enamel. *Biochem. J.* 131: 471.
Fincham, A. G., Burkland, G. A. and Shapiro, I. M. (1972). Lipophilia of enamel matrix. *Calc. Tiss. Res.,* 9: 247.
Frank, M. R. and Nalbandian, J. (1967). Ultrastructure of amelogenesis. In – *Structural and chemical organisation of teeth.* Vol. I. A. E. W. Miles (ed.). Academic Press, London. P. 399.
Kallenbach, E. (1968). Fine structure of rat incisor ameloblasts during enamel maturation. *J. Ultrastruct. Res.,* 22: 90.
Katchburian, E. and Holt, S. J. (1972). Studies on the development of ameloblasts. *J. cell Sci.,* 11: 415.
Matthieson, M. E. and von Bülow, F. A. (1969). The ultrastructure of human secretory ameloblasts. *Z. Zellforsch.,* 101: 232.
Reith, E. J. (1970). The stages of amelogenesis as observed in molar teeth of young rats. *J. Ultrastruct. Res.,* 30: 111.
Reith, E. J. and Butcher, E. O. (1967). Microanatomy and histochemistry of amelogenesis. In – *Structural and chemical organisation of teeth.* Vol. I. A. E. W. Miles (ed.). Academic Press, London. P. 371.
Ronholm, E. (1962). The amelogenesis of human teeth as revealed by electron microscopy. II. The development of the enamel crystallites. *J. Ultrastruct. Res.,* 6: 249.
Warshawsky, H. and Smith, C. E. (1974). Morphological classification of rat incisor ameloblasts. *Anat. Rec.,* 179: 423.
Weinstock, A. (1972). Matrix development in mineralizing tissues as shown by radioautography: formation of enamel and dentine. In – *Developmental aspects of oral biology.* H. S. Slavkin and L. A. Bavetta (eds.). Academic Press, New York. P. 266.

Dentinogenesis and pulp formation
Bevelander, G. and Hiroshi, N. (1966). The formation and mineralization of dentine. *Anat. Rec.,* 156: 303.
Eisenmann, D. R. and Glick, P. L. (1972). Ultrastructure of initial crystal formation in dentine. *J. Ultrastruct. Res.,* 41: 18.
Finn, S. B. (ed.). (1968). *Biology of the dental pulp organ.* University of Alabama Press, Alabama.
Gotjamanos, T. (1969). Cellular organization in the subodontoblastic zone of the dental pulp. II. Period and mode of development of the cell-rich layer in rat molar pulps. *Archs oral Biol.,* 14: 1011.
Kawasaki, K. and Fearnhead, R. W. (1975). On the relationship between tetracycline and the incremental lines in dentine. *J. Anat.,* 119: 49.
Moss, M. L. (1974). Studies on dentine. I. Mantle dentine. *Acta anat.,* 87: 481.
Owens, P. D. A. (1972). Light microscopic observations on the formation of the layer of Hopewell-Smith in human teeth. *Archs oral Biol.,* 17: 1785.
Sisca, R. F. and Provenza, D. V. (1972). Initial dentine formation in human deciduous teeth. An electron microscope study. *Calc. Tiss. Res.,* 9: 1.
Symons, N. B. B. (1967). The microanatomy and histochemistry of dentinogenesis. In – *Structural and chemical organisation of teeth.* Vol. I. A. E. W. Miles (ed.). Academic Press, London. P. 285.
Symons, N. B. B. (ed.). (1968). *Dentine and pulp.* Livingstone, Edinburgh.
Takuma, S. (1967). Ultrastructure of dentinogenesis. In – *Structural and chemical organisation of teeth.* Vol. I. A. E. W. Miles (ed.). Academic Press, London. P. 285.
Takuma, S. and Nagai, N. (1971). Ultrastructure of rat odontoblasts in various stages of their development and maturation. *Archs oral Biol.,* 16: 993.
Weinstock, M. and Leblond, C. P. (1973). Radioautographic visualization of the deposition of a phosphoprotein at the mineralization front in the dentine of the rat incisor. *J. Cell Biol.,* 56: 838.
Whittacker, D. K. and Adams, D. (1972). Electron microscopic studies on Von Korff fibres in the human developing tooth. *Anat. Rec.,* 174: 175.
Yoshiki, S. and Kurahaski, Y. (1971). A light and electron microscopic study of alkaline phosphatase activity in the early stages of dentinogenesis in the young rat. *Archs oral Biol.,* 16: 1143.

Development of the root
Atkinson, M. E. (1972). The development of the mouse molar periodontium. *J. periodont. Res.,* 7: 255.
Cutright, D. E. (1970). The morphogenesis of the vascular supply to the permanent teeth of *Macaca rhesus. Oral Surg.,* 30: 284.
Freeman, E. and Ten Cate, A. R. (1971). Development of the periodontium: an electron microscope study. *J. Periodont.,* 42: 387.
Freeman, E., Ten Cate, A. R. and Dickinson, J. (1975). Development of a gomphosis by tooth germ implants in the parietal bone of the mouse. *Archs oral Biol.,* 20: 139.
Gaunt, W. A. (1960). The vascular supply in relation to the formation of roots on the cheek teeth of the mouse. *Acta anat.,* 43: 116.
Grant, D. A., Bernick, S., Levy, B. M. and Dreizen, S. (1972). A comparative study of periodontal ligament development in teeth with and without predecessors in marmosets. *J. Periodont.,* 43: 162.
Kenny, E. B. and Ramfjord, S. P. (1969). Cellular dynamics in root formation of teeth in rhesus monkeys. *J. dent. Res.,* 48: 114.
Ooë, T. (1973). A propos de la formation de la bifurcation ou tripartition des racines des molaires humaines. *Acta anat.,* 82: 512.
Owens, P. D. A. (1974). A light microscope study of the development of the roots of premolar teeth in dogs. *Archs oral Biol.,* 19: 525.
Selvig, K. A. (1964). Ultrastructural study of cement formation. *Acta odont. scand.,* 22: 105.
Ten Cate, A. R. (1969). The development of the periodontium. In – *Biology of the periodontium.* A. H. Melcher and W. H. Bowen (eds.). Academic Press, London. P. 53.
Tonge, C. H. (1963). The development and arrangement of the dental follicle. *Trans. Eur. Orth. Soc.* P. 118.
Trott, J. R. (1962). The development of the periodontal attachment in the rat. *Acta anat.,* 51: 313.

Development of occlusion
Berkovitz, B. K. B. (1975). Mechanisms of tooth eruption. In – *Applied physiology of the mouth.* C. L. B. Lavelle (ed.). Wright, Bristol. P. 99.
Boyde, A. and Lester, K. S. (1967). Electron microscopy of resorbing surfaces of dental hard tissues. *Z. Zellforsch.,* 83: 538.
Engler, W. O., Ramfjord, S. P. and Hiniker, J. J. (1965). Development of epithelial attachment and gingival sulcus in rhesus monkeys. *J. Periodont.,* 36: 44.
Fletcher, G. G. T. (1963). A cephalometric appraisal of the development of malocclusion. *Trans. Brit. Soc. Orthodont.* P. 124.
Friel, S. (1954). The development of ideal occlusion of the gum pads and the teeth. *Amer. J. Orthodont.,* 40: 196.
Furseth, R. (1968). The resorption processes of human deciduous teeth studied by light microscopy, microradiography and electron microscopy. *Archs oral Biol.,* 13: 417.
Garn, S. M. and Burdi, A. R. (1971). Prenatal ordering and postnatal sequence in dental development. *J. dent. Res.,* 50: 1407.
Glavind, L. and Anader, H. A. (1970). Dynamics of dental epithelium during tooth eruption. *J. dent. Res.,* 49: 549.
Graber, T. M. (1972). The development of the dentition. In – *Orthodontics.* 3rd ed. Saunders, Philadelphia. P. 86.
Kraus, B. S. and Jordan, R. E. (1965). *The human dentition before birth.* Lea and Febiger, Philadelphia.
Magnusson, B. (1968). Tissue changes during molar tooth eruption. *Trans. R. Schs. Dent. Stockh. Umea.* No. 13.
Morita, H., Yamashiya, H., Shimizu, M. and Sasaki, S. (1970). The collagenolytic activity during root resorption of bovine deciduous tooth. *Archs oral Biol.,* 15: 503.
Moss, J. P. (1976). A review of the theories of approximal migration of teeth. In – *The eruption and occlusion of teeth.* Colston Papers No. 27. D. F. G. Poole and M. V. Stack (eds.). Butterworths, London. P. 205.
Ness, A. R. (1964). Movement and forces in tooth eruption. In *Advances in oral biology.* Vol. 1. P. H. Staple (ed.). Academic Press, London. P. 33.
Van der Linden, F. P. G. M. and Duterloo, H. S. (1976). *Development of the human dentition.* Harper and Row, Maryland.

Comparative dental anatomy

Evolution of jaws and teeth
Crompton, A. W. (1972). The evolution of the jaw articulation of cynodonts. In – *Studies in vertebrate evolution*. K. A. Joysey and T. S. Kemp (eds.). Oliver and Boyd, Edinburgh. P. 231.
Hildebrand, M. (1974). *Analysis of vertebrate structure*. Wiley, London. P. 125.
Hopson, J. A. (1966). The origin of the mammalian middle ear. *Am. Zool.*, 6: 437.
Miles, A. E. W. (1972). *Teeth and their origins*. Oxford biology readers. No. 21. Oxford University Press, London.
Romer, A. S. (1969). Cynodont reptile with incipient mammalian jaw articulation. *Science*, 166: 881.
Romer, A. S. (1970). *The vertebrate body*. 4th ed. Saunders, Philadelphia. P. 210.

Comparative histology of the dental tissues
Boyde, A. (1965). The structure of developing mammalian dental enamel. In – *Tooth enamel*. I. M. V. Stack and R. W. Fearnhead (eds.). Wright, Bristol. P. 163.
Cooper, J. S. and Poole, D. F. G. (1973). The dentition and dental tissues of the agamid lizard, *Uromastyx*. *J. Zool., Lond.*, 169: 85.
Grady, J. E. (1970). Tooth development in *Latimeria chalumnae*. *Smith. J. Morph.*, 132: 377.
Halstead, L. B. (1974). *Vertebrate dental hard tissues*. Wykeham, London.
Kerr, T. (1955). Development and structure of the teeth of the dogfish *Squalus acanthias* L and *Scyliorhinus canicula* (L). *Proc. zool. Soc. Lond.*, 125: 95.
Kerr, T. (1960). Development and structure of some actinopterygian and urodele teeth. *Proc. zool. Soc. Lond.*, 133: 401.
Lavelle, C. L. B., Shellis, R. P. and Poole, D. F. G. (1977). *Evolutionary changes to the primate skull and dentition*. Thomas, Illinois.
Meredith Smith, M. and Miles, A. E. W. (1969). An autoradiographic investigation with the light microscope of proline – H^3 incorporation during tooth development in the crested newt (*Triturus cristatus*). *Archs oral Biol.*, 14: 479.
Meredith Smith, M. and Miles, A. E. W. (1971). The ultrastructure of odontogenesis in larval and adult urodeles: differentiation of the dental epithelial cells. *Z. Zellforsch.*, 121: 470.
Poole, D. F. G. (1967). Phylogeny of tooth tissues: Enameloid and enamel in recent vertebrates, with a note on the history of cementum. In – *Structural and chemical organisation of teeth*. Vol. I. A. E. W. Miles (ed.). Academic Press, London. P. 111.
Poole, D. F. G. (1971). An introduction to the phylogeny of calcified tissues. In – *Dental morphology and evolution*. A. A. Dahlberg (ed.). University of Chicago Press, Chicago. P. 65.
Schmidt, W. J. and Keil, A. (1971). *Polarising microscopy of dental tissues*. Pergamon Press, Oxford.
Shellis, R. P. and Berkovitz, B. K. B. (1976). Observations on the dental anatomy of piranhas (*Characidae*) with special reference to tooth structure. *J. Zool., Lond.*, 180: 69.
Shellis, R. P. and Miles, A. E. W. (1976). Observations with the electron microscope on enameloid formation in the common eel (*Anguilla anguilla*; Teleostei). *Proc. R. Soc. Lond.*, B. 194: 253.

Types of tooth attachment
Kvam, T. (1960). The teeth of *Alligator mississipiensis* Daud. VI. Periodontium. *Acta odont. scand.*, 18: 67.
Miller, W. A. (1968). Periodontal attachment apparatus in young *Caiman sclerops*. *Archs oral Biol.*, 13: 735.
Mummery, J. H. (1924). *The microscopic and general anatomy of the teeth*. 2nd ed. Oxford University Press, Oxford. P. 447.
Noble, H. W. (1969). The evolution of the mammalian periodontium. In – *Biology of the periodontium*. A. H. Melcher and W. H. Bowen (eds.). Academic Press, London. P. 1.

Tooth replacement
Berkovitz, B. K. B. (1975). Observations on tooth replacement in piranhas (Characidae). *Archs oral Biol.*, 20: 53.
Berkovitz, B. K. B. and Moore, M. (1975). Tooth replacement in the upper jaw of the rainbow trout (*Salmo gairdneri*). *J. Exp. Zool.*, 193: 221.
Cooper, J. A. (1966). Tooth replacement in the Slow worm (*Anguis fragilis*). *J. Zool. Lond.*, 150: 235.
Edmund, A. G. (1969). Dentition. In – *Biology of the reptilia*. Vol. I. C. Gans, A. d'A. Bellairs and T. S. Parsons (eds.). Academic Press, London. P. 117.
Lawson, R. (1965). The development and replacement of teeth in *Hypogeophis rostratus* (Amphibia, Apoda). *J. Zool., Lond.*, 147: 352.
Miller, W. A. and Rowe, D. J. (1973). Preliminary investigation of variations in tooth replacement in adult *Necturus maculosus*. *J. Morph.*, 140: 63.
Moss, S. A. (1967). Tooth replacement in the lemon shark, *Negaprion brevirostris*. In – *Sharks, skates and rays*. P. W. Gilbert, R. F. Mathewson and D. P. Rall (eds.). Hopkins Press, Baltimore. P. 319.
Osborn, J. W. (1971). The ontogeny of tooth succession in *Lacerta vivipara* Jacquin (1787). *Proc. R. Soc. Lond.*, B, 179: 261.
Osborn, J. W. (1973). The evolution of dentitions. *Am. Scient.*, 61: 548.
Poole, D. F. G. (1961). Notes on tooth replacement in the Nile crocodile *Crocodilus niloticus*. *Proc. zool. Soc. Lond.*, 136: 131.

Features of vertebrate dentitions
Berkovitz, B. K. B. (1968). The early development of the incisor teeth of *Setonix brachyurus* (Macropodidae: Marsupialia) with special reference to the prelacteal teeth. *Archs oral Biol.*, 13: 171.
Cooper, J. S., Poole, D. F. G. and Lawson, R. (1970). The dentition of the agamid lizards with special reference to tooth replacement. *J. Zool., Lond.*, 162: 85.
Crompton, A. W. (1971). The origin of the tribosphenic molar. In – *Early mammals*. D. M. Kermack and K. A. Kermack (eds.). Academic Press, London. P. 65.
Edmund, A. G. (1969). Dentition. In – *Biology of the reptilia*. Vol. I. C. Gans, A. d'A. Bellairs and T. S. Parsons (eds.). Academic Press, London. P. 117.
Green, H. L. H. H. (1938). The development and morphology of the teeth of *Ornithorynchus*. *Phil. Trans. R. Soc.* 228B: 367.
Gregory, W. K. (1959). *Fish skulls*. Lundberg, Florida.
Hiiemae, K. M. (1976). Masticatory movements in primitive mammals. In – *Mastication*. D. J. Anderson and B. Matthews. Wright, Bristol. P. 105.
James, W. W. (1960). *The jaws and teeth of primates*. Pitman, London.
Lavelle, C. L. B., Shellis, R. P. and Poole, D. F. G. (1977). *Evolutionary changes to the primate skull and dentition*. Thomas, Illinois.
Miles, A. E. W. and Poole, D. F. G. (1967). The history and general organisation of dentitions. In – *Structural and chemical organisation of teeth*. Vol. I. A. E. W. Miles (ed.). Academic Press, London. P. 3.
Mummery, J. H. (1924). *The microscopic and general anatomy of the teeth*. 2nd ed. Oxford University Press, Oxford.
Noble, H. W. (1973). Comparative functional anatomy of temporo-mandibular joint. In – *Temporomandibular joint function and dysfunction*. I. Oral science reviews. 2. Munksgaard, Copenhagen. P. 3.
Peyer, B. (1968). *Comparative odontology*. University of Chicago Press, Chicago.
Pilbeam, D. (1972). *The ascent of man*. Collier-Macmillan, London.
Poole, D. F. G. (1976). Evolution of mastication. In – *Mastication*. D. J. Anderson and B. Matthews (eds.). Wright, Bristol. P. 1.
Poole, D. F. G. and Shellis, R. P. (1976). Eruptive tooth movements in non-mammalian vertebrates. In – *The eruption and occlusion of teeth*. Colston Papers No. 27. D. F. G. Poole and M. V. Stack (eds.). Butterworths, London. P. 65.
Schour, I. and Massler, M. (1949). The teeth. In – *The rat in laboratory investigation*. E. J. Farris and J. Q. Griffith Jr. (eds.). Lippincott, Philadelphia. P. 104.
Simons, E. L. (1972). *Primate evolution*. Collier-Macmillan, London.
Swinder, D. R. (1976). *Dentition of living primates*. Academic Press, London.

Index

Index

Aardvark (*Orycteropus afer*), dentition, 212
Abrasion, 91
Acini (see Glands, salivary)
Adder,
– dentition of viper (*Vipera berus*), 200
– fang of puff-adder (*Bitis arietans*), 201
Adenoids, 56
Aegyptopithecus zeuxis,
– dentition, 219
– evolution, 223
Age changes in:
– cementum, 107, 111
– dentine, 94, 100, 101
– pulp, 34, 100, 102, 104, 105, 168
Age determination from teeth and jaws, 176–179
Agnatha, 182
– dentitions, 195
Air sinuses and cells (see Sinuses, air)
Alignment of teeth, 35–37
– anatomical (normal), definition, 35
Alkaline phosphatase,
– in amelogenesis, 159
– distribution in enamel organ, 156
Alligator (*Alligator mississippiensis*), dentition, 200
Alveolar bone (see Bones, alveolar)
Amelogenesis, 158–163
– ameloblasts,
– – appearance associated with aprismatic enamel, 84, 159, 187
– – development, 156, 158, 163
– – maturation stage, 161, 162, 163
– – secretory granules of, 159
– – secretory stage, 159, 160, 163
– – striated border during maturation stage, 161, 162, 163
– – terminal bar apparatus, 160
– – Tomes' process, 160, 161, 163
– cross-striation formation, 161
– crystallite orientation and prism formation, 160
– induction, 156, 159
– matrix of enamel during, 159, 161
– maturation stage, 161, 162
– primary enamel cuticle, 162, 163
– reduced enamel epithelium, 162, 163
– rhythm, 161
– rôle of stellate reticulum during, 156, 159
– rôle of stratum intermedium during, 156, 159
– striae of Retzius formation, 85, 161
Amphibia, 182
– aprismatic enamel, 187, 188
– dentitions, 198
– enameloid, 188
Amphistyly, 182, 183
Angler fish (*Lophius piscatorius*), dentition, 197
Ankylosis, 191
– acrodont, 193, 199
– in amphibia, 198
– in fish, 197
– in humans, 175
– pleurodont, 193, 199
– in reptiles, 199, 200
Anteater (*Myrmecophagidae*), 212
Anthropoidea, 212
– dentitions, 215–222
Anthropometric landmarks (see Cephalometry)
Antrum (see Sinus, air, maxillary)
Aperture, piriform, 13
Apes (see Anthropoidea)
Aponeurosis, palatine, 14, 49, 50
Arches,
– branchial,
– – first, 44, 144, 148, 151, 152 (see also Cartilage, Meckel's)
– – fourth, 152
– – second, 48, 144, 145, 152
– – third, 152
– dental, 35–41
– gill arch derivatives in evolution of jaws, 182, 183
– palatoglossal (anterior pillar of fauces), 10, 11, 12, 49, 50, 54, 56, 57, 58
– palatopharyngeal (posterior pillar of fauces), 10, 11, 50, 54, 56, 57, 58
– zygomatic, 47, 61, 65, 70, 71, 73
Armadillo (*Dasypodidae*), dentition, 212
Arterial supply to:
– cheek, 55
– face, 54
– gingiva, 55
– lips, 55
– palate, 55
– periodontal ligament, 119
– pulp, 104, 105, 168
– teeth, 54, 55
Arteries,
– anterior superior dental, 54, 55, 119
– buccal, 54, 55
– dorsal nasal branch of ophthalmic, 54
– external carotid, 54, 57, 60
– facial, 47, 54, 55, 59
– greater (anterior) palatine, 11, 13, 14, 50, 55, 119, 133
– incisive, 54
– inferior dental, 15, 16, 54, 60, 119
– infraorbital, 13, 54, 55
– internal carotid, 57, 58
– làbial, 55
– lesser (posterior) palatine, 14, 55, 119
– lingual, 54, 55, 60, 119
– maxillary, 13, 54, 55, 60
– mental, 15, 54
– middle superior dental, 54, 119
– mylohyoid, 54
– nasopalatine, 55
– posterior superior dental, 54, 55, 119
– superficial temporal, 54, 59, 60
– superior labial, 59
– vertebral, 57
Arteriodactyla, dentitions, 209, 210
Astomia, 145
Attachment, types of tooth,
– ankylosis, 193
– fibrous, 191
– gomphosis, 191, 192
– hinged, 192
– thecodont gomphosis, 191, 192, 200
Attrition, 91, 94, 111, 176, 180
Australopithecus, 219, 220, 221
– *africanus*, 220
– *boisei*, 220
– evolution, 223
– *robustus*, 220
Autostyly, 182, 183
Axis vertebra, 57
Axolotl, enameloid, 188
Aye-aye (*Daubentonia madagascariensis*), dentition, 214

Band,
– Hunter-Schreger (see Enamel)
– primary epithelial, 153
– vestibular, 153
Basket cells (see Glands, salivary)
Bats,
– common vampire (*Desmodus rotundus*), 206
– fruit bat (*Pteropus*), 205
– South American spear-nosed (*Phyllostomus hastatus*), 205
Bear (*Ursus*), dentition, 209
Bicuspid (see Premolars)
Bilophodont teeth
– manatee (*Trichechus manatus*), 212
– Old World monkey, 216

Blood supply (see Arterial supply)
Bone, histological appearance of (see Bones, alveolar)
Bones, individual
-alveolar
--alveolar crest, 14, 72, 73
--alveolar crypt, 174
--alveolar process (alveolus) of mandible, 15, 16, 68, 120
--alveolar process (alveolus) of maxilla, 13, 14, 16, 68, 151
--angulation of teeth within, 36
--bundle bone, 122
--canaliculi, 121
--cancellous bone (spongy bone), 16, 121, 123
--collagen fibre orientation, 121, 122
--compact bone, 16, 121, 122
--composition and properties, 120
--development, 123, 148, 149, 150, 151, 170, 171
--distribution around teeth, 16, 73, 78, 120
--function, 120
--fundus, 14
--Haversian systems in, 121, 122, 123
--Howship's lacunae, 118, 123
--interdental (interalveolar) septa, 14, 16, 120, 149
--interradicular septa, 14, 16, 120, 149
--lacunae, 121, 122
--lamellae, 121
--lamina dura, 120, 122, 123
--lines, structural, 123
--marrow spaces, 121
--osteoblasts, 116, 117, 121, 122, 149, 171
--osteoclasts, 116, 117, 118, 121, 149
--osteocytes, 121, 122
--osteoid, 122, 149
--plasticity, 120
--plates, buccal or labial (outer), lingual or palatal (inner), 14, 16, 120
--radiographic appearance, 73
--repair, 112
--resorption, 14, 118, 123
--reversal lines, 123
--Sharpey's fibres, 114, 122, 123
--sockets, 14, 16, 120
--transalveolar fibres, 123
--Volkmann's canals, 120
--woven bone, 121
-angular, 183, 184
-articular, 184
-columella, 183
-conchae, nasal, 61
-coronoid, 183
-dentary, 183, 184
-frontal, 13, 68, 149, 183
-hyoid, 49, 57, 58, 63
-incus, 149, 184
-jugal, 183
-lacrimal, 13, 183
-malleus, 149, 184
-mandible, 15, 16, 49, 57, 58, 60, 62, 63
--alveolar plates, 16
--angle, 15, 44, 47
--anthropometric landmarks (see Cephalometry)
--body, 15, 49, 58, 62, 63, 65, 66, 149, 150, 151
--canal,
---incisive, 16, 53, 76
---mandibular, 15, 16, 52, 73, 76
---mental, 16, 52, 76
--canine eminence, 15
--chin, 15, 150
--condylar cartilage, 149, 150, 151
--condylectomy, 151
--coronoid cartilage, 149
--development, 148–151
--digastric fossa, 15
--foramen,
---mandibular, 15, 16, 44, 52, 54, 55, 76
---mental, 15, 52, 53, 55, 65, 70, 73, 76, 148
--functional matrices of, 151
--genial tubercles (spines), 15, 49, 73, 75
--growth, 150, 152
--incisive fossa, 15
--lingula, 15, 44, 149

--mandibular joint (see Joint, temporomandibular)
--mandibular nerve, course within, 52
--mandibular notch, 15
--movements of, 41, 44, 45, 46, 47
--mylohyoid,
---groove, 15
---line, 15, 44, 73, 76
--oblique lines,
---external, 15, 16, 73, 76
---internal, 15, 44, 73, 76
--processes,
---alveolar, 15, 16, 68, 120
---condyle, 15, 38, 43, 44, 45, 46, 47, 59, 60, 61, 65, 66, 67, 70, 71, 137, 149, 150, 151
---coronoid, 15, 47, 61, 66, 67, 70, 71, 151
--radiographic appearance, 65, 66, 67, 70, 71, 72, 73, 75, 76
--ramus, 11, 15, 44, 46, 47, 52, 58, 60, 62, 137, 149, 150, 151
--rest position, 35, 42
--retromolar region, 11, 52
--retromolar triangle, attachment of pterygomandibular raphe, 15, 44
--symphysis, 15, 75, 148, 149, 150
--temporal crest, 15, 47
-maxilla, 13, 14, 149
--anterior nasal spine, 13, 53, 67, 69
--anthropometric landmarks (see Cephalometry)
--antrum of (see Sinus, air, maxillary)
--body of, 13
--canine fossa, 13, 62, 63
--development, 147, 151
--foramen,
---incisive, 11, 14, 53, 55, 73, 74, 147
---infraorbital, 13, 48, 65
--growth, 151, 152
--infraorbital canal, 53
---foramen, 13
--lacrimal sulcus, 13
--orbital plate, 13
--palatine groove, 13, 16
--processes,
---alveolar, 13, 14, 16, 68, 151
---frontal, 13, 151
---palatine, 13, 14, 151
---zygomatic, 13, 66, 151
--radiographic appearance, 65, 66, 67, 70, 72, 73, 74, 75
--superior dental nerves, course within, 53
--sutures of,
---intermaxillary, 13, 73
---median palatine, 14, 73, 74
---transverse palatine, 14
--tuberosity, 13, 47, 54, 60, 63, 73, 75
--zygomaticoalveolar (jugal) crest, 13
-nasal, 13, 68, 183
--conchae, 61
-occipital, 149
-palate, hard, 11, 14, 50, 57, 58, 63, 67, 146, 147
-palatine bone,
--development, 147
--horizontal plate, 14
--lesser palatine foramen, 14, 53
--perpendicular plate, 13
--posterior nasal spine, 14, 69
--pyramidal process, 47
-parietal, 149, 183
-postfrontal, 183
-postorbital, 183
-prearticular, 184
-prefrontal, 183
-premaxilla, 183
--in humans, 151
-quadrate, 182, 183, 184
-sphenoid,
--greater wing, 47
--pterygoid hamulus, 44, 50, 75
--pterygoid plates, 47, 50, 75
--scaphoid fossa, 50
--spine of, 44, 149
-splenial, 184
-squamosal, 183, 184
-stapes, 183

—surangular, 183, 184
—temporal,
——articular eminence, 43, 44, 45, 46, 150
——glenoid fossa, 15, 38, 43, 45, 59, 137, 150
——petrous part, 43, 50
——processes,
———mastoid, 65, 67, 70
———postglenoid, 43
———styloid, 44, 49
———zygomatic, 43
——squamous part, 60, 149
——tympanic plate, 43
—zygoma, 47, 65
—zygomatic arch, 47, 61, 65, 70, 71
Bony attachments (see Ankylosis)
Bony fishes (see Osteichthyes)
Branchial arches (see Arches, branchial)
Buccal pad of fat, 57, 58, 62
Buccal salivary glands (see Glands, salivary)
Bunodont teeth, 209

Calcification,
—cementum, 172
—dates for calcification of teeth, 176
—dentine, 98, 99, 100, 164, 165, 166, 167
—enamel, 158, 159, 160, 161, 162
—pulp, 106
Calcium phosphate,
—amorphous, 91, 93
—fluorapatite, 186
—hydroxyapatite, 79, 80, 91, 92, 107, 158, 159, 160, 172
—octocalcium phosphate, 91, 93
Calcospherites, 100, 166, 167
Calculus, dental, 91
Callitrichidae, 212
—dentitions, 216
Canal,
—carotid, 50
—gubernacular, 174
—Haversian (see Bone, alveolar)
—incisive, 16, 53, 76
—infraorbital, 53
—mandibular, 15, 16, 52, 54, 73, 76
—mental, 16, 52, 76
—nasolacrimal, 13, 73, 74
—nutrient, 73, 75
—palatine, 13
—root, 34, 102
—for superior dental nerves, 53
—Volkmann's, 120
Canaliculi,
—in bone, 121
—in cementum, 108, 109
Canines,
—angulation of, in alveolus, 36
—blood supply, 54, 55
—chronology of development, 176–179
—crown form, 17, 24
—dimensions, 33
—innervation, 52
—morphology of human,
——deciduous mandibular, 25
——deciduous maxillary, 25
——permanent mandibular, 25
——permanent maxillary, 24
—pulp morphology, 34
Capsule,
—otic, 148
—of temporomandibular joint (see Joint, temporomandibular)
Caries, dental, 73, 88, 91
Carnassial teeth, 208
Carnivora, dentitions, 208, 209
Cartilage,
—condylar, 137, 149, 150, 151
—coronoid, 149
—Meckel's, 44, 148, 149, 150, 154, 182, 196
—palatoquadrate, 182
—symphyseal (mandibular), 149
—thyroid, 50

Cartilaginous fishes (see Chondrichthyes)
Cat (*Felis catus*), dentition, 208
Cavity, nasal, 10, 13, 14, 61, 65, 66, 73, 74, 146
Cavity, oral
—boundaries of, 10 (see also Mouth)
—development, 144–147
Cavity, oro-nasal, 146
Cebidae, 212
—dentitions, 215
Cementogenesis, 169, 170, 172
Cementum, 107–111
—acellular (primary), 98, 107, 108, 110, 172
—age changes, 107, 111
—canaliculi, 108, 109
—cellular (secondary), 107, 108, 109, 110, 172
—cementoblasts, 108, 109, 116, 117, 170, 171, 172, 175
—cementoclasts, 116, 117
—cementocytes, 107, 108, 109, 172
—cemento-dentinal junction, 91, 108, 109
—cemento-enamel junction, 79, 107
—chemical composition, 107
—coronal cementum, 210
—crystallites, 107, 172
—development (see Cementogenesis)
—distribution, 78, 107
—fibre orientation, 110
—function, 107
—hypercementosis, 111
—intermediate, 109
—junctional epithelium, association with, 131
—lacunae, 108, 109
—lines, incremental and structural, 108, 109, 110, 172
—matrix, in developing cementum, 172
—physical properties, 107
—precementum, 107, 108, 109, 110, 117, 172
—radiographic appearance, 73
—remodelling, 110
—reparative, 111, 175
—resorption, 107
—response to attrition, 111
—reversal lines, 110
—Sharpey's fibres, 109, 110, 111, 114, 172
—thickness, 107
Cephalometry (with lateral skull radiographs), 68, 69, 70
—angles used, 69, 70
—anthropometric landmarks used, 68
—planes used, 69, 70
Cercopithecidae, 212
—dentitions, 216
Cetacea, dentitions, 211
Chamaeleon (*Chamaeleo chamaeleo*)
—dentition, 199
—tooth replacement, 193
Chamber, pulp, 34
Cheek, 10, 11
—blood supply, 55
—innervation, 51, 54
—linea alba, 11
—minor salivary glands, 128, 142
—mucosa, 128, 136
—muscles, 48
—sebaceous glands (Fordyce spots), 11, 128
Chewing cycle of mammals, 202
Chimaeroids, jaw articulation, 182
Chimpanzee (*Pan troglodytes*), dentition, 217, 218
Chin, 15, 150
Chiroptera,
—dentitions, 205, 206
—enamel prism pattern, 188
Chondrichthyes, 182
—dentitions, 196, 197
——monk fish (*Squatina squatina*), 196
——ray, eagle (*Myliobatis aquilla*), 197
——ray, thornback (*Raia clavata*), 196
——shark, blue (*Prionace glauca*), 196
——shark, Porbeagle (*Lemna nasus*), 196
—placoid scales, 185
—tooth attachment, 191
—tooth replacement, 191, 196

Chondrocranium, 182, 183
Chronology of tooth development, 176–179
Cingulum, definition, 17
Cleft,
– lip, 144, 145, 147
– mandible, 145
– oblique facial, 145
– palate, 147
Coelacanth (*Latimeria chalumnae*), enamel, 187
Collagen (see Fibres, collagen)
Commissures, labial, 10, 11
Continuously erupting teeth, 203, 206, 207, 209, 210, 212, 214
Cord,
– enamel, 155, 157
– gubernacular, 174
Cornu (horns) of pulp, 34
Cow (*Bos tauros*), dentition, 210
Crest,
– alveolar, 14, 72, 73
– neural, 153, 155, 170
– sagittal,
– – of ape skull, 219
– – of *Australopithecus*, 220
– temporal, 15, 47
– zygomaticoalveolar (jugal), 13
Crevice, gingival, 90, 130, 131, 173
Crocodile (*Crocodilus*)
– dentition, 200
– enamel, 187
– tooth replacement, 193
Cro-magnon man, dentition, 222
Crossopterygian fish, plicidentine, 190
Crown,
– anatomical, definition, 17
– clinical, definition, 17
– dimension of, 33
– evolution of mammalian molar crown form, 201
– investments (see Enamel, investing organic layers on)
– morphologenesis, 155
– morphology (see individual teeth)
Crypt,
– alveolar, 174
– of lingual follicles, 135
– tonsillar, 11, 51, 57
Crystallites (hydroxyapatite),
– in aprismatic enamel, 187
– in cementum, 107, 172
– in dentine, 80, 87, 92, 165
– in enamel, 79, 80, 81, 82, 84, 87, 88, 159, 160
– in enameloid, 185, 186
– in plaque, 91
Cupola, of developing tongue, 152
Curvatures of teeth, 37
Curve,
– catenary, of dental arches, 35
– Monson, 37
– Spee, 37
– Wilson, 37
Cusp, definition, 17
– morphology (see individual teeth)
Cuticle, enamel (see Enamel, investing organic layers on)
Cynarioides, lower jaw, 184
Cynognathus, lower jaw, 184
Cysts, 118, 155

Daubentoniidae, 212
– dentition, 214
Deciduous teeth, human, 17, 19, 175, 180 (see also Dentitions)
– dimensions, 33
– morphology (see Canines, Incisors, Molars)
– occlusion, 180
– pulp morphology, 34
Dendritic cells (see Melanocytes)
Dental age, 176–179
Dental shorthand for tooth identification, 18
Denteons, in osteodentine, 190
Denticles, dermal, 185
Dentinal tubules (see Dentine)
Dentine, 91–101

– age changes, 94, 100, 101
– amelodentinal junction, 86, 87, 91, 92, 98
– calcospherites, 100, 166, 167
– cemento-dentinal junction, 91, 108, 109
– chemical composition, 92
– circumpulpal, 97, 98, 100, 166, 167
– crystallites, 80, 87, 92, 165
– dead tracts, 100
– dentinal thorns, 105
– development (see Dentinogenesis)
– distribution, 78, 91
– granular layer, 92, 97, 98, 108, 109, 167
– hyaline layer, 97, 98, 108, 167
– innervation, 95, 96, 97, 105, 168
– interglobular, 98, 100, 167
– intermediate, 98
– intertubular, 93
– ivory, 211
– lines, structural and incremental, 99, 100, 101, 167
– mantle, 97, 98, 164, 165, 166
– matrix of developing dentine, 166
– mineralisation, 98, 99, 100, 164, 165, 166, 167
– mineralising lines, 99
– neonatal line, 100
– odontoblast processes, 92, 93, 95, 96, 97
– – development, 165, 166
– – extent, 95, 96
– – function, 95
– – minor processes in pulp, 103
– – relationships to nerves, 97
– orthodentine, 91–101, 189
– osteodentine, 190
– Owen's line, 99, 101
– peritubular, 93, 94, 101, 165
– physical properties, 92
– plicidentine, 190
– predentine, 96, 97, 98, 102, 103, 156, 166, 167
– primary, 97, 101
– radiographic appearance of, 73
– reaction to stimuli, 94, 100, 101
– regional variations, 97
– resorption, 175
– of root, 98, 167
– Schreger line, 99
– sclerotic (translucent), 100, 101
– secondary dentine, 97, 100, 101
– sensitivity, 96, 97
– tubules,
– – branching, 92, 98
– – contents, 92, 93, 94, 95, 96, 97
– – curvatures, 92, 99
– – in dead tracts, 100
– – development, 166
– – diameter, 92, 93, 94, 96
– – direction, 92, 101
– – in enameloid, 185
– – formation, 166
– – through interglobular dentine, 100
– – in ivory, 211
– – nerve fibres, 95, 96, 97, 105
– – numbers and concentration of, 92, 93
– – in osteodentine, 190
– – periodontoblastic space, 95
– – in plicidentine, 190
– – in pulp stones, 106
– – in sclerotic dentine, 101
– – in secondary dentine, 101
– – in vasodentine, 189
– vasodentine, 189
– von Ebner lines, 99
Dentinogenesis, 164–167
– calcospherites, 166, 167
– circumpulpal dentine, 166, 167
– dentinal tubules, 166
– granular layer, 167
– hyaline layer, 167
– induction, 156, 158, 164
– interglobular areas, 167
– lines, incremental, 167

–mantle dentine, 164, 165, 166
–matrix, 164, 165, 166
–matrix vesicles, 165, 166
–mineralisation, 165, 166, 167
–odontoblast differentiation, 156, 164
–odontoblast movement, 166
–peritubular dentine, 165, 167
–predentine, 166
–rhythmicity, 167
–root, 167, 170
–secondary, 167
–subodontoblastic cells, rôle in, 164
–Von Korff's fibres, 164, 165, 166
Dentition,
–comparisons between human deciduous and permanent dentitions, 19
–deciduous (primary), 17
–development, 173–179
–permanent (secondary), 17
–vertebrate, 195–223
Development,
–amelogenesis, 158–163
–cementogenesis, 172
–dentinogenesis, 164–167
–dentitions, 173–179
–dentogingival junction, 173
–face, 144, 145
–mandible, 148–151
–maxilla, 151
–mouth, 144, 145
–nose, 144, 145
–occlusion, 180
–palate, 146, 147
–periodontal ligament and root, 169–172
–pulp, 168
–skull, 152
–temporomandibular joint, 150
–tongue, 152
–tooth (early stages), 153–157
Diastema in animals, 203, 210, 213, 216, 217
Dimetrodon, lower jaw, 184
Diphyodonty, 195, 201
Dog (*Canis familiaris*), dentition, 208
Dogfish (*Scyliorhinus canicula*), enameloid, 186
Dolphin (*Delphinus delphis*), dentition, 211
Drift, mesial, 37, 178, 180
Dryopithecus,
–cusp pattern, 30, 32, 219
–*dryopithecus,* 219
–*proconsul,* 219
–*sivapithecus,* 219
Duct,
–collecting, 138, 139, 140, 141, 142
–intercalated, 138, 139, 140, 141, 142
–nasolacrimal, 145
–parotid, 11, 47, 48, 59, 71, 139
–striated, 138, 139, 140, 141, 142
–sublingual, 142
–submandibular, 12, 141

Edentata, dentitions, 212
Eel (*Anguilla anguilla*)
–enameloid, 185, 186
–tooth attachment, 191
Egg tooth in reptiles, 199, 200
Elasmobranchii (see Chondrichthyes)
Elastic fibres (see Fibres, elastic)
Elephant,
–dentition of African (*Loscodonta africana*), 211
–dentition of Indian (*Elephas maximus*), 211
Eminence,
–articular, of temporal bone, 43, 44, 45, 46, 150
–canine, of mandible, 15
Enamel, 79–88
–ameloblast (see Amelogenesis)
–amelodentinal junction, 79, 80, 86, 87, 91
–aprismatic, 84, 88, 159, 187, 199
–brochs, 88
–cemento-enamel junction, 79, 107
–chemical composition, 79
–cross-striation, 84, 85, 161
–crystallites, 79, 80, 81, 82, 84, 87, 88, 159, 160, 187
–deciduous compared with permanent, 19
–demineralisation, effects on prisms of, 82
–development (see Amelogenesis)
–distribution, 78, 79
–gnarled, 83
–Hunter-Schreger bands, 83, 161
–integument (see below, investing organic layers on)
–interprismatic substance, 80
–investing organic layers on, 89–91
––acquired pellicle, 91
––calculus, 91
––enamel cuticle, primary, 88, 89, 90, 91, 162, 163
––enamel cuticle, secondary, 90
––Nasmyth's membrane, 89
––plaque, 90, 91
––reduced enamel epithelium (see Epithelium, enamel)
–lamella, 86, 87
–lines, incremental, 84, 85, 86, 88, 100, 161
–matrix in developing enamel, 158, 159, 160, 161, 162
–maturation (see Amelogenesis)
–neonatal line, 86, 100
–perikyma, 85, 86, 88
–physical properties, 79
–pores, 79, 81
–prisms, 79, 80, 81, 82, 83, 84, 86, 88, 160, 188
–prism sheath (boundary), 80, 81, 82, 160
–radiographic appearance, 73
–spindle, 86, 87
–striae of Retzius, 79, 84, 85, 88, 161
–surface features, 85, 86, 88
–surface integuments (see investing organic layers on)
–tubular, 185, 189, 203
–tufts, 86, 87
Enamel integuments (see Enamel, investing organic layers on)
Enamel organ,
–bell stage, 154, 155, 156, 158, 164, 168, 169
–bud stage, 154, 156
–cap stage, 154, 155
–cervical loop, 155
–development, 153–157
–enamel cord (septum), 155, 157
–enamel knot, 157
–enamel navel, 157
–enamel niche, 157
–epithelial rests (of Malassez), 116, 118, 170
–epithelial root sheath (or Hertwig), 118, 169, 170, 172
–layers,
––enamel strands, 157
––external enamel epithelium, 154, 155, 157, 169
––internal enamel epithelium, 154, 155, 156, 157, 158, 163, 164, 169
––stellate reticulum, 154, 155, 156, 157, 159
––stratum intermedium, 156, 157, 159, 160
–reduced enamel epithelium, 89, 130, 162, 163, 173
–of successional teeth, 156
Enameloid, 185, 186, 188, 196
Entoconid, 201, 202
Epiglottis, 12, 54, 58
Epithelium,
–enamel,
––external, 154, 155, 157, 169
––internal, 154, 155, 156, 157, 158, 163, 164, 169
––reduced, 89, 130, 162, 163, 173
–––appearance during eruption, 173
–––formation, 162, 163, 173
–––origin of interdental papilla lining, 132
–junctional, 90, 130, 131, 173
–olfactory, 144
–oral, 124–136
–respiratory, 133
Eruption, tooth
–active, 173, 176
–alveolar bone growth, 120, 176
–blood pressure, 176
–cell proliferation, 176
–changes in overlying tissue, 173
–collagen contraction theory, 115, 176
–of continuously growing rat incisor, 206

– date for each tooth, 176
– definition, 176
– and development of junctional epithelium, 173
– forces, 176
– as a function of periodontal ligament, 112
– functional phase, 173, 178
– gubernacular cord and canal, 174
– onset in relation to root development, 169, 173
– overeruption, 176
– passive, 173, 176
– phases, 173
– pre-eruptive phase, 173
– prefunctional phase, 173
– rate, 176
– resistance to eruptive forces, 176
– rôle of overlying tissues, 173
– root growth, 176
– theories, 176
– tissue fluid pressure, 116, 176
Eutheria, dentitions, 205–222
Evolution,
– of jaws, 182–184
– of mammalian molars, 201, 202
– of man, 223
– of teeth, 184
External enamel epithelium (see Epithelium, enamel)

Face
– blood supply, 54
– cutaneous innervation, 51
– development, 144, 145
– growth, 152
– lymphatic drainage, 56
– muscles, 48, 54, 59, 63, 145
– superficial dissection of, 59
– venous drainage, 55
Fang, snake, 200, 201
Fascia, of neck, 57, 58, 62, 63, 138
– temporal, 47
Fauces, pillars of (see also Muscles or Arches, palatoglossus and palatopharyngeus), 10, 11, 12, 49, 50, 54, 56, 57, 58
Fédération Dentaire Internationale system for identifying teeth, 18
Fibres,
– collagen,
– – alveolar bone, 121, 122
– – cementum, 107, 109, 110, 172
– – dentine, 92, 96, 98, 99, 164, 165, 166
– – enameloid, 186
– – eruption, contribution to, 115, 176
– – gingiva, 129, 132, 133
– – mucosa, oral, 136
– – periodontal ligament, 112, 113, 114, 115, 116, 117, 170, 171
– – pulp, 104, 168
– – Sharpey's,
– – – alveolar bone, 114, 122, 123
– – – cementum, 109, 110, 111, 114, 172
– – – mineralisation of, 110
– – temporomandibular joint, 137
– elastic,
– – mucosa, oral, 136
– – periodontal ligament, 112, 115
– – pulp, 104
– – temporomandibular joint, 137
– oxytalan, periodontal ligament, 112, 115
– reticulin, periodontal ligament, 112, 115
– Sharpey's (see Fibres, collagen)
– Von Korff (see Dentinogenesis)
Fibroblasts (fibrocytes)
– in periodontal ligament, 112, 116, 117, 170
– in pulp, 102, 103, 168
Fin, nasal, 144
Fishes (see Chondrochthyes and Osteichthyes)
Fissure,
– petrotympanic, 43
– squamotympanic, 43
– in teeth, definition, 17
Fistula, oro-antral, 74
Floor of mouth (see Mouth, floor of)
Fluorapatite, in dogfish enameloid, 186

Fluorine, in surface enamel, 88
Folds,
– fimbriated, 12
– glosso-epiglottic, 12
– lip, 10
– palatoglossal, 11
– palatopharyngeal, 11
– sublingual, 12, 142
– vestibular, 153
Follicle,
– dental, 89, 107, 111, 154, 169, 170, 171
– hair, of lip, 127
– lingual, 12, 135
Foramen,
– apical, of root, 34, 169
– caecum, on tongue, 12, 152
– greater palatine, 14, 53
– incisive, 11, 14, 53, 55, 73, 74, 147
– infraorbital, 13, 48, 65
– lesser palatine, 14, 53
– magnum, 66
– mandibular, 15, 16, 44, 52, 54, 55, 76
– mental, 15, 52, 53, 55, 65, 70, 73, 76, 148
Fordyce spots, 11, 128
Formula, dental, construction of, 17
Fornix vestibuli, 11, 128
Fossa, 17
– canine, of maxilla, 13, 62, 63
– canine, on premolar, 26
– cranial,
– – anterior, 67
– – middle, 43, 59, 67
– – posterior, 67
– digastric, of mandible, 15
– glenoid, 15, 38, 43, 45, 59, 137, 150
– hypophyseal, 67
– incisive, of mandible, 15
– infratemporal, 13, 46, 47, 52, 54, 55, 60 (see also Spaces, tissue, around jaws)
– mental, 73
– nasal, 13, 14, 61, 65, 66, 73, 74, 146
– pterygoid, 44
– pterygopalatine, 53, 54, 55
– scaphoid, 50
– submandibular, 73
– on teeth, definition, 17
– temporal, 47, 60
Freeway space, 35, 42
Frenum,
– labial, 11
– lingual, 12
Frog (*Rana temporaria*) dentition, 198
Furrow, naso-optic, 145

Ganglion,
– Gasserian (trigeminal), 97
– otic, 50, 54
– pterygopalatine, 53, 54
– submandibular, 54, 60
Gibbon, dentition, 216
Gingiva,
– attached, 129, 130, 136
– blood supply, 54, 55
– collagen fibre groups, 132, 133
– crevice (sulcus), 90, 130, 131, 173
– cuff, 130, 131, 132
– fluid, 131
– free, 129, 130, 132
– free gingival groove, 129, 130
– inflammation, 130, 131, 132
– innervation, 52
– interdental col, 132
– interdental papilla, 129, 132
– junctional epithelium, 90, 130, 131, 173
– lymphatic drainage, 56
– mucogingival junction, 129
– mucosa, 129, 130, 131, 132, 136
– pigmentation, 129
– stippling of, 129
– sulcular epithelium, 130, 131

– transseptal, 132, 133, 178
– venous drainage, 55
Glands,
– salivary, 138–142
– – acini (alveoli), 138
– – amylase (ptyalin), 138
– – canaliculi, secretory, 139
– – classification, 138
– – connective tissue stroma, 138
– – demilunes, 141, 142
– – ducts,
– – – collecting, 138, 139, 140, 141, 142
– – – intercalated, 138, 139, 140, 141, 142
– – – parotid, 11, 47, 48, 59, 71, 139
– – – striated, 138, 139, 140, 141, 142
– – – sublingual, 142
– – – submandibular, 12, 141
– – innervation, 51, 54
– – minor,
– – – alveolar, 129
– – – buccal, 128, 142
– – – labial, 127, 128, 142
– – – lingual, 135, 142
– – – palatal, 133, 142
– – – palatoglossal, 142
– – mucous salivary tissue, 138, 141, 142
– – myoepithelial (basket) cell, 141
– – parenchyma, 138
– – parotid, 47, 54, 57, 59, 60, 62, 138, 139
– – serous salivary tissue, 138, 139, 141, 142
– – sialography, 64, 71
– – stroma, 138
– – sublingual, 12, 54, 58, 63, 138, 142
– – submandibular, 54, 57, 59, 60, 63, 138, 141
– – Von Ebner's, 135, 142
– sebaceous, in oral mucosa (Fordyce spots), 11, 128
– – in skin of lip, 127
– sudorific (sweat), 127, 128
– thyroid, development, 12, 152
Glycosaminoglycans,
– in dentine, 98, 164, 166
– in developing tooth, 154, 155, 156, 159
– in periodontal ligament, 116
– in pulp, 104, 168
Gnathion, 68, 69
Gomphosis, 112, 191, 192, 200
Gonion, 68, 69
Gorilla, lowland (*Gorilla gorilla*), dentition, 218
Granular layer (of Tomes) (see Dentine)
Granules,
– kerato-hyaline, 124
– in Langerhans' cells, 126
– melanin, in gingiva, 129
– melanosome, 126
– in Merkel cells, 126
– mucigen, 141
– zymogen, 139
Groove,
– free gingival, 129, 130
– labiomarginal (sulcus), 10
– labiomental, 10
– mylohyoid, 15
– nasolabial, 10
– naso-optic, 145
– palatine, 13
Ground substance (see also Glycosaminoglycans)
– of periodontal ligament, 116
– of pulp, 104
Growth,
– planes and angles used in assessing human cranial growth, 69
– of mandible, 150, 152
– of maxilla, 151, 152
– of skull, 152
Gubernaculum, 174, 218
Guinea pig (*Cavia*), dentition, 207
Gum pads, 180

Hake (*Merluccius merluccius*),
– hinged tooth attachment, 192

– vasodentine, 189
Hamulus, pterygoid, 44, 50
Haplodont teeth, 197, 198, 199
Hedgehog (*Erinaceus europeus*), dentition, 205
Heidelberg man, 222
Herbivores (see Arteriodactyla and Perissodactyla)
Heterodonty,
– in fish, 197
– in mammals, 201
Hinged tooth attachment, 192, 197
Hippopotamus (*Hippopotamus amphibius*), dentition, 210
Histiocyte, in dental pulp, 103
Holostyly, 182
Hominidae, 212, 223
– dentitions, 219–222
Homo,
– *erectus*, 221, 223
– *habilis*, 221, 223
– *sapiens*, 222, 223
– *sapiens neanderthalensis*, 222, 223
Homodont dentitions, 198, 199, 200
Horse (*Equus caballus*), dentition, 210
Hyaenidae, dentition, 209
Hyaline layer (of Hopewell-Smith) (see Dentine)
Hydroxyapatite (see Crystallites, hydroxyapatite)
Hylobatidae, 212
– dentition, 216
Hyostyly, 182
Hypocone, 201, 216
Hypoconid, 201
Hypoconulid, 201, 216
Hypsodonty, 210
Hyracoidea; dentition, 212

Iguana (*Iguana iguana*), dentition, 199
Incisor,
– angulation of, in alveolus, 36
– blood supply, 54, 55
– chronology of development, 176–179
– classification of malocclusions, 41
– continuously growing, 203, 206, 210, 211, 214
– crown form, 17, 20
– dimensions, 33
– innervation, 52
– lip posture and inclination of incisors, 10
– morphology of human teeth,
– – deciduous mandibular first, 23
– – deciduous mandibular second, 23
– – deciduous maxillary first, 22
– – deciduous maxillary second, 22
– – permanent mandibular first, 21
– – permanent mandibular second, 22
– – permanent maxillary first, 20
– – permanent maxillary second, 20
– pulp morphology, 34
– relationships, 70
– – in anatomical centric occlusion, 39, 40, 41
Inclination of teeth, 36
Incremental lines (see Lines, incremental)
Indriidae, 212
– dentitions, 214
Infection, spread around jaws, 62, 63
Inflammation,
– around root apex, 111
– in gingiva, 130, 131, 132
– in periodontal ligament, 118
– in pulp, 97, 103
Innervation of:
– cheek, 51, 54
– dentine, 95, 96, 97, 105, 168
– face, cutaneous, 51
– floor of mouth, 54
– gingiva, 52
– lip, 51, 54, 145
– muscles,
– – mastication, 47
– – palate, 50
– – tongue, 49
– palatal mucosa, 53

– periodontal ligament, 112, 119
– pillars of fauces, mucosa of, 54
– pulp, 97, 102, 104, 105, 106, 168
– salivary glands, secreto-motor, 51, 54
– teeth, 52, 53
– tongue, 54, 152
Insectivora, dentitions, 205
Internal enamel epithelium (see Epithelium, enamel)
Investments of crown (see Enamel, investing organic layers on)
Isthmus,
– maxillary, 144
– oropharyngeal, 49, 51
Ivory, 211

Joint,
– quadrate-articular, 184
– squamosal-surangular, 184
– temporomandibular, 15, 43, 44, 45, 46, 137
– – articular eminence, 43, 44, 45, 46, 150
– – capsule, 43, 47, 137, 150
– – condyle, mandibular, 15, 38, 43, 44, 45, 46, 47, 59, 60, 61, 65, 66, 67, 70, 71, 137, 149, 150, 151
– – development, 150
– – disc, 43, 45, 47, 59, 137, 150
– – evolution, 182, 183, 184
– – glenoid fossa, 15, 38, 43, 45, 59, 137, 150
– – histology, 137
– – ligaments, 43, 44
– – movements, 43, 44, 45, 46
– – postglenoid process, 43
– – radiographic appearance, 71
– – relationships, topographical, 59
– – synovial membrane, 43, 137
Junction,
– amelodentinal, 79, 80, 86, 87, 91, 92, 98
– cemento-dentinal, 91, 108, 109
– cemento-enamel, 79, 107
– dentogingival, 130, 131, 132, 173
– gap, 103, 106, 121, 158
– mucogingival, 129
Junctional epithelium (see Gingiva)

Kangaroo, red (*Macropus rufus*)
– dentition, 204
– tooth replacement, 204
– tubular enamel, 189
Kinesis in reptile skulls, 199
KNM-ER, 1470 cranium, 221, 223
Knot, enamel, 157
Kuehneotherium, molar, 201

Labyrinthodonts, plicidentine, 190
Lacunae,
– in alveolar bone, 121, 122
– in cementum, 108, 109
– Howship's, 118, 123, 149
– – in dentine, 175
Lagomorpha, dentition, 207
Lamina,
– dental, 148, 153, 155, 156, 157, 174
– dura, 73, 120, 122, 123
– propria, 124, 136
– vestibular, 153
Lamprey, sea (*Petromyzon marinus*), dentition, 195
Laryngopharynx, 58
Lathyrogens, effects on tooth morphogenesis, 155
Lemur, ring-tailed (*Lemur calta*), dentition, 213
Lemuridae, 212
– dentitions, 213
Leucocytes, in pulp, 103
Ligament,
– accessory of temporomandibular joint, 44
– cushioned hammock, 171
– periodontal (see Periodontal ligament)
– septopremaxillary, 151
– sphenomalleolar, 149
– sphenomandibular, 44
– stylomandibular, 15, 44, 62
– temporomandibular, 43

Line,
– external oblique of mandible, 15, 16, 73, 76
– incremental,
– – in alveolar bone, 123
– – in cementum, 108, 109, 110, 172
– – in dentine, 99, 100, 101, 167
– – in enamel, 84, 85, 86, 88, 100, 161
– internal oblique (mylohyoid) of mandible, 15, 44, 73, 76
– neonatal,
– – in dentine, 100
– – in enamel, 86
– reversal,
– – in bone, 123
– – in cementum, 110
Lining mucosa (see Mucosa, oral)
Lip, 10, 58
– anterior oral seal, 10
– blood supply, 55
– cleft, 144, 145, 147
– commissures, 10, 11
– competency, 10
– development, 144, 145
– frena, 11
– grooves, associated with, on face, 10
– innervation, 51, 54, 145
– intermediate zone, 128
– lymphatic drainage, 56
– minor salivary glands, 127, 128, 142
– mucosa, 127, 128, 136
– muscles, 48
– philtrum, 10, 48
– red zone, 10, 127, 128
– sebaceous glands, 127
– sexual dimorphism, 10
– shape, 10
– skin, 127
– sweat glands, 127
– tubercle, 10
– venous drainage, 55
– vermilion border, 10, 127, 128
– zones, 10, 127, 128
Lizard,
– bearded (*Amphibolurus barbatus*)
– – dentition, 199
– – skull, 183
– egg tooth in rainbow lizard (*Agama agama*), 199, 200
– green (*Lacerta viridis*),
– – developing enamel, 187
– – tooth replacement, 193, 194
– kinesis in, 199
– monitor (*Veranus*), plicidentine, 190
– rainbow (*Agama agama*),
– – changing tooth morphology with replacement, 199
– – egg tooth, 199, 200
– Sardinian wall lizard (*Lacerta bedriagae sardoa*), tooth replacement, 194
– spiny-tailed (*Uromastyx hardwicki*), prismatic enamel, 188
Loop, cervical, 155
Lophs (lophodont teeth), 204, 212, 216
Loris, African slow (*Perodicticus potto*), dentition, 214
Lorisidae, 212
– dentition, 214
Lungfish, aprismatic enamel, 187
Lymphatic drainage,
– of face, 56
– of gingiva, 56
– of lips, 56
– of palate, 56
– of teeth, 56
– of tongue, 56
Lymphatics,
– in dental pulp, 56, 105
– in periodontal ligament, 56, 119
– Waldeyer's tonsillar ring, 56 (see also Tonsil)
Lymph nodes,
– buccal, 56
– jugulodigastric, 56
– paratracheal, 56
– pharyngeal, 56
– submandibular, 56

–submental, 56
Lymphocytes,
–in oral epithelium, 124, 126
–in pulp, 103

Macaque, stump-tailed (*Macaca arctoides*), dentition, 216
Macrophage, in pulp, 103
Macropodidae, prism pattern, 188
Macrostomia, 145
Malocclusion (see occlusion)
Mammals,
–chewing cycle, 202
–dentitions, 203–222
–evolution of molar, 201, 202
–evolution of temporomandibular joint, 182, 183, 184
Mammal-like reptiles, 184
Mammelons, 20, 21, 22, 23, 24
Man, evolution of, 219–223
–Cro-magnon, 222
–Heidelberg, 222
–*Homo* species (see Homo)
–Neanderthal, 222
–Swanscombe, 222
Manatee (*Trichechus manatus*), dentition, 212
Mandible (see Bones, individual)
Mandibular posture, 42
Margin,
–cervical,
––definition, 17
––morphology (see individual teeth)
–incisal,
––definition, 17
––morphology (see individual teeth)
Marmoset, dentition, 216
Marsupials,
–dentitions, 203, 204
–enamel prism pattern, 188
–tooth replacement, 203, 204
–tubular enamel, 189
Mastication,
–chewing cycle in mammals, 202
–dysfunction, 35
–muscles of, 46, 47
–and occlusion, 35
Masticatory mucosa (see Mucosa, oral)
Maxilla (see Bones, individual)
Meatus, external auditory, 43, 59, 60, 61, 70, 71
Melanin, 126, 129
Melanocyte, 125, 126
Melanosomes, 126
Membrane,
–bucconasal, 144
–Nasmyth's, 89
–oropharyngeal, 144
–pulp-limiting, 171
Menton, 68, 69
Merkel cell, 125, 126
Mesenchymal cells,
–in periodontal ligament, 116
–in pulp, 103
–in tooth development, 153, 154, 156, 158, 164
Mesial drift, 37, 178, 180
Metacone, 201
Metaconid, 201
Metatheria, dentitions, 203, 204
Micro-organisms, in dental plaque, 91
Microstomia, 145
Molars,
–Angle's classification of malocclusions, 39, 40
–angulation of, in alveolus, 36
–blood supply, 54
–chronology of development, 176–179
–crown form, 17, 28
–dimensions, 33
–evolution of mammalian, 201, 202
–innervation, 52
–morphology of human,
––deciduous mandibular first, 32
––deciduous mandibular second, 32
––deciduous maxillary first, 31
––deciduous maxillary second, 32
––permanent mandibular first, 30
––permanent mandibular second, 31
––permanent mandibular third, 31
––permanent maxillary first, 29
––permanent maxillary second, 29
––permanent maxillary third, 30
–occlusal relationships, 39, 40
–pulp morphology, 34
–taurodont, 222
Monkeys,
–Callitrichidae, 212
––marmoset, dentition, 216
––tamarin, dentition, 216
–Cebidae, 212
––squirrel monkey (*Saimiri sciureus*), dentition, 215
–Cercopithecidae, 216
––macaque, stump-tailed (*Macaca arctoides*), dentition, 216
–New World, 215, 216
–Old World, 216
Monophyodont dentition, 193, 195, 199, 206
Mouse (*Mus musculus*)
–dentition, 207
–prism pattern, 188
Mouth,
–anterior boundary, 10 (see also Lip)
–development, 144–147
–floor, 10, 12, 15, 57, 58, 142
––blood supply, 55
––innervation, 54
––mucosa, 134, 136
––topographical relationships, 57, 58
–functions, 10
–lateral walls, 10 (see also Cheeks and Retromolar region)
–posterior boundary, 10 (see also Oropharynx)
–roof, 10 (see also Palate)
–vestibule, 10, 11, 128, 153
Movements of mandible, 44, 45, 46, 47
Mucin, 138
Mucosa, oral, 124–136
–alveolar, 128, 129, 136
–buccal (cheek), 128, 136
–epithelial cell types, 124, 125, 126
––keratinocytes, 125
––Langerhans' cell, 125, 126
––melanocyte, 125, 126
––Merkel cell, 125, 126
––non-specific dendritic cell, 125, 126
–epithelial layers, 124
––stratum corneum (cornified layer), 124, 125, 126, 127
––stratum germanitivum (basal layer), 124, 125
––stratum granulosum (granular layer), 124, 125
––stratum lucidum (clear layer), 124
––stratum spinosum (prickle cell layer), 124, 125
–floor of mouth, 134, 136
–Fordyce spots, 11, 128
–gingiva, 129, 130, 131, 132, 136 (see also Gingiva)
–gustatory, 127, 136
–keratinization, types of,
––hyperkeratosis, 127
––non-keratinized, 127
––orthokeratosis, 127
––parakeratosis, 127
–lamina propria, 124, 136
–lining, 127, 136
–lip (labial), 127, 128, 136
–masticatory, 127, 136
–palate, 124, 133, 136
–pigmentation, 126, 129
–regional variations, 126, 127, 136
–specialised mucosa, 127, 136
–submucosa, 124, 136
–tongue, 134, 135, 136
–vestibule, 128
Mucous glands (see Glands, salivary)
Mud-puppy (*Necturus maculatus*)
–dentition, 198
–tooth replacement, 193, 198

Muscle,
- buccinator, 11, 44, 48, 50, 52, 57, 58, 59, 60, 61, 62, 178
- circumoral facial muscles, 48
- depressor anguli oris, 48, 57, 59
- depressor labii inferioris, 48
- depressor labii superioris, 48, 57
- digastric, 15, 52, 57, 58, 63
- facial, 48, 54, 59, 63, 145
- genioglossus, 15, 49, 57, 58, 60, 63
- geniohyoid, 15, 58
- hyoglossus, 49, 52, 57, 60, 63
- levator anguli oris, 48, 59
- levator labii superioris, 48, 59, 63
- levator labii superioris alaque nasi, 48
- levator palati, 46, 50, 51
- masseter, 15, 46, 47, 48, 54, 57, 58, 59, 60, 61, 62, 63, 151
- of mastication, 46, 47
- mentalis, 48
- mylohyoid, 10, 12, 15, 52, 57, 58, 62, 63
- orbicularis oculi, 48
- orbicularis oris, 10, 48, 59, 62, 63, 127
- at oropharyngeal isthmus, 51
- palatoglossus, 11, 49, 50, 51
- palatopharyngeus, 11, 50, 51, 58
- Passavant's, 50
- pharyngeal constrictors, 44, 46, 50, 51, 57, 58, 60, 61, 62
- platysma, 48, 58
- postvertebral, 57
- prevertebral, 57
- pterygoids,
-- lateral, 43, 44, 46, 47, 52, 54, 59, 60, 61, 137, 151
-- medial, 15, 46, 47, 52, 57, 59, 60, 61, 62, 63, 151
- risorius, 48
- salpingopharyngeus, 50
- of soft palate, 50, 133
- sternocleidomastoid, 57, 59, 60
- styloglossus, 49, 57, 60
- stylohyoideus, 57
- styloid group of muscles, 57, 58
- stylopharyngeus, 57
- temporalis, 15, 46, 47, 59, 60, 61, 151
- tensor palati, 14, 46, 50, 51
- of tongue, 49, 152
- in uvula, 50
- zygomaticus major, 48, 59, 63
- zygomaticus minor, 48, 63
Mustelidae, dentition, 209
Myoepithelial cell (see Glands, salivary)
Mystatoceti, dentition, 211

Narwal (*Monodon monoceros*), dentition, 211
Nasion, 68
Nasmyth's membrane (see Enamel, investing organic layers on)
Nasopharynx, 50, 56, 57, 58
Navel, enamel, 157
Neanderthal man (*Homo sapiens neanderthaliensis*), 222, 223
Nerves, individual,
- accessory, 49, 50
- anterior palatine, 11, 13, 14, 50, 52, 53, 133
- anterior superior dental, 52, 53
- auriculotemporal, 51
- buccal, 51, 52, 54, 60
- chorda tympani, 43, 52, 54, 152
- external nasal, 51
- facial, 48, 51, 53, 54, 59, 60, 152
- glossopharyngeal, 51, 53, 54, 152
- great auricular, 51, 59
- greater superficial petrosal, 54
- hypoglossal, 49, 60, 152
- incisive, 52, 53
- inferior dental (alveolar), 11, 15, 16, 46, 52, 60, 148
- infraorbital, 13, 51, 52, 53, 54, 145
- infratrochlear, 51
- lacrimal, 51
- lesser superficial petrosal, 54
- lingual, 11, 46, 52, 54, 60, 152
- mental, 15, 51, 52, 53, 54, 148
- middle superior dental, 52, 53
- mylohyoid, 52, 60
- nasopalatine, 11, 14, 52, 53
- posterior palatine, 14, 53
- posterior superior dental, 13, 52, 53
- superior laryngeal, 54, 152
- supraorbital, 51
- supratrochlear, 51
- trigeminal, 47, 50, 51, 52, 53, 54, 60, 97, 105, 119, 145 (see also individual branches)
- vagus, 54, 57, 58
- zygomaticofacial, 51
- zygomaticotemporal, 51
Nerve supply (see innervation)
Neural crest, 153, 155, 170
Neutral zone, 35
Newt, enameloid, 188
Niche, enamel, 157
Nose,
- development, 144-147
- external, innervation, 51
- nasal fossa, 13, 14, 61, 65, 66, 73, 74, 146
- piriform aperture, 13

Occlusal surface,
- definition, 17
- morphology (see individual teeth)
Occlusion, 35-41 (see also Alignment of teeth, and Posture, mandibular)
- anatomical (normal), definition, 35
- centric, 38, 39, 40
- of deciduous dentition, 180
- development, 180
- edge-to-edge bite,
-- in centric occlusion, 40
-- in deciduous dentition, 180
-- in protrusive occlusal position, 41
- ideal, 35
- malocclusion, 35, 39, 40, 41
-- Angle's classification, 39, 40
-- classification by incisor relationship, 41
- overbite, 39, 180
- overjet, 38, 39, 40
- post-normal molar relationship, 40
- pre-normal molar relationship, 40
- tooth contacts,
-- in centric position, 39
-- in lateral position, 41
-- in protrusive position, 41
Odontoblast (see Pulp, dental)
Odontoblast process (see Dentine)
Odontoceti,
- dentitions, 211
- enamel prism pattern, 188
Odontoclasts, 175
Opossum, Virginian (*Didelphis virginianis*), dentition, 203
Oral cavity (see Mouth)
Orang-utan (*Pongo pygmaeus*), dentition, 218
Orbit, 13, 53, 61, 65, 66, 67, 68
Orbitale, 68, 69
Organ,
- enamel (see Enamel organ)
- resorbing, of Tomes, 175
Oropharynx, 10, 49, 50, 51, 56, 57, 58
Orthodentine (see Dentine)
Ossification,
- mandible, 148, 149, 150
- maxilla, 151
- palate, 147
Osteichthyes, dentitions,
- angler fish (*Lophius piscatorius*), 197
- piranha (*Serrasalmus rhombeus*), 198
- rainbow trout (*Salmo gairdneri*), 197
- sheepshead fish (*Sargus ovis*), 197
Osteoblast, osteoclast, osteocyte (see Bone, alveolar)
Osteodentine, 190
Overbite, 39, 180
Over-closure, 42
Overjet, 38, 39
- reverse, 40
Over-opening, 42
Oxytalan fibres (see Fibres, oxytalan)

Paget's disease, hypercementosis, 111
Palate, 10, 11, 50, 57
– aponeurosis, 14, 49, 50
– blood supply, 55
– cleft, 147
– development, 146, 147
– glands, 133, 142
– hard, 11, 14, 50, 57, 58, 63, 67, 146, 147
– incisive papilla, 11
– innervation, 50, 53
– lymphatic drainage, 56
– mucosa, 124, 133, 136
– muscles, 50, 51
– primary, 146, 147
– raphe, 11, 133
– rugae, 11
– secondary, 146, 147
– soft, 11, 14, 50, 51, 57, 58, 147
– tonsil, 11, 56, 62
– topographical relationships, 57
– uvula, 11, 50, 147
– venous drainage, 55
Pangolin (*Maris*), dentition, 212
Papilla,
– dental, 91, 102, 154, 155, 156, 157, 158, 164, 168, 169, 170
– dermal, 124, 136
– incisive, 11
– interdental, 129, 132
– sublingual, 12, 141
– of tongue (see Tongue)
Pappotherium, molar, 201, 202
Paracone, 201
Paraconid, 201
Pellicle, acquired, 91
Peramus, molar, 201, 202
Periodontal ligament (membrane), 111–119
– attachment to bone, 78, 112, 114, 120, 122, 123
– attachment to cementum, 78, 109, 110, 111, 112, 114, 172
– blood vessels, 112, 119
– cementoblasts, 116, 117
– cementoclasts, 116, 117
– collagen fibres, 112, 113, 114, 115, 116, 117, 170, 171
– – development, 171, 172
– – function, 113, 115
– – indifferent fibre plexus, 114
– – intermediate plexus, 113, 114
– – principal fibre groups, 113
– – Sharpey's fibres, 109, 110, 111, 114, 122, 123, 172
– comparison with other connective tissues, 112
– defence cells in, 116
– development, 111, 169, 170, 171
– distribution, 78, 111
– elastic fibres, 112, 115
– epithelial rests (of Malassez), 116, 118, 170
– eruption, rôle in, 112, 115, 116, 176
– fibroblasts, 112, 116, 117, 170
– functions, 112
– gomphosis, 112, 191, 192
– ground substance, 116
– innervation, 112, 119
– intermediate plexus, 113, 114
– lymphatics, 119
– mesenchymal cells, 116
– osteoblasts, 116, 117
– osteoclasts, 116, 117, 118
– oxytalan fibres, 112, 115
– radiographic appearance, 73
– reattachment of, during resorption of teeth, 175
– reticulin fibres, 112, 115
– tissue fluid, 116
– tooth support, rôle in, 112, 113, 116
– venous drainage, 119
Periodontal space, 111
Periodontium, 78
Perissodactyla, dentitions, 210
Permanent teeth, human, 17, 19, 175, 180 (see also Dentitions)
– alignment, 35, 36, 37
– development, 156
– dimensions, 33

– eruption, 176, 177, 178, 179
– morphology (see Canines, Incisors, Premolars and Molars)
– occlusion, 38, 39, 40, 41, 180
– pulp morphology of, 34
Permeability of dental tissues,
– dentine, 92
– enamel, 79, 81
– cementum, 107
Pharynx,
– laryngopharynx, 58
– nasopharynx, 50, 56, 57, 58
– oropharynx, 10, 49, 50, 51, 56, 57, 58 (see also Muscles)
Pholidota, 212
Pig, dentition, 209
Pillars, of fauces, 10, 11, 12, 49, 50, 54, 56, 57, 58
Piranha, dentition, 198
– enameloid, 185
– tooth attachment, 191
– tooth replacement, 193, 195
Pits, nasal, 144
Placode,
– nasal, 144
– optic (lens), 144
Placodermi, jaws, 182
Placoid scales, 185
Plane,
– Bolton, 69, 152
– Frankfort, 69
– mandibular, 69
– maxillary, 69
– occlusal, 36, 37
– sella-nasion, 69
– Y-axis, 69
Plaque, dental, 90, 91
Plasma cells, in dental pulp, 103
Plates,
– alveolar (see Bones, alveolar)
– orbital (see Bones, maxilla)
– palatine (see Bones, palatine bone)
– pterygoid (see Bones, sphenoid)
– tympanic (see Bones, temporal)
Pleurodont ankylosis, 193, 199
Plexus,
– incisor, nervous, 53
– intermediate, of periodontal ligament, 113, 114
– marginal, of dental pulp, 105
– pharyngeal, nervous, 49, 50
– pharyngeal, venous, 55
– pterygoid, venous, 55, 60
– Raschkow's, of dental pulp, 97, 105, 168
– subodontoblastic capillary, 104, 105, 168
– subodontoblastic, neural (see Raschkow's)
– of superior dental arteries, 55
– of superior dental nerves, 53
Plicidentine, 190
Point,
– A (subspinale), 68, 69
– B (supramentale), 68, 69
– Bolton, 68
– Registration, 69, 152
– S (sella), 68, 69
Polymorphonuclear leucocytes,
– in dental pulp, 103
– in gingival fluid, 131
Polyphyodonty, 193, 196, 198, 199
Pongidae, 212
– dentitions, 217, 218
Posture,
– lips, 10
– mandibular, 42
Premolars,
– angulation of, in alveolus, 36
– blood supply, 54
– chronology of development, 176–179
– crown form, 17, 26
– dimensions, 33
– function, 26
– innervation, 52
– morphology of human

243

– – mandibular first premolar, 27
– – mandibular second premolar, 28
– – maxillary first premolar, 26
– – maxillary second premolar, 27
– pulp morphology, 34
Primates, 212
– dentitions, 213–222
Primordia, of face and teeth (see Development)
Prism, enamel (see Enamel)
Probainognathus, jaw evolution, 184
Proboscidea, dentitions, 211
Process, alveolar (see Bone, alveolar),
– condylar, of mandible, 15, 38, 43, 44, 45, 46, 47, 59, 60, 61, 65, 66, 67, 70, 71, 137, 149, 150, 151
– coronoid, of mandible, 15, 47, 61, 66, 67, 70, 151
– frontal, of maxilla, 13, 151
– fronto-nasal, 144, 145, 146, 151
– nasal,
– – lateral, 144, 145
– – medial, 144, 145
– mandibular, 144, 145
– mastoid, of temporal, 65, 67
– maxillary, 144, 145, 146, 151
– odontoblastic (see Dentine)
– palatine, of maxilla, 13, 14, 151
– postglenoid, 43
– pyramidal, of palatine bone, 47
– styloid, 44, 49
– zygomatic, of maxilla, 13, 66, 151
– zygomatic, of temporal, 43
Propliopithecus, 219, 223
Prosimii, 212
– dentitions, 213, 214, 215
Protocone, 201
Protoconid, 201
Prototheria, dentitions, 203
Protuberance, mental, 15
Pulp, dental, 102–106
– age changes, 34, 100, 102, 104, 105, 106, 168
– blood supply, 102, 104, 168
– calcification, 106
– cell free zone (of Weil), 102
– cell rich zone (of Weil), 102, 168
– collagen fibres, 104, 168
– composition, 102
– defence cells, 102, 103, 168
– development, 102, 168
– distribution, 34, 78, 102
– elastic fibres, 104
– fibroblast, 102, 103, 168
– fibrocyte, 103
– function, 102
– ground substance, 104, 168
– histiocyte, 103
– inflammation, 97, 103
– innervation, 97, 102, 103, 104, 105, 106, 168
– lymphatics, 105
– lymphocytes, 103, 168
– macrophages, 103, 168
– marginal plexus, 105
– mesenchymal (undifferentiated) cells, 103
– morphology, 19, 34
– odontoblasts, 95, 97, 98, 101, 102, 103, 106, 164, 165
– – degeneration in crowding, 100
– – and dentine formation, 156, 158, 159, 164, 165, 168, 169, 170
– – desmosomes, 103, 106, 165
– – differentiation, 156, 168, 170
– – function, 102
– – movement during dentinogenesis, 165
– – organelles, 103
– – processes (see Dentine)
– – rôle in early mineralisation, 165
– – sensory function, 106
– pericytes, 168
– plasma cells, 103
– polymorphonuclear leucocytes, 103
– radiographic appearance, 73
– Raschkow's plexus, 97, 105, 168
– reaction to stimuli, 94, 100, 101

– sensation, 105, 106
– stones, 106
– subodontoblastic capillary plexus, 104, 105, 168
– subodontoblastic nervous plexus (see Raschkow's plexus)
– tissue fluid, 102, 104
– veins, 102, 104, 168
– zones, 102
Python (*Python*),
– dentition, 200
– tooth replacement, 200

Rabbit (*Oryctolagus cuniculus*), dentition, 207
Radiographic appearance of:
– alveolar crest, 72, 73
– alveolus, 73
– anterior cranial fossa, 67
– anterior nasal spine, 65, 67
– Bolton plane, 69
– Bolton point, 68
– coronoid process of mandible, 66, 67, 70, 71, 75
– dental hard tissues, 73
– developing teeth, 76
– ethmoidal air cells, 66
– external auditory meatus, 68, 70, 71
– external oblique line of mandible, 76
– external occipital protuberance, 67
– foramen magnum, 66
– Frankfort plane, 69, 70
– frontal air sinuses, 65, 66, 67
– genial tubercles, 75
– Gnathion, 68
– gonion, 68
– hypophyseal (pituitary) fossa, 67
– incisive foramen, 74
– infraorbital foramen, 65
– internal oblique line of mandible, 76
– lambdoid suture, 65, 66, 67
– lamina dura, 73
– mandible, 65, 66, 67, 70, 72, 73, 75, 76
– mandibular canal, 76
– mandibular condyle, 65, 66, 67, 70, 71
– mandibular dentition, 65, 66, 67, 70, 72
– mandibular plane, 69, 70
– mandibular symphysis, 75
– mastoid air cell, 66, 71
– mastoid process of temporal bone, 65, 67, 70
– maxilla, 65, 66, 67, 70, 72, 73, 74, 75
– maxillary air sinuses (antrum), 65, 66, 67, 70, 74, 75
– maxillary dentition, 65, 66, 67, 72
– maxillary plane, 69
– maxillary tuberosity, 70, 74, 75
– median palatine suture, 74
– meningeal vessels, 67
– mental foramen, 65, 70, 76
– menton, 68
– middle cranial fossa, 67
– nasal bones, 66, 67
– nasal fossae, 65, 66, 70, 74, 75
– nasal septum, 65, 66
– nasion, 68
– nasolacrimal duct, 74
– nutrient canals, 73, 75
– orbit, 65, 66, 67
– orbitale, 68
– palate, 67, 74
– periodontal ligament, 73
– periodontal space, 73
– petrous ridge, 65, 67
– pogonion, 68
– porion, 68
– posterior cranial fossa, 67
– pterygoid hamulus, 75
– pterygoid plates, 75
– pulp, 73
– registration point, 69
– salivary glands, 71
– sella-nasion plane, 69
– sella point, 68
– skull, 65, 66, 67, 68, 69, 70

– sphenoid air sinus, 67
– sphenoid ridge in middle cranial fossa, 65
– subspinale (A point), 68
– supramentale (B point), 68
– temporomandibular joint, 70, 71
– vertebral column, 70
– y-axis, 69
– y of Ennis, 75
– zygoma, 65, 66, 70, 71, 75
– zygomatic process of temporal bone, 66
– zygomatic process of frontal bone, 65
Radiographic projections of skull, jaws and teeth, 64
– antero-posterior view of skull, 64, 65
– cephalometric analysis from lateral skull radiographs, 64, 68, 69, 70
– intra-oral radiographs, 64, 73–76
– – bitewings, 64, 72
– – periapical, 64, 72, 73, 74, 75, 76
– – mandibular occlusal, 64, 72, 75
– – maxillary occlusal (nasal), 64, 72
– – maxillary occlusal (oblique), 74
– – maxillary occlusal (vertex), 64, 72
– lateral oblique view of jaws, 64, 70
– lateral view of skull, 64, 67
– occipitomental view of skull, 64, 66
– orthopantomogram, 64, 70
– postero-anterior view of skull, 64, 65
– reverse Towne's view of mandibular condyles, 64, 66
– sialogram, 64, 71
– transcranial temporomandibular joint, 64, 71
Radiolucency, definition, 64
– of oro-dental tissues, 73
Radio-opacity, definition, 64
– of oro-dental tissues, 73
Ramapithecus, 219, 220, 223
Ramus of mandible (see Bones, mandible)
Raphe,
– palatine, 11, 133
– pterygomandibular, 11, 44, 48
Rat (*Rattus norvegicus*), dentition, 206, 207
Ray,
– eagle (*Myliobatis aquilla*),
– – dentition, 197
– – osteodentine, 190
– thornback (*Raia clavata*),
– – dentition, 196
– – tooth attachment, 191
– – tooth replacement, 191
Receptors,
– in periodontal ligament, 112, 119
Replacement of teeth in animals, 193–195
– alligator, 200
– amphibians, 198
– cartilaginous fish, 196
– chamaeleon, 193
– crocodile, 193
– diphyodonty, 195
– horizontal, in elephant, 211
– iguana, 199
– kangaroo, 204
– lizard, 194
– marsupial, 203, 204
– mud-puppy, 193, 198
– piranha, 193
– python, 200
– ray, 191, 196
– reptiles, 199, 200
– shark, 193, 196
– slow worm, 194
– trout, 193
Replacement of teeth in man, 174, 175
Reptiles, 182
– dentitions, 199
– enamel, 187
– evolution of jaws, 183, 184
– tooth replacement, 199
Resorption,
– of alveoli, 14, 118, 123
– of cementum, 107
– of deciduous teeth, 175

– of dentine, 175
Rests, epithelial,
– from dental lamina, 155
– of Malassez, 116, 118, 170
Reticulin, fibres (see Fibres, reticulin)
Retromolar region of mouth, 10, 11
Retzius, striae of (see Enamel)
Ridge,
– marginal, on tooth, definition, 17
– mylohyoid, 15
– Passavant's, 50
– on tooth, definition, 17
Rodentia, dentitions, 206, 207
Root, anatomical (definition), 17
– clinical (definition), 17
– development, 169, 170, 171, 172
– dimensions of, 33
– form, in relation to that of alveolus, 14, 16
– fracture repair, 111
– morphology (see individual teeth)
Root canals, 34, 102
– accessory (lateral), 102, 104
– apical foramina, 34, 104, 169
– in deciduous teeth, 19
– shape and size, 34
Root diaphragm, 169, 170
Rugae, palatine, 11

Salamander, enameloid, 188
Saliva,
– composition, 138
– function, 138
Salivary ducts (see Ducts)
Salivary glands (see Glands, salivary)
Seal, Californian (*Zalophus californianus*), 209
Selenodont teeth, 210, 212
Septum,
– enamel, 155, 157
– interdental, 14, 120
– interradicular, 14, 120
– lingual, 49
– nasal, 48, 61, 65, 66, 73, 146, 147
– primary nasal, 146
– secondary nasal, 146, 147
Serous salivary glands (see Glands)
Sexual dimorphism,
– ape canine, 217
– human lips, 10
Shark,
– blue (*Prionace glauca*),
– – dentition, 196
– – osteodentine, 190
– lemon (*Negaprion brevirostris*), tooth replacement, 193
– Porbeagle (*Lemna nasus*), dentition, 196
Sharpey's fibres (see Fibres, Sharpey's)
Sheath,
– carotid, 60
– epithelial root, 118, 169, 170, 172
– prism (Boundary), 80, 81, 82, 160
Shedding of deciduous teeth, 175
Shelf,
– palatal, 146, 147
– simion, 217, 218
Shrew, long-tailed (*Sorex araneus*), dentition, 205
Siamang, dentition, 216
Sinus, air,
– ethmoidal, 61, 66
– frontal, 65, 66, 67
– mastoid, 59, 66, 71
– maxillary (antrum), 13, 14, 16, 53, 54, 61, 65, 66, 67, 72, 73, 74, 75, 151
– sphenoid, 67
Sirenia,
– dentitions, 212
– enamel prism pattern, 188
Skin, of lip, 127
Skull,
– appearance, anterior view, 16
– appearance, lateral view, 16
– cephalometric landmarks, 68, 69, 70

—growth, 152
—radiographic appearance, 65, 66, 67, 68, 69, 70
Sloth, two-toed (*Choloepus didactylus*), dentition, 212
Slow worm (*Angius fragilis*), tooth replacement, 194
Snake, dentitions, 200, 201
Socket, tooth (see Bones, individual, alveolar)
Soft palate (see Palate)
Somites, occipital, 152
Spaces, tissue, around jaws,
—buccal, 62
—canine fossa, 62, 63
—infratemporal, 62, 63
—lateral pharyngeal, 60, 62, 63
—palatal, 62, 63
—parotid, 62
—peritonsillar, 62
—pterygomandibular, 11, 46, 52, 62, 63
—around ramus, 62
—sublingual, 62, 63
—submandibular, 15, 62, 63
—submasseteric, 62
—submental, 62, 63
Specialised mucosa (see Mucosa, oral)
Spine,
—anterior nasal, 13, 53, 67, 69
—genial, 15, 49, 73, 75
—posterior nasal, 14, 69
—sphenoid, 44, 149
Squirrel (*Sciuridae*), dentition, 207
Stellate reticulum, 154, 155, 156, 157, 159
Stomodeum, 144, 146
Strands, enamel, 157
Strata of oral mucosa (see Mucosa, oral)
Stratified squamous epithelia,
—collecting ducts of salivary gland, 140
—oral mucosa (see Mucosa, oral)
Stratum intermedium, 156, 157, 159, 160
Striae of Retzius (see Enamel)
Sturgeon (*Acipenser*), 197
Stylocone, 201
Submerged teeth, 175
Submucosa (see Mucosa, oral)
Subspinale, 68, 69
Sulcular epithelium (see Gingiva)
Sulcus,
—gingival, 90, 130, 131
—labiomarginal, 10
—lacrimal, 13
—terminalis, 12, 135
—vestibular, 11, 128
Supramentale, 68, 69
Surfaces of teeth,
—definition, 17
—morphology (see individual teeth)
Suture,
—intermaxillary, 13, 73
—lambdoid, 67
—median palatine, 14, 73, 74, 147
—transverse palatine, 14, 147
Swanscombe man, 222
Swellings, lateral lingual, 152
Symphysis, mandibular, 15, 75, 148, 149, 150

Tadpole (*Rana temporaria*), 198
Talon, 29, 30
Talonid, 202
Tarsiidae, 212
—dentition, 215
Tarsius (*Tarsius banconus*), 215
Taste buds, 134, 135
Taurodont molars, 222
Teeth,
—for description of the morphology of human teeth, see Canines, Incisors, Molars and Premolars,
—for teeth of animals, see animal concerned
—alignment in alveolus, 35, 36, 37
—arterial blood supply to, 54, 55
—attachment to jaws (see Attachment of teeth)
—curvatures, 37
—development (see Development)
—dimensions,
— —deciduous, 33
— —permanent, 33
—evolution, 182, 185
—histological appearance of teeth *in situ*, ground and decalcified sections, 78
—innervation, 52, 53
—lymphatic drainage, 56
—mandibular,
— —relationship to alveoli, 16
— —relationship to mandibular canal, 16
—maxillary,
— —relationship to alveoli, 14, 16
— —relationship to antrum, 16
—numbers in dentition, 17
—occlusion of, 38–41
—radiographic appearance of, 73
—replacement (see Replacement of teeth)
—submerged, 175
—succession, 17
—venous drainage, 55
Teleosts (see Osteichthyes)
Thylacine wolf (*Thylacinus cynocephalus*), 204
Tissue fluid,
—dental pulp, 104
—pressure in periodontal ligament, 116
Tissue spaces (see Spaces, tissue)
Tomes' granular layer (see Dentine)
Tomes' process (see Ameloblast)
Tongue, 10, 12
—blood supply, 55
—development, 152
—dorsum, 12, 51, 54, 134, 135, 136
—fimbriated fold, 12
—foramen caecum, 12, 152
—frenum, 12
—inferior (ventral) surface, 12, 134, 136
—innervation, 54, 152
—lingual tonsil, 12, 134, 135
—lymphatic drainage, 56
—mucosa, 134, 135, 136
—muscles, 49
—papillae,
— —circumvallate, 12, 54, 134, 135
— —filiform, 134
— —fungiform, 134
—relationship to tissue spaces, 63
—septum, 49
—sulcus terminalis, 12, 135
—taste bud, 134, 135
—thrust, 10, 35
—topographical relationships, 58
—venous drainage, 55
Tonsil,
—crypt of, 11, 51, 57
—lingual, 12, 56, 134, 135
—palatal, 11, 56, 62
Tonsillar ring of Waldeyer, 56
Tooth development, 153–172
—bell stage, 149, 154, 155, 156, 157, 158, 164, 168, 169
—bud stage, 154, 156
—cap stage, 154
—chronology, 176
—enamel cord, 155, 157
—enamel knot, 157
—enamel niche, 157
—enamel strands, 157
—lamina, dental, 148, 153, 155, 156, 157, 174
—permanent tooth anlage, 156
—primary epithelial band, 153
Tooth morphology (see Canines, Incisors, Molars, Premolars)
Tree shrew (*Tupaia glis*), dentition, 213
Trigon, 29, 30
Trigonid, 201
Tube, Eustachian (auditory), 50, 51
Tubercle,
—genial, 15, 49, 73, 75
—of lip, 10
—postglenoid, 43

– of tooth, definition, 17
Tuberculum impar, 152
Tumours and epithelial rests, 118
Tupaiidae, dentition, 213
Tusk,
– elephant, 211
– narwal, 211
– walrus, 209

Unerupted teeth,
– dead tracts in, 100
– periodontal space of, 111
Ungulates,
– dentitions, 209–210
– prism pattern, 188
Urodeles, enameloid, 188
Uvula, 11, 50, 57, 147

Vasodentine, 189
Vein,
– buccal, 55
– common facial, 55
– deep lingual, 55
– external jugular, 57
– facial, 47, 55, 59
– greater palatine, 11, 14, 50, 55, 133
– inferior dental, 16, 55
– inferior labial, 55
– internal jugular, 55, 57, 58
– lesser palatine, 14
– nasopalatine, 55
– pterygoid, 55
– retromandibular, 55, 60
– sublingual, 12
– superficial temporal, 59
– superior dental, 55
– superior labial, 55
– supraorbital, 55
– supratrochlear, 55
Venous drainage,
– of face, 55
– of gingiva, 55
– of lips, 55
– of palate, 55
– of periodontal ligament, 119
– of pulp, 104
– of teeth, 55
– of tongue, 55
Vertebrates, classification, 182
Vesicle, matrix, in developing dentine, 165
Vestibular fornix (sulcus), 11, 128
Vestibule, 10, 11, 128, 153
Viverridae, dentition, 209
Von Ebner lines (see Dentine)
Von Korff fibres (see Dentinogenesis)

Waldeyer's tonsillar ring, 56
Walrus (*Odobenus rosmarus*), dentition, 209
Whale, sperm (*Physeter catodon*), 211
Wombat (*Phascolomis ursinus*), 203
– dentition, 203
– enamel, 189
Wrasse (*Labrus bergylta*), enameloid, 186

X-rays, 64

Y-axis, 69
Y-of-Ennis, 75

Zone, neutral, 35
Zsigmond system for tooth identification, 18